Core Paediatrics and Child Health

Edited by

Diab Farhan Haddad MD MRCP(Paed)
Consultant Paediatrician, The Paediatric Unit, St Peter's Hospital, Chertsey, UK

Stephen A. Greene MB BS FRCP
Senior Lecturer in Child Health, Tayside Institute of Child Health, University of Dundee, Ninewells Hospital and Medical School, Dundee, UK

Richard E. Olver MB BS BSc MRCPCH FRCP FRCPE
Professor of Child Health, Tayside Institute of Child Health, University of Dundee, Ninewells Hospital and Medical School, Dundee, UK

Foreword by

Professor Sir Cyril Chantler MA MD FRCP FRCPCH
Children Nationwide Professor of Paediatric Nephrology, and Dean, Guy's, King's and St Thomas' Medical and Dental School, King's College, London, UK

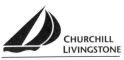

CHURCHILL
LIVINGSTONE

EDINBURGH LONDON NEW YORK PHILADELPHIA ST LOUIS SYDNEY TORONTO 2000

CHURCHILL LIVINGSTONE
An imprint of Harcourt Publishers Limited

© Harcourt Publishers Limited 2000

⚓ is a registered trademark of Harcourt Publishers
Limited

First published 2000

ISBN 0 443 05916 0

British Library Cataloguing in Publication Data
A catalogue record for this book is available from the
British Library.

Library of Congress Cataloging in Publication Data
A catalog record for this book is available from the
Library of Congress.

Medical knowledge is constantly changing. As new
information becomes available, changes in treatment,
procedures, equipment and the use of drugs become
necessary. The editors, contributors and the publishers
have, as far as it is possible, taken care to ensure that the
information given in this text is accurate and up to date.
However, readers are strongly advised to confirm that
the information, especially with regard to drug usage,
complies with current legislation and standards of
practice.

The
publisher's
policy is to use
**paper manufactured
from sustainable forests**

Printed in China

Foreword

'A system of medical education that is actually calculated to obstruct the acquisition of sound knowledge and to heavily favour the crammer and the grinder is a disgrace' wrote Thomas Huxley in 1877. Similarly in 1915, Sir William Osler remarked that 'to an inquisitive mind, the study of medicine may become an absorbing passion ... but the spirit is taken out of instruction and teachers and taught alike go down into the Valley of Ezekial where they stay among the dry bones'.

At last, and many would say, not before time, a major revolution is taking place within medical schools in the United Kingdom to improve the quality of medical education. The key components of these changes include the recognition that we are all students of medicine and continue to learn throughout our medical lifetime. Medical students are starting the journey and it is important that they are encouraged or even inspired to learn and understand. Courses are now designed to encourage deep learning strategies rather than the superficial acquisition of knowledge.[1] They encourage a problem-orientated approach to learning. A sound understanding of biomedical science is still the foundation of safe practice, but the importance of the social sciences is now appreciated.

To some extent learning to practice medicine has some similarities to learning a language. An adequate knowledge of grammar and vocabulary is vital, but it does not enable you to speak the language, that requires practice. Likewise, understanding the scientific basis of medicine is important but it needs to be coordinated with the acquisition of clinical skills throughout the course. The recognition that learning continues throughout one's career and that the aim is to acquire the right skills and competencies for the clinical practice that is to be undertaken at various stages in that career has directed educators to attempt to define the core knowledge, attitudes and competencies required to become a preregistration house officer and to limit the amount of factual knowledge to be understood during the undergraduate course to this core. At the same time, special study modules and intercalated bachelor degrees are designed to develop a spirit of enquiry and deep learning strategies.

This book sets out the core for paediatrics and child health and then explores it at different levels. It will need to be read with intelligence and not learnt by rote. A particular feature is the emphasis on the scientific basis to the clinical problem which is then explored, and the enticement to become engaged at a deeper level with the problem under consideration. It is perhaps important to emphasise that the successful student will not need to know everything in this book but he or she will need to have an adequate knowledge of the key problems and the key diagnoses.

The authors are to be congratulated on this approach and I believe the book will be useful not only for medical students but for all students of medicine who are engaged with the health and healthcare of children.

C. CHANTLER

[1] McManus I C et al 1998 Clinical experience, performance in final examinations, and learning style in medical students: prospective study. British Medical Journal 316: 345–350

Preface

The idea of this book had its origins in the General Medical Council's document *Tomorrow's Doctors*,[1] which created a demand for new teaching resources to reflect its new thinking about the scope and content of medical education in the UK. Central to the GMC recommendations was the need to address the problem of factual overload in the medical curriculum (a problem which had first engaged the attention of the Council as early as 1863!). As a result, the concept of a 'core curriculum' was introduced, to be supplemented by 'special study modules' in which students were to be encouraged to explore selected topics in depth.

Although it is easy to subscribe to the concept of a core curriculum, it is much more difficult to define what is 'core' and what is not, i.e. what must be included in the curriculum for all students and what can be left out or made optional. In Scotland, the Child Health departments of the four clinical medical schools set about the task of defining core material according to certain criteria[2] and developed a 'Core Curriculum in Paediatrics and Child Health'.[3] The scope of this book is very much defined by this new curriculum, which forms the basis of the teaching of paediatrics and child health in the Scottish medical schools.

When deciding what to include in this book as core, we have applied the criteria used to design the Core Curriculum. Thus, any condition or topic which has been included has one or more of the following features: it is common; potentially serious in its impact on a child's health (particularly important if preventable by early and appropriate intervention); the subject of a screening programme or public health programme such as immunization; of ethical or legal importance; of interest to the public. At a practical level, our intention is to provide sufficient knowledge to make it possible to embark on a junior training post involving children, for example, a GP trainee, A&E or paediatric house officer, with a reasonable degree of confidence and competence.

Other key elements in the GMC recommendations which we have attempted to reflect in this book is the need to demonstrate the relevance of science to clinical practice and that learning medicine should be a process of inquiry and understanding rather than rote. Furthermore, teaching should be relevant to medical practice in real life and not based on artificial divisions between disciplines and between hospital- and community-based clinical practice.

We have maintained a system-based organization but largely adopted a problem-orientated approach. The chief presenting features of disease within a system are dealt with as a 'Key problems' and each is used as a starting point for the discussion of possible aetiology and the approach to clinical management before considering the 'Key diagnosis' in detail. Important differential diagnoses are included under 'Related topics'. To allow for the coverage of the major embryological, anatomical and physiological features specific to paediatrics, most chapters of the book include a section on 'Essential background'. A 'Clinical methods' section emphasizes aspects of history taking and physical examination relevant to the disorders of the particular system. We have tried where appropriate to highlight community child health and primary care perspectives, and the emphasis on 'Key diagnoses' has not been made at the expense of common minor complaints.

It is inevitable that some difference of opinion will arise regarding the range of topics included in a textbook. To address this point and cater for different needs, interests and aptitudes, we have given ourselves the option of including 'Beyond core' material. Another feature is the inclusion of sections titled 'Highlights and hypotheses'. Cutting edge research, landmark papers and areas of controversy all can feature under this heading. Such material, it is hoped, will raise the level of interest and foster curiosity. In a sense, these additional components together represent our own 'special study modules'.

Finally, in this age of rapid developments in medicine and instant communication, it is likely that some aspects of even the most up to date books will be out of date when published.

Mindful of this fact, we attempted to devote particular attention to general principles governing the approach to clinical problems. Although we believe that this strategy will prolong the useful life of this book, we realise we can only delay the inevitable. Even what is called a principle today will no doubt be dismantled and superseded by the relentless arrival of tomorrow.

2000
D. F. Haddad
S. A. Greene
R. E. Olver

[1] General Medical Council 1993 Tomorrow's Doctors

[2] Haddad D, Robertson K J, Cockburn F, Helms P, McIntosh N & Olver R E 1997 What is core? Guidelines for the core curriculum in paediatrics. Medical Education 31: 354–358

[3] Scottish Child Health Group. A Core Curriculum in Paediatrics and Child Health; http://w3.abdn.ac.uk/umi2/

Acknowledgements

The editors wish to thank the Wellcome Trust Medical Photographic Library and Teaching At Low Cost (TALC) for allowing the use of their rich collection of slides.

We wish to thank all our colleagues for their support, with special acknowledgements to Dr Jean Bowyer, Dr Gavin Main, Dr Alan McCulloch and Mr Arthur Morris for their help and contribution of slides.

We are indebted to Mrs Vera Murray for her highly professional and skilful secretarial support.

Contributors

Kenneth J. Aitken MA(Hon) Mphil(ClinPsy) PhD
Independent Consultant Child Clinical
Psychologist, Edinburgh, UK

Robert Carachi MD PhD FRCS
Senior Lecturer in Surgical Paediatrics, University
of Glasgow; Honorary Consultant Paediatric
Surgeon, The Royal Hospital for Sick Children,
Yorkhill NHS Trust, Glasgow, UK

Anthony Costello MA FRCP
Consultant Paediatrician and Reader in
International Child Health, Institute of Child
Health and Great Ormond Street Hospital for
Children NHS Trust; Honorary Consultant to the
Hospital for Tropical Diseases, London, UK

David Goudie MB ChB
Consultant in Clinical Genetics, Dundee Teaching
Hospitals; Honorary Senior Lecturer, Dundee
University, Dundee, UK

Stephen A. Greene MB BS FRCP
Senior Lecturer in Child Health, The University of
Dundee, Ninewells Hospital and Medical School,
Dundee, UK

Alex Habel MB ChB FRCP MRCPCH
Consultant Paediatrician, West Middlesex
University Hospital; Honorary Consultant
Paediatrician, Great Ormond Street Hospital for
Children, London, UK

Diab Farhan Haddad MD MRCP (Paed)
Consultant Paediatrician, The Paediatric Unit, St
Peter's Hospital, Chertsey, UK

Helen Hammond MA(Oxon) BM BCh FRCP(E) FRCPCH
MSc
Consultant Paediatrician (Community Child
Health), West Lothian NHS Trust; Honorary
Senior Lecturer, Department of Child Life and
Health, Edinburgh University, Edinburgh, UK

Peter J. Helms MB BS PhD FRCP FRCPCH
Professor of Child Health, University of Aberdeen;
Honorary Consultant Paediatrician, Royal
Aberdeen Children's Hospital, Aberdeen, UK

Simon C. Ling MB ChB MRCP(UK)
British Digestive Foundation, Research Fellow and
Senior Registrar, Department of Child Health and
Royal Hospital of Sick Children, Glasgow, UK

Richard E. Olver MB BS BSc MRCPCH FRCP FRCPE
Professor of Child Health, University of Dundee,
Ninewells Hospital and Medical School, Dundee,
UK

D. D. Ratnasingh MB BS MRCP MRCPCH
Consultant Paediatrician, Paediatric Department,
West Middlesex University Hospital, Isleworth,
UK

Eric Shinwell LRCP MRCS
Director of Neonatology, Kaplan Medical Center,
Rechovot, Israel

Lawrence T. Weaver MA MD FRCP DCH
Professor of Child Health, University of Glasgow
and Royal Hospital for Sick Children, Glasgow

Contents

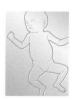

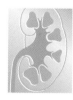

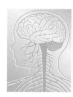

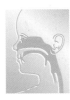

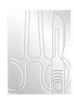

CHAPTER 1

The scope and practice of child health

R. E. Olver

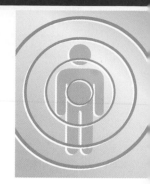

INTRODUCTION

What is child health?

Child Health is an age-related speciality which encompasses birth and puberty but has an upper age limit which is relatively ill defined. Sixteen is the usually accepted cut-off point, but 16 year olds are not necessarily adults emotionally or physically. Furthermore, the period of dependency on parents is lengthening, both as a result of an increased duration in full-time education and lack of opportunities for youth employment and housing.

The term 'child health' is frequently used synonymously with 'paediatrics'. This is not strictly correct, but these complementary disciplines can be thought of as two sides of the same coin, with child health reflecting an emphasis on the maintenance of health, essentially preventative in its focus, whilst paediatrics is concerned more with the diagnostic and therapeutic aspects of managing established disease. In practice there is a great deal of overlap, and, increasingly, clinicians working in the field are engaged in both aspects of care.

Childhood is characterized by growth and development: physical, cognitive and psychosocial. It is this rather than the virtual absence of degenerative disease which differentiates child health and paediatrics from adult medicine. Many of the important conditions which affect children are developmental in as much as they are due to disordered development (congenital disorders) or incomplete development (immaturity). Congenital disorders, whether genetically determined (e.g. Down syndrome, cystic fibrosis) or acquired

in utero (e.g. rubella, teratogenic effects of drugs) and those related to birth itself (e.g. birth asphyxia) may be detected antenatally or be present at birth or in infancy. Almost by definition, diseases related to immaturity become clinically apparent according to age.

The following are some examples:

Newborn
Respiratory distress syndrome, peri-intraventricular haemorrhage, and hypoglycaemia in the preterm infant (see Ch. 4) with immature organ systems

Infant
Respiratory (see Ch. 6) and gastrointestinal infection (see Ch. 5) due to immaturity of the immune system; sudden infant death syndrome (see Ch. 15)

Preschool child
Exanthems and other infections (see Ch. 14) due to lack of immunity, as the child mixes with other children; accidents (see Ch. 15) as a result of increased mobility and curiosity coupled with lack of judgement

School age child
Cognitive disorder may become apparent (see Ch. 17); liability to accidents remains, with road traffic accidents prominent, particularly in boys; in adolescence, sexual and emotional difficulties may develop (see Ch. 18)

The stage of development a child has reached will influence how he or she understands and responds to illness and its management.

Why is child health important?

As enshrined in the United Nations Convention on the Rights of the Child (Table 1.1), children have the same rights to health as adults, and it can be argued that it is the mark of a civilized

Table 1.1   United Nations Convention on the Rights of the Child (1989)
This embodies the right of every child to:
• Equality regardless of race, nationality or sex
• Special protection for full physical, intellectual, moral, spiritual and social development in a healthy and normal manner
• A name and nationality
• Adequate nutrition, housing and medical services
• Special care if handicapped
• Love, understanding and protection
• Free education, play and recreation
• Priority for relief in times of disaster
• Protection against all forms of neglect, cruelty and exploitation
• Protection from any form of discrimination, and the right to be brought up in a spirit of universal brotherhood, peace and tolerance

society that it cares for and protects those, such as its children, that are most vulnerable. Furthermore, children represent the economic future of a country and failure to nurture this resource is wasteful as well as uncaring. As indicated below, the likelihood of a child fulfilling his or her full potential to be a healthy adult is significantly influenced by environmental factors.

The processes underlying growth and development (see Chs 2 and 3), like those involved in the expression of disease, are subject to a complex interplay between an individual's genes and the environment. Increasingly we are becoming aware that health in early life, or the lack of it, may have important long-term effects on health in adult life. Thus, exposure during fetal life and infancy to adverse environmental events may programme an individual to be susceptible to subsequent disease (see Highlights and Hypotheses: early influences on later health).

However, it is not just the effects of early life which are important. In addition to the interplay between genetic and environmental factors, there is also an interplay between early and late influences. Thus, both poor fetal growth and adult obesity both predispose (see Highlights and Hypotheses: early influences on later health) to the development of type 2 diabetes. These

observations introduce the idea that children are born with a potential for health and that there are opportunities to intervene to maintain health both early and later in life. It is the objective of those working in child health to help children achieve their full potential.

Organization of child health services

Those parts of the clinical services concerned principally with health maintenance (health education, surveillance of growth and development, and immunization), which were once the responsibility of paediatricians working in the community child health service, are now provided in the community by general practitioners. This change parallels a reorganization of the community child health services to provide a specialist service (see Ch. 17), particularly in the areas of complex neurological disability and child protection (managing child abuse). Both the community child health service and hospital-based paediatric service provide so-called secondary care – receiving referrals from general practitioners who provide primary care. Some large children's hospitals provide tertiary care; that is to say that

HIGHLIGHTS AND HYPOTHESES

EARLY INFLUENCES ON LATER HEALTH

Genetically or environmentally determined?

In order to account for the worldwide explosion in coronary heart disease, hypertension, obesity and type 2 diabetes (syndrome X), Neel (1962) put forward the 'thrifty phenotype' hypothesis. This proposes that populations highly susceptible to syndrome X are equipped with ancestral genes which are selectively advantageous to the hunter–gatherer lifestyle because they allow efficient utilization and conservation of food energy during periods of prolonged starvation. However, in an environment characterized by abundance, this thrifty metabolism predisposes to hyperglycaemia, hyperfibrinogenaemia and hypertriglyceridaemia. Humans may therefore be equipped with genes that cannot handle the modern Western diet.

Another hypothesis was proposed In the late 1980s by Professor David Barker and his colleagues, who demonstrated a highly significant relationship between birth weight (and weight at 1 year) with the risk of cardiovascular and respiratory disease (Fig. 1.1), and with type 2 diabetes in adult life. Additionally, they reported that lower respiratory tract infection in infancy, while the lung is still growing rapidly, results in reduced adult respiratory function. They suggested that these adverse events in early life induce (programme) permanent changes in structure, physiology and metabolism. Suggested mechanisms for programming include changes in gene expression, reduced cell number, imbalance between cell types (Fig. 1.2), changes in the pattern of hormonal release and the resetting of hormonal responses.

Further testing of both the thrifty phenotype and Barker hypotheses is needed. However, they are not necessarily mutually exclusive, and both mechanisms may to a variable extent underly the observed effects of early environmental influences on health in later life.

---

they receive referrals from other hospitals in certain highly specialized areas (e.g. paediatric cardiac surgery, renal dialysis).

The fact that many children with diseases previously fatal in childhood now survive requires continuity of care into adolescence and young adulthood. The UK is somewhat behind Scandinavia and North America in this respect, but there are good examples of cooperation between paediatricians and adult physicians to

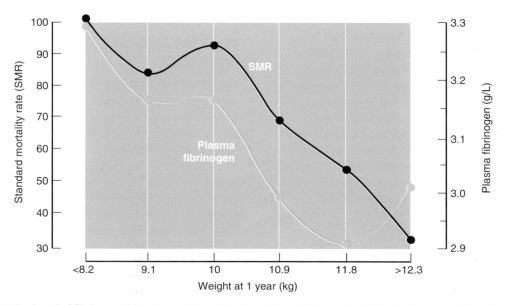

Figure 1.1   Level of fibrinogen (a major predictor of ischaemic heart disease) and standardized mortality rates for chronic obstructive pulmonary disease in a cohort of men born between 1911 and 1930 versus body weight at 1 year of age; data collated and analysed in the late 1980s. (From Barker D 1991 Journal of the Royal College of Physicians)

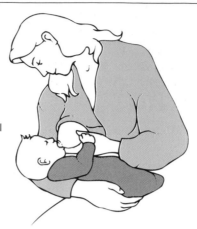

How does programming work?

The body's cells must have some way of "remembering" nutrition and other early environmental influences but how does this happen?

It could be. . .

| by affecting long-term activity of certain genes | **or** | changing the proportions of certain cells in different body tissues | **or** | giving preferential treatment to certain types of cells |

Figure 1.2 Possible mechanisms of programming in early life for health or disease. (Adapted from Lucas A 1996 MRC News)

provide an adolescent service for the management of chronic diseases such as diabetes and cystic fibrosis.

The dependency of the child within the family and the centrality of the family environment in shaping the child's cognitive, emotional and social development cannot be overemphasized. This has two important consequences. Firstly, when a child presents with a health problem it is the family as a unit that must be 'managed', not just the child. Secondly, adverse external factors, particularly economic, may impact on a child's health via their effect on the family unit as a whole. Thus, poverty and deprivation (emotional and physical, including abuse) are major environmental influences on the health of the developing child. After the family, school is the most important component of a child's environment, and school has a particularly important role in meeting the special needs of children with disabilities due to chronic illness or neurological disorder (see Ch. 17). Thus, coordination of hospital and community child health services with each other and with the non-

medical agencies such as social work and education is crucial if the ideal of a holistic approach to the child and family is to be achieved.

What is health and how is it measured?

Other than a general agreement that health is not just the absence of ill-health, it is virtually impossible to find a consensus definition of health. However, the following quotation from Katherine Mansfield provides a definition which seems to encapsulate the positive aspects of health: 'By health I mean the possibility of living life to the full, an adult life in close contact with everything I love ... I want to be everything that I am able of being'. Although written in an adult context, this quotation does bring out the idea of an individual's potential for health, an idea which is central to the practice of paediatrics.

As for the question of how we measure health, the short answer is that we don't. What we do is measure the rate of ill health in a population by means of mortality and morbidity statistics, and make the assumption that where mortality and morbidity rates are low, the population is generally healthy, and vice versa. Each measure has its own strengths and weaknesses. Death is a definite endpoint, and mortality data are routinely collected with reasonable accuracy. However, mortality measures only the most extreme form of ill health and in childhood, other than in the newborn period, death is uncommon. Furthermore, mortality statistics do not measure pain, discomfort or handicap and consequent loss of potential for health. Less than 0.1% of the child population dies each year whereas it has been estimated that up to 3% of children have a significant disability, i.e. a condition that limits normal activity. The efforts of the child health services are more appropriately geared towards preventing morbidity, but the difficulty here is that these data are not routinely collected and, when they are, they may be difficult to interpret because of variations in the criteria used.

CHANGING PATTERNS OF DISEASE IN CHILDHOOD

Population trends and family structure

The dramatic increase in life expectancy seen in the UK during the twentieth century is typical of the developed world, and has been accompanied by a halving of the birth rate (Table 1.2) due to social and economic forces. As a consequence, the UK population profile has been transformed by an increase in the proportion of the middle-aged and elderly and a progressive decline in the proportion of children (Fig. 1.3). This decline has now bottomed out, and it is expected that children will continue to form a stable 20% of the population for the next 30 years or so. By virtue of their young age, children represent a disproportionately large (30%) share of the population's life expectancy, and there is a correspondingly greater impact of death in childhood in terms of years of life lost.

The overall pattern of demographic change seen in the UK has not occurred uniformly

Table 1.2	Life expectancy at birth (UK)		
		Year	
		1901	1991
Life expectancy (years)			
Male		45	73
Female		49	79
Birth rate (per 1000 population)		28	14

Sources: Registrar General's statistical reviews 1841–1971; Office of Population Censuses and Surveys, population estimates 1981 and 1991

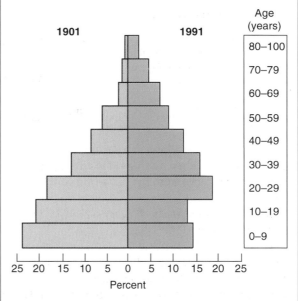

Figure 1.3 Population profile: 1901 versus 1991. (Source: Office of Population Census and Surveys)

throughout the world. Thus, in the non-industrialized nations, children form up to 50% of the total population, a pattern which is reflected in some ethnic communities within the UK. For example, children constitute 46 and 44% respectively of the Bangladeshi and Pakistani UK populations. Although there is a correlation between the proportion of children in a population and childhood mortality rate in global terms, no such simple relationship exists across ethnic groups in the UK. For example, the risk of death during infancy is substantially higher than the UK average in Pakistani children but lower than average in those of Bangladeshi parentage.

The changes in population structure described above have been accompanied by changes in the structure of the family unit. Although two-parent families remain the norm, the number of single-parent families now exceeds 20%. This is important because children living in poverty are at increased risk of poor health (see Ch. 20) and children with only one parent are at increased risk of poverty. Children with lone parents most commonly have a divorced mother, but the steepest increase is in never-married mothers who tend to be younger and are more likely to have a preschool child, both of which factors reduce earning capacity.

Family structure varies with ethnic group. Compared with white children, Bangladeshi and Pakistani children have more siblings and fewer grandparents and are less likely to live with a single parent. A survey carried out in 1990 showed that approximately 50% of Caribbean children lived with a lone parent compared with 15% of white children and less than 10% of children in families from the Indian subcontinent.

MORTALITY AND MORBIDITY

The term 'mortality rate' refers to deaths over a defined period of time expressed as a proportion of the population of the relevant age or, as in infancy, as a proportion of births (Fig. 1.4). Morbidity covers all forms of ill health, both acute and chronic.

The increase in life expectancy discussed in the previous section is, of course, a reflection of the spectacular decline in mortality rates in childhood (Fig. 1.5). This decline, which has been observed at all ages but particularly in infancy, began as a result of a number of factors related to the economic prosperity of the late Victorian era: better nutrition, housing (less overcrowding), sanitation and education. For the most part, improvements in medical care, such as the use of antibiotics (1940s) and widespread implementation of effective immunization programmes (1950s/1960s) came later. However, there are examples of early improvements in clinical practice such as the phasing out of the unqualified handwoman by the Midwives Act of 1902 with the consequent improvement in the management of labour.

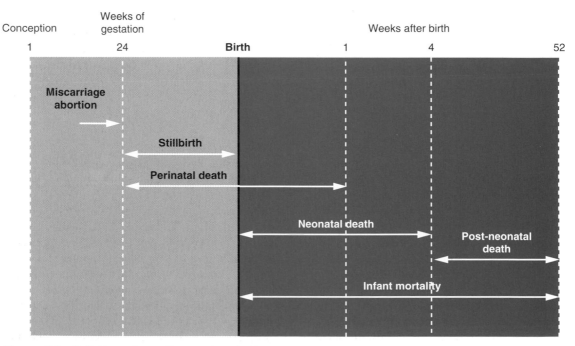

Figure 1.4 Definitions of mortality rates in early life

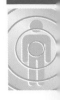

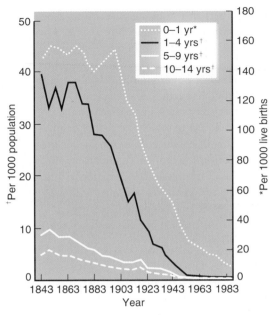

Figure 1.5 Trend in mortality in children aged 0–14 years 1841/5 to 1986/90

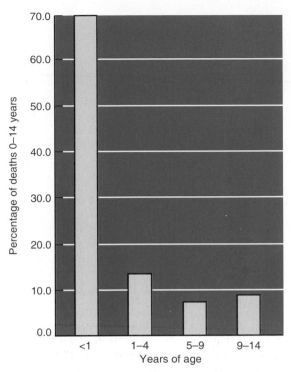

Figure 1.6 Deaths in age groups as a percentage of all deaths in children 0–14 years of age in 1993 (England and Wales)

Infant mortality

Deaths occurring in the first year of life have long been accepted as an indicator of the health of the population generally. At the turn of the twentieth century, 150 children out of every 1000 live births died before their first birthday; since then infant mortality has fallen consistently, dropping below 100 deaths per 1000 live births in the 1920s and reaching single figures in 1984 (Fig. 1.5). Subsequently, infant mortality has fallen every year bar one, although the rate of decline has necessarily slowed. Even at the levels of less than 7 per 1000 live births reached in the 1990s, the total number of lives lost in the first year of life accounts for 70% of all deaths in children between birth and 14 years (Fig. 1.6). The fact that infant mortality rates are significantly lower in Japan and Scandinavia demonstrates that further improvements in the UK rates (6.1 in 1996) are possible.

Neonatal and postneonatal deaths

For epidemiological purposes, infant mortality is subdivided into *neonatal deaths* (birth to 1 month) and *postneonatal deaths* (1 month to 1 year); the

major causes are shown in Figure 1.7. Congenital abnormalities account for approximately half of all infant deaths (of which about half are due to congenital heart disease) spread more or less equally between the neonatal and post neonatal periods. Deaths related principally to immaturity (e.g. the respiratory distress syndrome) occur predominantly in the first month of life, and there is a very strong inverse relationship between neonatal mortality and birth weight – with the risk of death in babies less than 1500 g some 200-fold higher than in those weighing 3000 g or more at birth (Fig. 1.8). The incidence of sudden infant death syndrome (SIDS) has fallen dramatically over the past decade, but remains the most important cause of postneonatal death. The fall in deaths from SIDS provides an example of how health education can be effective in reducing mortality (see Fig. 15.15). Thus, public awareness of the factors underlying SIDS – sleeping in the prone position before the infant is old enough to roll over, over-wrapping (leading to

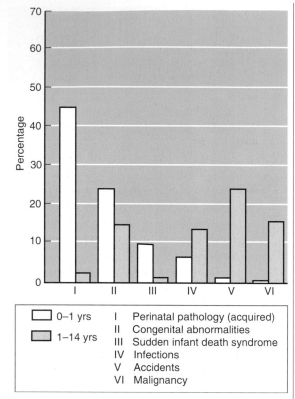

Figure 1.7 Causes of death in childhood expressed as a percentage of all deaths in age groups: England and Wales (1992-3) and Scotland (1994) combined (see Ch. 4 for Perinatal pathology)

overheating) and smoking – has been associated with a reduction in the incidence of SIDS from nearly 50% to about 30% of all postneonatal deaths.

The effect of poverty on health, alluded to in the previous section, is seen clearly in the infant mortality rates, particularly in the postneonatal period in which the risk of death is 80% higher in babies born to mothers in social class V (unskilled manual) compared with social class I (professional). A maternal age of less than 20 years is associated with a $2\frac{1}{2}$-fold increase of the postneonatal mortality compared with those born to mothers aged 25–34 years.

Child mortality beyond infancy

Death beyond the first year of life has become uncommon as the prevalence of serious infectious disease has declined. In the 1930s, before the introduction of immunization and antibiotics, one in every two childhood deaths was attributable to one of five diseases: pneumonia, tuberculosis, diphtheria, measles and whooping cough. By the 1990s these diseases accounted for 1 in 150 deaths. Mortality rates between 1 and 15 years are now lower than in any other period of life.

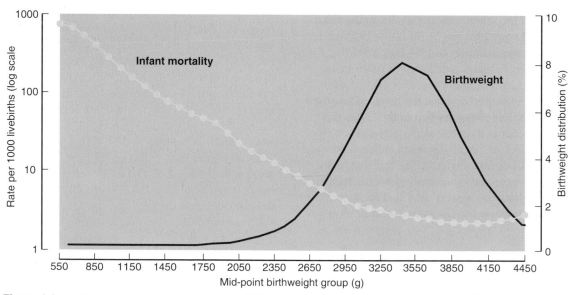

Figure 1.8 Infant mortality versus birth weight: 1989–91 England and Wales. (From Botting 1995)

As death from infectious disease has declined, so other causes have assumed greater importance (Fig. 1.7). Injuries and poisoning now account for one-third of all deaths in childhood (half of which are road accidents; see Ch. 15) and malignant disease (see Ch. 11) accounts for about one-third of the remainder, even though mortality rates for malignant disease have halved over the past 25 years. Infections (see Ch. 14), although much less common than previously, together account for approximately 15% of childhood deaths.

Morbidity

Definitions

Ill health in a population can be defined in terms of incidence and prevalence:

> **Incidence:**
> The number of new cases of a disease occurring in a defined population (e.g. size, age range, ethnic group) per unit time (usually a year)

> **Prevalence:**
> The most often used measure of prevalence is *point prevalence*, the number of cases of a particular disease in a defined population at a point in time, but *period prevalence* (number of cases present in a population over a period of time) is also used.

Quantifying morbidity

As indicated earlier, accurate assessment of the amount of ill health in the population is difficult. There is no single source of routinely collected data which provides a comprehensive picture of the range of illnesses from which children (or adults for that matter) suffer. Sources of data include questionnaire-based surveys of households, surveys undertaken in general practice, computer-based records of hospital activity and specialized databases for specific diseases (for further details see Beyond core: sources of morbidity data in childhood).

Acute and chronic illness

General practitioners are the initial point of contact with the health services for the majority of

---

BEYOND CORE

SOURCES OF MORBIDITY DATA IN CHILDHOOD

Sources of data include:

- The General Household Survey (GHS), an annual review of about 12 000 households which includes questions for parents about their children's health
- The National Morbidity Survey of General Practice (MSGP), the latest of which (1991/2) involved 60 practices in England and Wales, in which details of each patient contact are recorded
- Hospital information systems (HISs) which record details of individual patient admissions
- Disease-specific registers and databases, such as those for cancer and cystic fibrosis

Together these sources provide a window on the state of the population's health although each alone has particular weaknesses as well as strengths. Thus, the GHS suffers from the problem that errors may be introduced by forgetfulness, differing perceptions of illness or inappropriate use of diagnostic labels, but on the positive side it covers minor and major illness and counts both declared (i.e. that which brings the child into contact with the health services) and undeclared illness. Although the data collected by the MSGP and by HISs may be more accurate diagnostically, the former is not based on a random sample of practices and the latter is limited by the variable standard of the clinical information recorded and the completeness of returns. Registers and databases may collect better quality data but are available for only a limited number of conditions, most of which are chronic. None of the sources records unrecognized illness.

The GHS, MSGP and HISs all identify respiratory disease as the most common cause of illness in childhood (Table 1.4).

children with acute illnesses. Children make up approximately 30% of general practice workload and consulting rates are high, particularly in the 0–4 years age range (Table 1.3). The majority of children seen in general practice do not have serious disease, and less than 10% are referred on to hospital. More than half of all general practitioner consultations involve respiratory disease, and this is true at all ages although the aetiology may vary, acute respiratory infections predominating in the 0–4 years age group and asthma in the 5–15 years age group. Preventative care accounts for approximately 20% of consultations in the 0–5 years age group, reflecting the shift of this activity from community child health into primary care. Respiratory disorders also head the list of diagnoses of children admitted to hospital (Table 1.4), although they make up a smaller proportion of the total than in general practice, with injuries and poisoning relatively more prominent, particularly in the 5–15 years age group. Surprisingly, as the population's health has improved, annual admission rates have risen (Fig. 1.9). The reason for this is not clear but it may reflect changes in parental expectation and a lower threshold for general pratitioners to refer and for paediatric units to admit. In inverse proportion to the rise in admission rates is the duration of hospital stay, which has now fallen to under 3 days. This may reflect factors related to the higher admission rates (e.g. less severe cases being admitted) and more effective treatments being available.

In spite of the rise in hospital admissions (Fig. 1.9), patient days (number of admissions ×

duration of stay) has fallen by a third between 1954 and 1994, and is likely to fall further as the policy of treating children in their homes ('hospital at home') is implemented wherever practicable. However, for the most part, this involves chronic diseases. A key element of the strategy to deliver care in the child's home is the specialist nurse. The specialist nurse has skills in managing a particular disease (e.g. cystic fibrosis, diabetes, asthma) and provides the link between hospital and home, supporting the family while care is delivered at home (often by the parents or the child, depending on age and the disorder being treated). Although the impact of specialist nurses has yet to be fully evaluated, there is already evidence that their involvement in care can reduce the number of admissions and the duration of stay needed. Inevitably, the strategy of avoiding hospital admission also places more emphasis on outpatient and day care.

Children attending as outpatients generally have non-urgent or chronic conditions. Typically, children attending fall into one of three categories:

1. New referral from general practice requiring further investigation and treatment. Common examples include:
   - Urinary tract infection/enuresis (see Chs 8 and 18)
   - Murmur picked up during routine surveillance
   - Failure to thrive
   - Recurrent headache/abdominal pain
   - Concern about neurodevelopment
   - Chronic constipation
   - Possible convulsion.

Table 1.3	Morbidity – some statistics
General practitioner's involvement[a]	**Hospital's involvement**[b]
Each child of 0–4 years consults general practitioner × 6 per year	For every 1000 children aged 0–14 years attending a general practitioner:
Each child of 5–15 years consults general practitioner × 2.5 per year	73 are referred on to outpatient or accident and emergency departments
Children = 30% of general practice workload	23 are admitted

[a] Source: Morbidity Statistics from General Practice 1991/2 (England and Wales)
[b] Source: Morbidity Statistics from General Practice 1993 (UK)

Table 1.4   Top ten diagnoses in children 0–16 years old admitted to the medical paediatric wards, Ninewells Hospital & Medical School, Dundee, 1995

Diagnosis	Percentage
Upper respiratory tract infection[a]	13.2
Lower respiratory tract infection	13.0
Asthma	9.8
Gastroenteritis	8.4
Non-specific viral illness	5.7
Convulsions[b]	4.1
Febrile convulsions	4.0
Malignancy	3.7
Accidental poisoning	3.4
Renal tract infection[c]	1.6

These data refer to individual periods of admission, and the rates in some categories, such as malignancy and convulsions, may partly reflect multiple admissions of particular children
[a] Includes otitis media and croup
[b] Convulsions other than febrile convulsions are mostly epilepsy
[c] Mostly cystitis but includes pyelonephritis

[2] Chronic disease for review, for example:
- Asthma
- Diabetes
- Cystic fibrosis
- Epilepsy
- Malignancy/hereditary anaemia.

[3] Ward follow-up to check that the condition for which the child was admitted has resolved, for example:
- Lower respiratory tract infection with chest X-ray changes and/or for further diagnostic work-up or therapeutic intervention, e.g.
- Conditions such as those listed in categories 1 and 2 above, diagnosed during the admission.

According to the General Household Survey (GHS), the prevalence of chronic disease in children 0–15 years old doubled between 1972 and 1991. This may, in part, be due to changing parental perceptions and expectations but also a real increase in the prevalence of chronic diseases such as asthma, cystic fibrosis (see Ch. 6) and

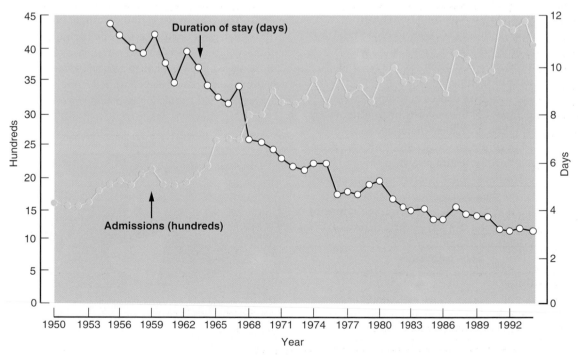

Figure 1.9   Annual medical admissions and duration of stay for the Royal Hospital for Sick Children, Edinburgh, 1950–1994

diabetes (see Ch. 9). In the 1991 GHS, nearly 8% of respondents reported respiratory disease (mostly asthma) while ear (mostly otitis media) and skin (mostly eczema) disorders were each reported by 2% and nervous/mental disorders by 1.5%. Long-standing illness which limited activity (i.e. disability) was reported in 4% of 0–4 year olds and 10% of 5–15 year olds.

Disability

Impairment is the child's medical problem (e.g. hemiplegia) and disability (Ch. 17) is the extent to which the child cannot perform the functions expected of, his or her peer group (e.g. a hemiplegic child unable to run or climb stairs). Thus, together with mortality, disability is a measure of the loss of potential for health referred to at the beginning of this chapter.

As with other forms of morbidity, there are no routinely collected data on childhood disability. The major survey of disability undertaken in 1975/6 was analysed on the basis of severity and function (Table 1.5). Approximately 3% of children aged 0–15 years were found to have severe disability, the rate being higher in boys than girls. The most common functional disabilities (i.e. those occurring in >1% of the 0–15 year old child population) were behaviour, communication, locomotion, continence and intellectual functioning).

In the summary of causes of severe disability shown in Table 1.5, the majority of children were thought unlikely to achieve independence and many had multiple handicaps (roughly one-third single, one-third two, and one-third three to five). Not only does multiple disability severely curtail function, and thus quality of life, it also curtails life expectancy. Thus, those children with three or more severe disabilities have a 50% chance of dying by 20 years of age.

Child abuse

The term 'child abuse' (see Chs 15 and 17) covers neglect and physical, sexual and psychological harm done to children (Fig. 1.10). It is an important category of morbidity which is not

Table 1.5 Causes of severe disability in children 0–15 years old	
Primary disorder	*% of total*
Mental retardation[a]	38
Neurological[b]	22
Special senses[c]	15
Psychiatric	6
Musculoskeletal	6
Respiratory	4
Other	9

Source: Dykes J 1978 Ten thousand severely handicapped children. Australian Publishing Service, Canberra
7/1000 children; 1.8 disorders/child
Principal diagnoses:
[a] Down's syndrome
[b] Epilepsy, cerebral palsy
[c] Deafness, visual defects, speech and hearing disorders

covered by any of the data sources previously mentioned and is thus very difficult to quantify. This is true particularly in respect of sexual abuse, which was rarely reported in the UK until the 1980s. Thus the increase in the number of children in this category coming to the attention of health and social services is almost certainly a reflection of increased professional and public awareness. National data have been compiled from local authority child protection registers since 1989 and

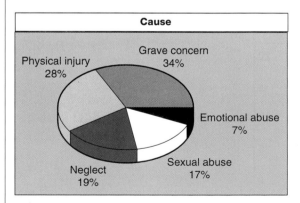

Figure 1.10 Reasons for children aged 0–17 years being on child protection registers in England, 1992

show that approximately 4 per 1000 children aged 0–15 years are included in the register at any one time, with girls three times more likely to be on the register for sexual abuse in the 10–15 years age group.

FURTHER READING

Botting B (ed) 1995 OPCS Series DS No. 11: the health of our children. HMSO, London

Donaldson R J, Donaldson L J 1993 Essential public health medicine. Kluwer, Dordrecht

Woodroffe C, Glickman M, Barker M, Power C (eds) 1993 Children, teenagers and health: the key data. Open University Press, Milton Keynes

Growth and sexual development

S. A. Greene

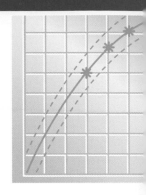

ESSENTIAL BACKGROUND

INTRODUCTION

While adults continue to develop and change physically, the process of growth in childhood is of such dramatic proportions that it is one of the defining differences between the adult and the child. An understanding of the normal growth process is essential, and all diseases in childhood must be considered against the background of the normal growth pattern. Children grow in a remarkably predicable pattern, despite the multifactorial and complex underlying controlling processes. Growth may be affected as part of a specific disease process involving the various systems controlling growth, or as a consequence of more generalized illness or physical deformity, as well as being influenced by the social circumstances of the child and its family. Growth

in a child serves as an indicator of well-being and state of health in general.

ANATOMY AND PHYSIOLOGY

Growth and development are defined as the process by which a fertilized ovum becomes an adult organism; they are driven by the genetic endowment and influenced by interaction with the environment. Growth is the change in size; development is the differentiation of form and change of function.

Every organ and system has to go through these processes of physical change and functional adaptation. The potential for growth and development is present from the time of conception, and thus inherent in the genetic make up of every normal child. Nevertheless, numerous factors, internal and external, exert their influence on these processes.

In summary, the term 'growth and development' encompasses the following aspects:

- Cellular differentiation, organogenesis and change in size
- Functional maturation and adaptation
- Neurodevelopment
- Psychosocial integration.

A discussion on specific neurodevelopment is given in Chapter 3.

Cell growth and organogenesis

The growth of cells is sustained by a combination of energy nutrients derived from food intake and hormonal actions on cell replication and cell size. A

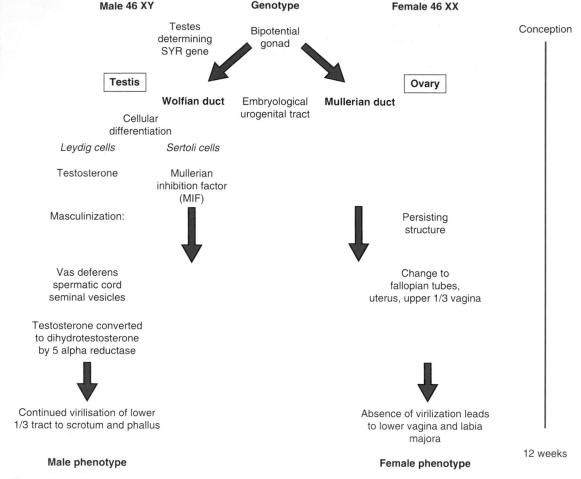

Figure 2.1 Development of the sexual phenotype

hormone is an intercellular messenger, i.e. a protein produced by a cell with an independent cellular metabolic action. Classically the hormone is produced by an endocrine gland and transported through the peripheral blood system by separate protein-binding hormones, to exert its action on cells in distant target glands. Some hormones, however, may act locally, being transported in interstitial tissue (paracrine), to adjacent cells (juxtacrine) or within the same cell (autocrine).

Cell differentiation into a defined organ structure (organogenesis) is completed by the end of the first trimester. This includes complete differentiation into the male and female sexual tracts (Fig. 2.1). Thereafter, organogenesis is concerned with increasing size (e.g. of the brain)

or atrophy (e.g. of the thymus gland) as the whole organism grows. The growth of the fetus is mainly driven by a nutrient supply reflecting maternal and placental function. Fetal insulin appears to be the most important growth factor early in gestation. Fetal insulin-like growth factor (IGF-1) is the primary hormone influencing fetal growth in later gestation.

Endocrine regulation of growth

The major hormones involved with growth are controlled through a hypothalamic–pituitary–target gland axis (Fig. 2.2). A portal circulatory blood system between the hypothalamus and the anterior pituitary gland provides a method of

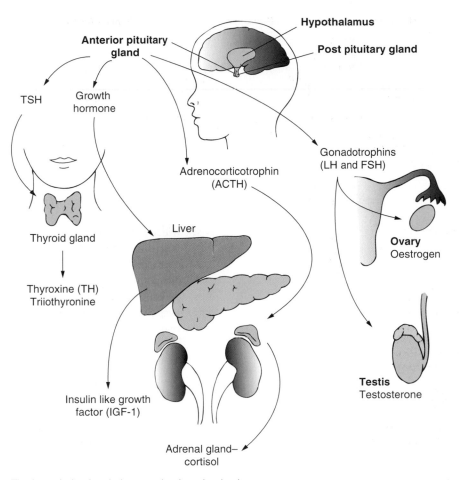

Figure 2.2   The hypothalamic–pituitary–endocrine gland axis

direct communication between the brain and the endocrine system. Hypothalamic releasing factors stimulate the anterior pituitary gland to release pituitary hormones into the peripheral circulation: cortisol-releasing factor (CRF); adrenocorticotrophin (adrenocorticotrophic hormone, ACTH); growth hormone-releasing hormone (GHRH); human growth hormone (hGH); gonadotrophin-releasing hormone (GnRH); luteinizing hormone (LH) and follicle-stimulating hormone (FSH); thyroid releasing hormone (TRH); and thyroid-stimulating hormone (TSH). These hormones act at their respective target organs by binding to specific cell receptors. hGH acts both peripherally to induce cellular growth, particularly at the bone growth plates, and also on receptors in the liver to

produce IGF-1, one of the major general cell growth factors. (Deficiency of the IGF-1 receptor is the cause of the African Pigmy.)

Physical growth of the child

A model of the factors involved in growth is given in Figure 2.3. The physical growth of the child after birth, through puberty to adulthood is dependent on the integration of many factors, leading to physical growth of the bones and lean body tissue. Ultimately stature is determined by the growth of the long bones and the spinal column. Lean tissue growth (ligaments, muscle) probably has a role in the rate of growth, 'setting' individual growth potential.

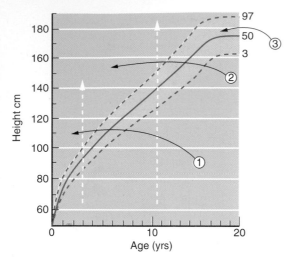

① Infancy period:
Growth mainly dependent on nutrition

② Mid childhood:
Growth mainly dependent on nutrition and specific growth factors especially hGH and thyroxine

③ Puberty:
Growth mainly dependent on nutrition growth factors and sex steroids (testosterone or oestrogen)

Figure 2.3 Model of predominant factors involved in growth

Height increases because of the dimensional changes in bones, particularly the long bones of the lower limbs. Receptors for hGH are found in high concentration on the chondrocytes of the epiphyseal growth plates of the long bones, and activation induces longitudinal growth of the bones. Thyroid hormones, IGF, oestrogens and androgens also stimulate proliferation and maturation of the chondrocytes, leading to epiphyseal cartilage growth and ultimately cartilage calcification and epiphyseal fusion. Maturation (i.e. cessation of growth) is achieved when all of the epiphyseal growth plates are fused.

Nutrition and growth

Poor nutrition resulting from poverty is the major cause of poor growth in the world. This is the case even in Western industrial societies. Severe and/or chronic illness may leave an effect on growth either acutely or chronically. For instance, acute infections (e.g. pneumonia, tonsillitis) will

slow growth, often severely. However, this is a temporary phenomenon, with a rapid 'catch-up' in growth occurring over the following weeks and months after resolution of the acute illness. A more chronic illness (e.g. cystic fibrosis) will have more permanent effects on growth, with periods of very slow growth during active phases of the illness and a failure to catch up adequately during the more quiescent periods of the illness. Indeed, even in a chronic illness which is cured there are likely to be permanent effects on growth with ultimately failure to achieve the expected final adult height (e.g. inflammatory bowel disease, post-cardiac surgery, renal failure and transplantation).

Adequate nutrition together with optimal metabolism are the building blocks of growth. An intact and efficient endocrine system is the engine that drives the normal growth pattern. Abnormalities in the endocrine system in children and adolescents are rare and account for a small proportion (<10%) of children referred to hospital for assessment of growth failure or an abnormally fast growth (see Ch. 9). While optimal nutrition is important throughout childhood and adolescence, the specific growth factors of hGH and IGF-1 become essential during childhood, with the sex steroids (testosterone in the male, oestrogen in the female) enhancing the effect during puberty (Fig. 2.3).

Central to normal growth is the integration of the actions of the growth factors. Any deficiency or imbalance will alter the speed of growth (see later), and, in severe disruption, lead to growth arrest. Protracted failure to gain weight or weight loss (failure to thrive) eventually leads to growth arrest in most cases, although height may continue to increase slowly for some time.

Puberty and adolescence

Puberty is the period of physical change during which a child attains secondary sex characteristics and at the end of which is fully fertile. Adolescence is the period encompassing puberty together with the cognitive, psychological and social behaviour characteristics that occur during this period. The physical changes of puberty are driven by distinct changes in the hormonal milieu secondary to changes in the circulating hormone concentration of gonadotrophins from the hypothalamus: LH and FSH. LH and FSH are in turn driven by changes in the balance of neurotransmitter hormones in the hypothalamus and median eminence of the brain. Activation of these neurotransmitters (usually by increasing frequency of their pulsatility) occurs some time before the appearance of the secondary sex characteristics, the latter starting to develop when there have been significant changes in circulating concentrations of either testosterone or oestrogen. The timing of the appearance of physical changes are shown in Figure 2.4.

The tempo of puberty (initial appearance and or duration) varies considerably, and is part of the constitutional variation of growth. An early onset of puberty is associated with an accelerated growth pattern, with puberty usually of a short duration associated with a high peak velocity during the growth spurt. Conversely, constitutional delayed growth is associated with a delayed onset of puberty, which often has a long duration and a lesser peak height velocity.

While adolescence itself must not be viewed as a problem, it is a period that has its own specific problems. In Western culture, adolescence is a time of increasing independence from parents and a correspondingly closer relationship to the peer

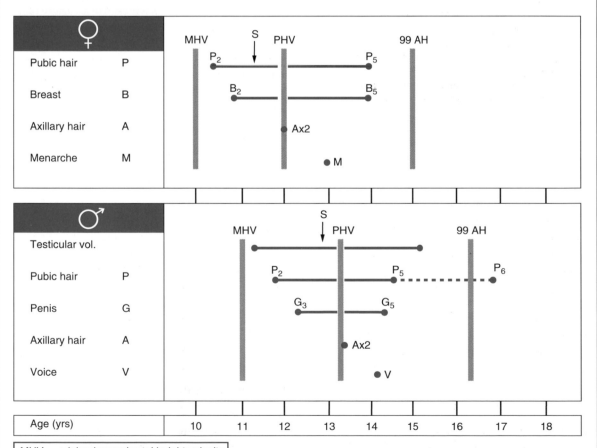

MHV = minimal prepubertal height velocity
PHV = peak height velocity
AH = adult height
S = sesamoid bone–X ray

Figure 2.4 Timing of events in puberty

group. A disabled young person may be further handicapped by the lack of facilities and opportunities for such individualization. However, there is still likely to be a reduction in the unquestioning acceptance of adult authority, together with increased size and possibly strength. Challenging behaviour can result.

NORMAL VALUES

Measurement of growth

Clinical practice requires the measurement either of supine length in the infant (<2 years of age) or standing height in the older child or adolescent, together with weight. Even with attention to detail and eradication of practical errors (Table 2.1), variations in the results of repeated frequent measurement of the child occur. This is due to variation in the child! Children are stretchy, with this elasticity influenced by fear, excitability, general well-being and time of day (children and adults appear to be on average 1 cm taller in the morning).

Speed of growth

The average growth of a child ranges from 14–16 cm/year during infancy, 7–12 cm/year in puberty to 4–6 cm/year during the mid-childhood years. In this latter period the average growth velocity is, therefore, around 0.5 cm per month. This value demonstrates one of the difficulties in transferring the physiological descriptions of growth into meaningful clinical practice. The accuracy in the measurement of growth limits the interpretation by the measurer, who must allow enough time to pass to obtain an accurate description of growth. Indeed, in assessing the effect of growth-promoting agents or the efficacy of changes to the therapy of chronic disease, most clinical studies use measurements over one or several years, and final outcomes require the measurement of adult height.

Various machines have been designed to measure as accurately as possible small changes in length or standing height. Short-term growth can be assessed with high accuracy using measures of lower limb (kneemometry); however, this measure is usually reserved for research studies. In clinical practice there are a variety of simple and robust measuring devices.

Accuracy of measurement

This depends on:

- Adopting a standard approach to the measurement of the child (see above)
- Standardization of the measuring device
- Accurate plotting of measurements on a growth chart (Table 2.2).

The growth chart

The height chart

This plots height (centimetres) against chronological age (Fig. 2.5). The growth chart is an integral part of the assessment of any child, and is considered to be part of the necessary documentation of the history of any illness; having obtained a height measurement it must be plotted on to a chart!

Table 2.1   A guide to accurate measuring
• Check the accuracy of the measuring device, using a standard (usually a metre rule)
• Remove the child's socks and shoes
• Stand the child flat against the measuring device with heels together, legs straight and shoulders relaxed
• Place the measuring arm on the top of the head, with the child looking straight ahead (with the lower margins of the eyes in the same horizontal plane as the external auditory meati). Ensure that the posture is correct by applying pressure to the mastoid processes to help stretch the child gently
• Read the height to the last complete millimetre
• Plot correctly on the appropriate growth chart

Table 2.2   Accurate plotting on a growth chart
• Check that the chart is for the appropriate sex
• Check the age
• Some charts use decimal age for which a nomogram is supplied
• Use a single point: ●

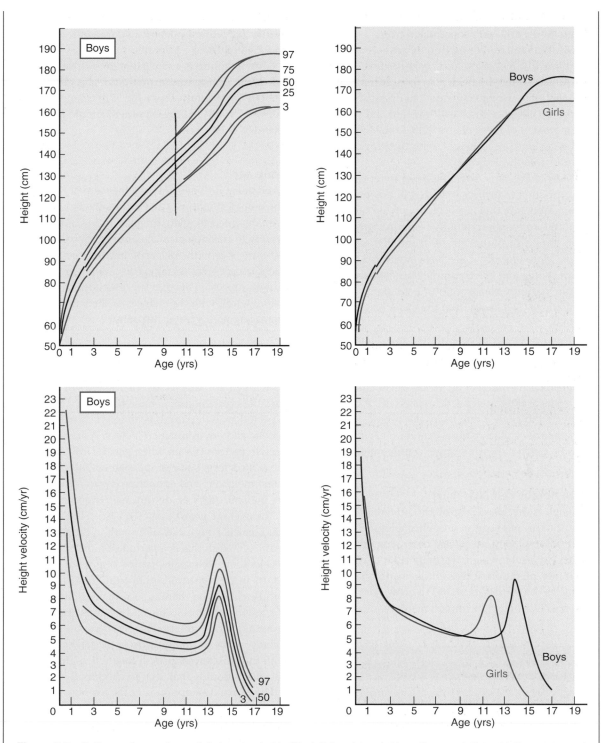

Figure 2.5 Patterns of normal growth in boys and girls. The left-hand panels show the population variation expressed as centiles for height and height velocity in boys only. The right-hand panels show the 50th centile for height and height velocity for boys and girls

The most frequently used charts over the last 30 years in the UK were constructed from measurements from a mixture of cross-sectional and longitudinal population cohorts developed by James Tanner. In 1995, data from seven cohort studies were used to construct an updated cross-sectional UK growth chart for height and weight. Comparison of these charts with Tanner charts show an increase in height, with the previous 10th centile now the 3rd centile.

Most charts have been designed to represent the variation in growth expected in a population. Conventionally this has been drawn as 'centiles', with the convention initially being to show the 3rd, 10th, 25th, 50th, 75th, 90th and 97th centile lines. More recently it has been suggested that the 0.4th centile and 99.6th centile lines be used (these mathematically correspond to 3 standard deviations (SD) away from the mean height value).

The genetic variation expected in a child's final height can be plotted on the chart as the target height and range (Table 2.3). This allows the interpretation of the child's cross-sectional height in terms of ultimate genetic expression. A child is expected to grow along his or her centile, and discrepancies require investigation (i.e. current centile position beyond target centile range).

The height velocity chart

This plots the speed of growth, conventionally in centimetres per year against chronological age (Fig. 2.5). As with the height chart, it is divided into centiles. However, it is important to realize that interpretation of the centile position is not the same as for the height chart. To grow normally, irrespective of genetic endowment, requires that over time the height velocity is around the 50th centile. For clinical purposes between the 25th and 75th centile is acceptable.

Growth failure is a persistent growth velocity below the 25th centile; growth excess is growth velocity persistently above the 75th centile. Conventionally, the measurement should be recorded over 1 year.

Bone age

Assessment of 'bone age' is a measure of physiological maturity. Several methods have been designed to relate the maturation of bone growth to chronological age, thus giving another measure of growth. Disparity between bone age and chronological age suggests a delay in the growth process. This may be constitutional or pathological, with the chances of the latter increasing with greater disparity.

Patterns of normal growth

As with all human characteristics, growth is a variable expression of genetic potential. The expected growth pattern is an interaction between genetic and environmental factors. A normal growth pattern is seen when genetic influences (bone structure, body shape, parents' height, intact metabolic and endocrine enzyme pathways) are maximized by an optimum environment.

The average growth pattern is seen in Figure 2.5. There is a high rate of growth in the first 2–3 years, although this is a period of rapid deceleration. The fastest period of growth actually occurs in the last trimester of fetal life. During middle childhood there is a fairly constant period of growth, which is followed by a rapid period of growth during puberty. The growth spurt seen in puberty is the period outside of the fetal period with the most rapid growth rate, when growth velocity is double that seen in childhood.

The above description is of the average growth pattern, which, by definition, many children will exhibit. However, many children also have a marked variation in the tempo of growth, secondary to interactions between genetic and environmental factors. This is expressed as

Table 2.3 Calculation of adult target height and target centile range
Target height (TH) = [(father's height (cm) + mother's height (cm)) /2] ± 6.5 cm[a]
Target range (TR) = TH ± 8.5 cm
[a] Based on the average height difference between men and women = 13 cm

constitutional variation in growth, i.e. a growth pattern different from the expected. Occasionally, the constitutional differences in growth may be considered severe, especially in association with children who are genetically 'designed' to be at the extremes of expected genetic growth, e.g. familial short or tall stature (see p. 24). In this situation severe variation in the tempo of growth will cause concern. Either the normal variation is severe enough for medical carers to consider that there may be an underlying pathology (e.g. undiagnosed chronic illness or endocrinopathy) or children and/or parents themselves are concerned about their stature. The majority of 'abnormal growth' patterns are in fact extremes of normal variation, and the final height falls within the expected adult target height range (Fig. 2.6).

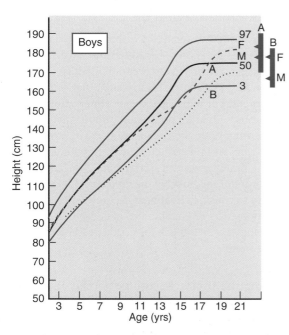

Figure 2.6   Patterns of constitutional delayed growth in puberty. The mid-parental height for boy A is on the 75th centile. The mid-parental height for boy B is on the 25th centile. Both boys showed similar delay throughout childhood. Boy A dropped just below the 3rd centile for only a short period of growth during puberty. Boy B is well below the 3rd centile from early childhood. Both boys with constitutional delay obtain a final stature appropriate to their parental height, and are normal for the population

CORE PROBLEMS

VARIATION OF GROWTH

As discussed earlier, normal growth requires the integration of normal genetic instructions with optimum environmental conditions and intact homoeostatic endocrine and metabolic systems. Abnormalities in these systems will give rise to an abnormal growth pattern, and the majority of these conditions will require treatment in their own right, with a few specific growth disorders requiring specific growth therapy (e.g. hGH, see Ch. 9).

Most of the growth problems encountered in clinical practice represent a normal variation in growth from the expected growth pattern. These are usually attributed to constitutional delay of growth and puberty (CDGP) or familial short stature (FSS) or a combination of both.

✳ KEY DIAGNOSIS

Constitutional delay of growth and puberty

Separation of CDGP and an abnormal growth pattern secondary to underlying pathology can be difficult. Ultimately CDGP is a diagnosis of exclusion made retrospectively with the knowledge of the final height. In clinical practice, however, it is not possible to wait until the period of growth is over, and some investigations will be required to exclude underlying pathology. The chance of underlying pathology in a child with a height between −2 and −3 SD (i.e. moderately below the 3rd centile) is less than 10%. This increases to 50% with a height <−3 SD and above 80% when <−4 SD.

The short and delayed child should be assessed carefully. The history may reveal symptoms of an underlying medical condition. Accurate information on the height potential of the child is determined from the parents' height. Growth failure may have to be excluded by repeat measurement of height and comparison of height velocity against standard charts. In severe cases, formal endocrine testing may be required even in

Table 2.4 Normal variants of growth
Familial short stature (FSS) Short stature (height <3rd centile) throughout childhood and adolescence Final height <3rd centile Normal height velocity (between 25th and 75th centile) Height within target range as defined by parent's height Bone age consistent with chronological age (within 2 SD)
Constitutional delay of growth and puberty (CDGP) Short stature (height <3rd centile) at some point in childhood and or adolescence Height below range defined by parents' height Retarded bone age (>2 SD below chronological age) Reduced height velocity in later childhood years (<25th centile) Delayed onset of puberty
Familial tall stature and constitutional growth acceleration Can be defined using 'tall' expressed as >97th centile and velocity >75th centile

the absence of specific symptoms. Guidelines for the approach to investigations of the short child are given in Chapter 9.

Familial short stature

By definition 3% of the population will be defined as short. Concern arises in short families when FSS combines with CDGP; the growth pattern of the child is often very worrying for that family, and they will request advice (see Table 2.4 for the specific differences between FSS and CDGP).

VARIATION IN SEXUAL DEVELOPMENT

Early puberty (precocious puberty) is defined by the onset of puberty before 8 years (girls) and 9 years (boys). It can be divided into 'true' (or 'central') early puberty and 'pseudo'-sexual precocity. True early puberty occurs when all of the events of normal puberty occurring early, whereas in pseudo-precocious puberty only some aspects of sexual development occur, depending on whether abnormal concentrations of androgens or oestrogens are present. In the latter, the puberty may be iso-sexual, i.e in the same sex or heterosexual (i.e. virilization of the female, feminization of the male).

The timing of the onset of puberty becomes earlier with improved population health. Concern has been expressed recently that puberty is earlier, particularly in girls, because of increased oestrogens in the environment and also because of increasing obesity in the population.

Late puberty is defined as absence of secondary sex deveopment by 14 years of age in girls and 15 years in boys. Because of the lack of the pubertal growth spurt, many of these teenagers will present with short stature. While the majority prove to be severe cases of CDGP, with or without FSS, it is mandatory to investigate their endocrine system (see Ch. 9).

✳ KEY DIAGNOSIS

Precocious puberty

This condition is relatively common in girls, where it is invariably idiopathic and a true integrated puberty. Very occasionally it is secondary to a central brain lesion, the commonest of which is damage after radiotherapy or surgery. Ovarian producing tumours are exceedingly rare. Precocious puberty in boys is very rare, and related to underlying pathology (e.g. a brain tumour or hamartoma). The earlier the onset of the puberty the greater the families' desire to consider treatment. LH-releasing hormone (LH-RH) analogues have been developed which block the action of LH-RH on the gonad.

Premature thelarche and pubarche

Premature thelarche is an isolated transient early breast development in girls, frequently seen in the neonatal and infancy period, with no other signs of secondary sexual development. Treatment is unnecessary. *Premature pubarche* is an isolated development of pubic and axillary hair, more common in girls. It is driven by activation of adrenal steroids, usually in mid-childhood, often accompanied by a small growth spurt.

2

Gynaecomastia

This is common in boys in early to mid-puberty, and frequently it is unilateral. It can be exacerbated in moderate simple obesity. It usually regresses spontaneously. Occasionally surgery may be indicated for cosmetic and emotional reasons.

FURTHER READING

Tanner J M 1978 Foetus into man. Open Books, London

CHAPTER 3

Neurodevelopment

D. F. Haddad

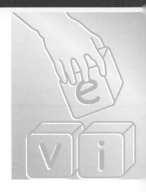

CORE PROBLEMS IN NEURODEVELOPMENT

CORE PROBLEMS	KEY DIAGNOSIS	RELATED TOPICS
• Global developmental delay	Mental handicap	Epilepsy[10] (Autism)
• Delayed walking	Normal variation	Cerebral palsy[10] Muscular dystrophy[10] Spinal lesion
• Delayed speech	Hearing loss	Normal variation Mental handicap Cerebral palsy[10] Stammering Autism

Where the primary location of a topic is in another chapter, this is indicated by a superscript

ESSENTIAL BACKGROUND

INTRODUCTION

The process of growth and development is central to paediatrics. It is said that a knowledge of the normal development of children is as fundamental for those providing care for children as anatomy is for surgeons.

The normal mechanisms driving the process of growth and development are numerous and complex. Whilst there are a number of disorders that directly involve these mechanisms, resulting in poor growth and failure to achieve a normal pattern of development, growth and development can also be undermined in a much wider range of disorders affecting various organ systems. It is fair to say that almost any pathology of any system, if severe enough, may influence a child's growth and interfere with his or her normal development. Thus, as was stated in the previous chapter, growth and development parameters in children can serve as indicators to their well-being and state of health in general.

Definitions

The various aspects of growth and development were defined in Chapter 2.

Though these different aspects of growth and development are closely interlinked, for clarity they are studied separately. Physical growth (increase in height and weight) has been addressed in the previous chapter. This chapter is devoted to the study of neurodevelopment. Psychosocial problems are addressed in Chapter 18 (behavioural disorders) and Chapter 17 (community paediatrics). Functional maturation is discussed in the physiological background for each system in the appropriate chapter.

SPHERES OF NEURODEVELOPMENT

Physical growth of the nervous system involves myelination of nerves and an increase in the number of connections between cells. In the brain, this is reflected in an increase in the size of the head. As the myelination progresses, the nervous control of various functions improves. The functional maturation of the somatic innervation is assessed by the conventional neurological examination. It is clear that intact nervous mechanisms are necessary in order for more complex functions to be achieved.

Neurodevelopment is the process of acquisition of learned skills. It involves the employment of intact motor and sensory systems, together with the centres of balance, coordination, motor planning and cognition in order to learn new skills, aided by observation, imitation and training. Social development integrates the motor, behavioural and intellectual skills and incorporates experiences and training to produce the individual as a full member of society.

The neurodevelopmental skills can be categorized into four groups:

- Gross motor
- Fine motor and vision
- Hearing, speech and language
- Social.

Because fine motor skills are dependent on visual control, clues to the stages of maturation of the visual pathways are listed with fine motor skills. Similarly, since normal hearing is essential for speech and language development, ways for obtaining evidence of normal hearing are listed together with skills of speech and language.

DEVELOPMENTAL MILESTONES

There are numerous skills to be learnt throughout childhood. Learning these skills is a continuous uninterrupted process. However, it is punctuated by the acquisition of major skills that are crucial for the child's progress in each of the four spheres of development. The ages at which these skills are acquired are called developmental milestones (Table 3.1).

The age at which a given skill is achieved is dependent on multiple intrinsic and environmental factors. It is thought that, at least for some skills, a critical period exists, when the intrinsic mechanisms reach a level of maturity allowing them to respond to extrinsic factors. Attempts at training prior to this are likely to be

futile, and absence of adequate stimulation during the critical period is likely to reduce the responsiveness to training; acquiring the skill then becomes more difficult.

The age at which a given skill is learnt follows a normal distribution pattern. In this text, most of the ages quoted for achieving milestones are those by which 95% of children will have achieved them. Hence, children unable to demonstrate these skills by the quoted ages qualify for further evaluation. Though the rate of progress in each sphere may vary, the sequence of acquisition of skills within a sphere is more or less constant.

Gross motor development

A head to foot progression occurs; thus the baby learns to control the head first, then to sit and stand.

First attempts at head control can be observed in a newborn baby. However, full head control is achieved at around 5 months of age (Fig. 3.1). A baby is expected to sit without support by 8 months of age, to stand by around 12 months and walk by 14 months. A toddler of 2 years of age should be able to kick a ball with either foot, to walk up and down stairs at around 3 years, and to hop and skip by the age of 4 years.

Vision and fine motor skills

Full-term newborn babies are able to fixate visually on objects brought into their line of vision. Interestingly, newborn babies display visual preference for female human faces. In the first few weeks, babies are able to follow objects of interest only for a short distance. At around 2–3 months of age, infants in the supine position follow objects by turning their heads and eyes through a complete arc of 180°.

Complete alignment of both eyes may not be achieved in the first few weeks. Mild intermittent squint is acceptable in this period (see Ch. 13). Objective clinical testing for visual acuity using cards with letters or shapes becomes possible at around 3 years of age.

Between 3 and 4 months of age babies display hand regard, when they spend a considerable

Table 3.1	Developmental milestones			
	8 weeks	8–9 months	2 years	3½ years
Gross motor	Partial head control	Prone: pivots, rolls to supine Sits without support	Walks and runs without falling Kicks a ball	Runs smoothly and fast Alternates feet going up stars
Vision	Intent regard of mother's face Follows objects past the midline			Shape recognition test
Fine motor	Hands held open for long periods	Grasps dangling object Picks up a pellet by raking, may use pincer grasp	Builds a tower of 5–6 cubes Imitates a straight line Turns pages singularly	Builds a tower of 7–8 cubes Completes a six-shape formboard Imitates a circle
Hearing	Startles to sudden noise Response to unseen mother's voice	Distraction test (see Fig. 13.6)		Word recognition test
Speech and language		Free varied vocalization 'Listens' to adult conversation	Names 3–5 pictures/ objects Joins 2 words together Vocalizes needs	Clear four-word sentences Recounts experiences
Social	Social smile	Awareness of strangers Chews food with bits in it	Uses toys meaningfully Uses cup and spoon Toilet awareness	Toilet trained by day Complete self-feeding Imaginative play

Adapted from the Scottish child health surveillance programme

amount of time looking at their own hands. This fascination with hand movements is thought to aid eye–hand coordination.

At 5 months of age babies reach for objects and grasp them by a whole hand grip. At 6 months they are able to transfer objects from one hand to another. At around 9 months babies begin to use a pincer grasp to pick up small objects (using the thumb and forefinger). They should be able to pull a ball attached to a string at around this age.

The ability to place 1 inch (2.5 cm) cubes above one another to make a tower is usually utilized to measure fine motor development in toddlers and young children. At 18 months of age a tower of three cubes is achieved; at 2 years six cubes, and at 3 years nine cubes or more can be stacked. A form board with six or more shapes is managed at around 3 years of age.

Pencil skills can be used for the same purpose. Thus, a 15 month old toddler is able to scribble, at 2 years to make a straight line, at 3 years a circle, at 4 years a square and at 5 years a triangle. Later on, fine motor development is judged from the ability at handwriting, drawing, doing up buttons and shoelaces, etc.

Hearing, speech and language

There is plenty of evidence that fetuses in utero are able to hear and even respond to sound. A newborn turns his or her head to the direction of the sound source and startles to a sudden loud noise. A baby 6–8 weeks of age responds to the unseen mother's voice.

Clues to an understanding of language can be obtained from early infancy. In the second half of the first year, babies start to respond to their own

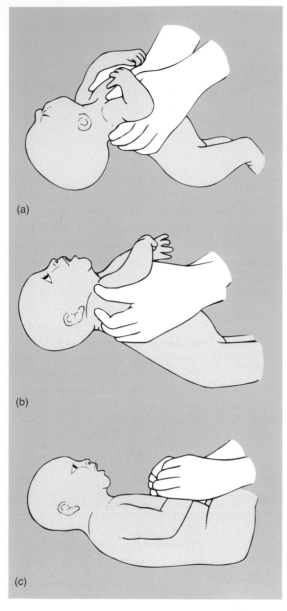

(a)

(b)

(c)

Figure 3.1 Development of head control

names, and later respond to 'no'. At 18 months of age, a baby is able to point to one or two body parts if requested. A 2 year old toddler understands simple commands, and at 3 years understands a few prepositions.

Coordination of sucking and swallowing in a full-term newborn should be fully developed. Infants at around the age of 8 months should be able to chew small lumps in their feeds. Difficulties with any of these skills may forecast trouble for articulation and speech production.

At about 4 months of age, a baby is able to make noises by producing vowel sounds. At 6 months monosyllables, for example 'ba', 'ma' and 'ta', can be pronounced. A baby of 1 year of age can say a few words, usually including 'mama' and 'baba'. An 18 month old toddler's vocabulary contains more than ten words used correctly. A child of 2 years is able to construct two-word sentences. At 3 years a child knows his or her name, age and sex, and can name a few colours.

At 4 years of age children are able to express themselves reasonably well and recount experiences. Five year olds should be able to know their full name and address. Their speech should be intelligible to strangers.

Social development

In early infancy the ability to interact with other people is used as a guide to social development. Later on, the acquisition of self-help skills and behavioural patterns that imitate adults and allow the child to act in a socially acceptable manner is utilized to assess progress in this sphere. Finally, in later childhood, the ability to enjoy social contact, whether through shared play or other activities, is used as a measure of social development.

One of the most useful and most frequently quoted milestones is social smile. Babies at around 6 weeks of age start to smile in the context of a social encounter with another person. A baby learns to laugh at around 4 months of age.

Stranger anxiety refers to fear and anxiety shown when an 8 month old infant is approached by a stranger. Separation anxiety is shown when the 8 month old infant is separated from his or her mother or other care-giver. Difficulties in putting babies to sleep may be experienced for the first time at this stage. By the end of the first year, babies wave 'bye-bye' when in the mood.

A child of 15 months attempts to feed with a spoon but is rather messy. During the second year children show willingness to take on some responsibility in self-help skills. They help in dressing by adopting appropriate body postures, and they may respond to toilet training. However, there is a significant variation in the age at which bowel and bladder control are achieved (see Toilet training).

Play as a social skill evolves from solitary play which involves mainly handling of objects during the second year of life, through parallel play (when a group of children gather together but each plays his or her own game), to the type of play when more than one child is involved. In the fourth year and beyond, role playing as part of a group is the main theme of play activity.

Cognition

The more complex 'higher' function of the human brain is cognition. Mental abilities include such diverse functions as abstract thinking, logical processing and memory, as well as visual–spatial orientation and sensory perception. A person's performance in these areas is not uniform; almost all of us have strengths in certain areas and weaknesses in others.

The nature of the thinking process changes with age. In infancy, thoughts are tied to immediate sensation and manipulation. Concrete thinking is operational in the preschool child when symbols (words) of tangible objects, experienced feelings and situations can be handled. Abstract thinking is not functional till later in childhood.

Above 7 years of age, certain aspects of cognition are amenable to assessment through the formal IQ (intelligence quotient) tests, which allow the ability to handle symbolic material and abstract thinking to be measured. At an earlier age this might be difficult because assessing cognition involves measuring the performance in communicative, adaptive and social skills. In early infancy, it is difficult to assess cognition directly: social skills and development in other spheres serve as crude indicators of cognition and intelligence.

As with other skills, the rate of progression in cognitive development can vary from child to child. This explains the limitations of the predictive value of the tests of cognitive functioning performed in childhood.

Toilet training

Voluntary sphincter control, as with other developmental skills, depends on the interaction of the maturation of the neurophysiological mechanisms with environmental factors, including efforts at toilet training (see also Ch. 18). However, the situation here is complicated by a number of issues:

- There is a great variation in the ages at which the maturation of the biological mechanisms for bowel and bladder control is attained. Though the majority reach this stage of development in the second half of the second year, a significant minority do not do so until late in childhood and even beyond. This means that parents' expectations can sometimes be totally unrealistic for a particular child.
- The inconveniences of looking after a child who has not achieved bowel and bladder control frequently creates a sense of tension and time pressure. Undue significance may be attached to the early attainment of sphincter control, and some parents may pursue toilet training with vigour and perseverance not seen elsewhere in child rearing.
- Exercising control over these physiological functions may require some commitment of time and attention on the child's part, and sometimes can be distressing. Thus, repeated emptying of the bladder or bowel may interrupt play activity. If constipation ensues, defaecation may become painful (see Ch. 5).
- Soiling, or wetting of pants, is one of the few tools of manipulation that a child possesses (see Ch. 18), and may be part of an attention seeking device or a way of exercising free will. It is important to note, and always to mention to parents, that this is done subconsciously and children should not be blamed for this.

In addition to efforts at toilet training, the major feature of the second year is mobility. This, combined with a heightened appetite to explore the world around them, results in toddlers being everywhere and into everything. Safety in the household becomes crucial. This exploratory behaviour attracts further measures of control and discipline. These experiences of cultural pressure and restrictions frequently generate frustration and anger in children, sometimes resulting in temper tantrums and breath-holding spells.

The primitive reflexes

These reflexes are not 'learned' developmental skills. They are, rather, innate reactions to stimuli observed at certain stages of brain development. There are several primitive reflexes (Table 3.2): the Moro reflex (Fig. 3.2), the sucking and rooting reflex and the asymmetrical tonic neck reflex (Fig. 3.3). However, their timed appearances and disappearances can serve as pointers to the stage of functional maturation of the nervous system attained.

As these reflexes involve involuntary symmetrical movements of the two sides of the body, they can be utilized, when present, in the physical and neurological examination of infants without the need for cooperation. Asymmetry of the response may suggest paralysis or bone fractures, etc. Absence of the reflexes is usually seen in states of central nervous system depression, while their persistence may suggest delayed maturation or structural lesions of the central nervous system.

DEVELOPMENTAL ASSESSMENT

Developmental assessment may be carried out in the context of one of the following:

- A generalized child health surveillance system/screening
- The general evaluation of a child conducted to address some other clinical problem
- To address a clinical suspicion of a developmental problem.

Developmental screening involves the routine developmental assessment at certain ages. In the UK, it is carried out as part of a comprehensive health surveillance programme, usually in a primary care setting (see Ch. 17).

When a more expert opinion is needed, developmental assessment is usually undertaken by a specialist (paediatric neurologist/community paediatrician). Sometimes the assessment is best conducted over the course of several days at a developmental centre by a multidisciplinary team (physiotherapist to assess muscle tone, gross motor development; occupational therapist to assess fine motor development; a child psychologist to measure cognitive abilities; a speech therapist; an orthoptist; a trained nursery nurse; etc.)

The aims of the developmental assessment include the following:

- Screening for developmental problems to allow early intervention
- To establish normality and allay parental anxiety
- As a legal requirement in certain cases, such as adoption and fostering
- To detect abnormal developmental patterns that may aid in the diagnosis of a mental or physical impairment or untoward environmental influences

Table 3.2	**The primitive reflexes**		
Reflex	Description	Appears	Disappears
Moro	Sudden lowering of the head of a supine baby results in extension and abduction of the arms followed by flexion and adduction (see Fig. 3.2)	Birth	2–4 months
Grasp	Gentle touching of the palm of the opened hand results in flexion of the fingers in a grasp movement	Birth	6 months
Parachute (propping reaction)	The gentle sideways push of the sitting infant, results in extension and abduction of the appropriate arm as if to avoid falling. There is an equivalent forward parachute	9 months	Persists

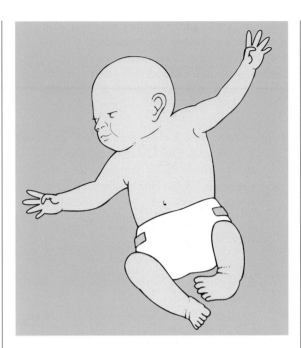

Figure 3.2 The Moro reflex

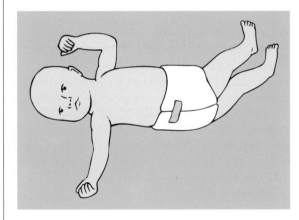

Figure 3.3 The asymmetrical tonic neck reflex

- To detect untoward effects of previous injury or potential injury, whether prenatal, natal or postnatal – this may carry a medicolegal value.

The developmental assessment should start by obtaining a developmental history. Parents are usually quite accurate in their accounts of their child's development. However, an element of denial or overinterpretation can sometimes be present. It is sometimes useful to ask parents to make a comparison with the child's elder siblings when they were at the same age, or to comment on the child's behaviour compared to peers.

There are a number of practical points that may be helpful in conducting developmental assessment:

- Always perform the assessment in the four spheres of development (gross motor, fine motor, language, social).
- Repeat assessments may be necessary. Children are not at their best when confronted by strangers, particularly in the environment of a clinic or hospital or during periods of illness. Regression in development is to be expected at times of stress and upheaval.
- It is reasonable to begin the assessment, in the chosen sphere, with the milestones appropriate for the presumed stage of development. A rough idea about the stage of development can be obtained from knowledge of the age of the child and the history, together with any other available information.
- Correction for prematurity should be done whenever necessary. Thus, for an 11 month old baby who was born at 32 weeks of gestation with nothing else to suggest major deviation from normal, it is reasonable to start with milestones appropriate for the age of 9 months. Depending on whether these are found to be achieved or not, one progresses to either the subsequent or preceding milestones.
- The need to correct for prematurity depends on its degree and on the chronological age of the child. As a rough guide, it is thought that by the age of 2 years, a premature baby (with normal development) would have caught up with a full-term baby born on the same day.

AETIOLOGY AND MECHANISMS OF DEVELOPMENTAL DELAY

The term 'developmental delay' is loosely used, and a precise definition is lacking. In this chapter, delay is defined as failure to acquire a particular developmental skill at an age when 95% of peers have done so. This definition hinges on the fact that the acquisition of developmental skills follows a normal distribution.

There are several patterns of delay: global (involving all spheres of development), partial (affecting certain spheres but not others), and delay in achieving some milestones within a particular sphere of development

Delay in the acquisition of a developmental skill can be caused by:

- Normal variation
- Lack of stimulation/lack of training
- The presence of physical or functional impairment
- The presence of cognitive difficulties (mental handicap).

Normal variation

The term 'normal variation' encompasses two concepts. Firstly, that people vary in their abilities, with strengths in certain areas and weaknesses in others. Secondly, that children vary in the rate of progression through their development. Some can display delayed maturation (slow starters/late developers). As long as the child eventually realizes his or her full potential, this variation in rate of development is considered normal.

Normal variation is the commonest cause of delay in acquiring a developmental skill, and can produce any of the patterns listed earlier. However, when the degree of delay is severe, the likelihood of other causes increases.

Lack of stimulation and training

This is a common cause of delay in development. However, the need for these inputs in order to acquire a developmental skill varies with the skill. Thus, minimal or no training is required in order to achieve head control while adequate opportunities for training are obviously required to learn how to ride a bike. The reasons why a child may not get the appropriate stimulation and training necessary to acquire a skill are numerous and diverse:

- Severe systemic illness, particularly if it involves repeated hospital admissions and

lengthy periods of confinement to bed, can deprive the child of the appropriate training and stimulation. These children are frequently globally delayed, but as their underlying illness improves, and with intensified training and stimulation, the majority of them catch up with their peers.
- Ignorance and lack of experience on the part of parents can sometimes be implicated in the failure to provide the environment for normal development. Family upheavals, financial hardships and lack of support for the family can all contribute to the unstimulating upbringing.
- The disadvantages conferred on the child's development by social deprivation are frequently compounded by the effects of malnutrition and ill health.
- A special case of social deprivation and under stimulation is child neglect, a form of child abuse. Developmental delay due to neglect is frequently associated with non-organic failure to thrive (see Ch. 5).

When there are sufficient grounds to suspect under-stimulation as a cause of developmental delay (whether due to neglect or not), confirmation can be obtained by offering the child a placement in a nursery or toddler group with adequate facilities and trained staff. Dramatic improvement and catch-up in development are usually seen if understimulation is the sole cause of the delay. However, if understimulation is diagnosed late, its sequelae may not be completely reversible.

Physical or functional impairment

The presence of a functional or neurological impairment may interfere with the learning or execution of certain skills. A classic example is the effect of deafness on development of speech and language. Another important example is the delay in walking in children with spinal lesions. Looking for such physical, functional or neurological impairments is an integral part of the evaluation of children with developmental delay.

Mental handicap

Neurodevelopmental skills are learned skills. As such they require a degree of mental processing which varies from skill to skill. The exclusion of mental handicap as an underlying cause is one of the main aims of assessment of children with developmental delay.

CORE PROBLEMS

Concerns regarding the development of children frequently arise. However, in the majority of cases the perceived problems fall into the category of normal variation, possibly combined with a degree of parental anxiety. The diagnostic work-up required is minimal and frequently involves little more than detailed assessment and periods of observation. Nevertheless, in certain cases more serious pathology has to be considered and the appropriate diagnostic steps taken.

The three most frequently encountered developmental problems are:

- Global developmental delay
- Delayed walking
- Delayed speech.

GLOBAL DEVELOPMENTAL DELAY

There is no one diagnostic scheme that is suitable for all children with global developmental delay. The approach should be individualized, taking into account issues such as the age at presentation, the severity of the delay and the presence of historical or other data that point towards one of the possible mechanisms of delay discussed earlier. The following points are helpful in structuring the diagnostic process:

- Repeat assessments, periods of observation and even empirical placements of children in supervised nurseries and groups can all be undertaken in the process of evaluation.
- The presence of dysmorphic features or other defects may suggest a particular condition or syndrome. However, it is important to realize that sometimes these findings may be incidental.

- It is not necessary to withhold therapeutic intervention while waiting to establish the precise aetiology of the delay; early institution of therapeutic measures is frequently required for maximal benefits to be achieved. Thus, services of speech or occupational therapists, etc, may be employed while still working on the diagnosis.
- The number of conditions and syndromes of which mental handicap is a feature is large. It is reasonable to withhold the investigations for these conditions until there is sufficient evidence that mental handicap is the underlying cause of the delay. However, certain treatable conditions should be checked for early in the diagnostic process, since delay in instituting treatment is potentially damaging. Hypothyroidism and phenylketonuria are two such conditions (in the UK, these conditions are routinely screened for as part of the Guthrie test; see Ch. 4).

✳ KEY DIAGNOSIS

Mental handicap

Recently introduced alternative terms for mental handicap are 'learning difficulties' and 'special educational needs'. The change in terminology reflects the recent dramatic shifts in the social attitude towards children with limited intellectual abilities. The new terms rightly place the emphasis on the support that the community should provide to the child in order to meet his or her individual needs rather than on the child's own deficiencies.

There is some confusion about the definition of mental handicap, and the issue is still being debated. Regardless of the precise wording, mental handicap implies mental impairment of a magnitude sufficient to require additional help and education. This definition allows for the fact that at the mild end of the spectrum of mental handicap there is an overlap with the normal range. Social and cultural attitudes, as well as the expectations from the child, influence the choice of label.

IQ tests provide an objective scale against which certain aspects of mental functioning can be measured. However, their use has some limitations; tests of certain faculties are not adequately represented and varied individual experiences, cultural differences and language difficulties may interfere with the accuracy of the scoring. Furthermore, an IQ score reflects the performance of a child at a certain point in time, and inferences about the child's potential are not always accurate.

The IQ is calculated from the mental age as a fraction of the chronological age and expressed as an absolute number by multiplying the fraction by 100. The performance on the IQ scale, which follows a normal distribution pattern (Fig. 3.4), has been utilized for classification of mental handicap.

Aetiology and pathogenesis

Mental handicap is not a disease; it is a state which reflects the outcome of interaction of multiple factors, both intrinsic and environmental (Table 3.3). In this sense, it may be less useful to talk about an aetiology or cause of mental handicap than to focus on the interplay of risk factors which result in the mental impairment. As an example, babies with phenylketonuria (see Ch. 16) are usually normal at birth; that is, they are born with their potential for mental development intact. Only if exclusion of phenylalanine from their diet is not implemented early enough to prevent accumulation of toxic metabolites does brain damage occur and mental handicap begin to develop (see Fig. 16.6).

This concept may not so neatly apply to some other situations. For example, a baby born with severe brain structural defects is destined to have severe mental handicap, no matter how safe and stimulating the environment may be. Even then, environmental factors may still have some modifying influence on the degree of mental impairment. It is important to remember that, in such a situation, the relative significance of minor changes in mental functioning increases.

Risk factors for mental handicap can be classified according to the stage of development at which they are determined. They may not necessarily be operational then, but exert their influence at a later stage.

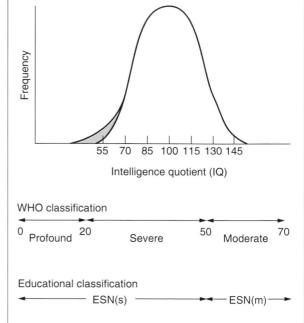

Figure 3.4 The population distribution of intelligence. ESN = Education Special Need; s = severe; m = moderate

Clinical features

The main feature of mental handicap is developmental delay. Severe mental handicap results in a global pattern of developmental delay which is evident from early infancy. Lesser degrees of learning difficulty exert variable influences on the different spheres of development, with social and communicative skills affected most and the gross motor skills disturbed least. Mild degrees of learning difficulty may have no appreciable effect on development, or may only interfere with certain skills requiring a certain level of sophistication. Such a pattern may not be recognized until later in childhood, when difficulties in reading, arithmetic or comprehension surface.

Other features relate to the symptoms and signs of the underlying conditions (Table 3.4), as well as to emotional and psychiatric complications. Children with mental handicap are at increased risk of neglect and abuse.

Diagnosis

There are two levels of diagnosis: first, to diagnose mental handicap as the cause of the

Table 3.3 'Causes' of mental handicap

Potential contributing factor	Important examples
Genetic	
Chromosomal disorders	Down's syndrome (see Fig. 16.4)
Inheritable disorders	Fragile X syndrome
Metabolic	Phenylketonuria (see Fig. 16.7)
Brain structural defects	Microcephaly
Prenatal	
Congenital infections	Congenital rubella
Teratogens	Alcohol, drugs
Intrauterine growth retardation	Placental insufficiency
Idiopathic congenital malformations	Hypothyroidism
Perinatal	
Extreme prematurity	Babies < 28 weeks of gestation
Hypoxic–ischaemic injury	Birth asphyxia
Metabolic	Hypoglycaemia, jaundice
Postnatal	
Infections	Meningitis/encephalitis
Trauma	Head trauma
Anoxia	Near-drowning
Metabolic	Hypoglycaemia
Psychosocial	
Malnutrition	
Unknown	20–50% of all cases

Many of these conditions can be listed as causes of cerebral palsy (CP); it is the timing, site and severity of the brain injury that determines whether the child will end up with CP, mental handicap or both

developmental delay; second, to establish a 'cause' for the handicap. The diagnosis of mental handicap is based on:

- Presence of significant developmental delay, particularly in communicative, social and adaptive behaviour
- Exclusion of other possible mechanisms for the delay in development or, when present, the demonstration that they are not of a degree that can explain the extent of the delay
- Demonstration of an IQ score of 70 or less.

Sometimes normal variation (as shown by late developers, for example) may not reliably be excluded until late in childhood. One should be prepared to revise the diagnosis and reassess the degree of mental handicap as the true situation declares itself with the passage of time. The same can be said about understimulation, which may not be suspected until the child's social circumstances change and an improvement is seen.

Certain conditions can contribute to developmental delay and be confused with mental handicap. The most important of these are cerebral palsy and epilepsy (see Ch. 10), deafness and autism (see p. 42 and Ch. 18, respectively); these conditions should always be checked for.

Establishing the presence of the conditions underlying mental handicap should be based on the clinical data and on the judicious use of laboratory investigations. The process can be difficult and laborious, and is not always successful. Mental handicap remains unexplained in one-fifth of severe cases and one-half of mild cases.

Because of the diversity of the possible causes or risk factors for mental handicap, a plan of investigation should be devised in accordance with the clinical findings and should follow a

Table 3.4 Investigations of children with mental handicap

Investigation	Indications
First line[a] Thyroid function Common metabolic disorders	Screening for relatively common and treatable conditions

Metabolic investigations[a]
 Urine
  Reducing substances
  Organic and amino acids
  Mucopolysaccharides
 Blood
  Sugar, gases, ammonia, amino acids, others
 Leucocytes/skin biopsy
 Study of cellular enzymes
	Features suggestive of metabolic disorder
	  Persistent vomiting
	  Poor feeding/failure to thrive
	  Periodic clouding of consciousness
	  Unexplained jaundice/hypoglycaemia
	  Hepatomegaly
	  Cataract
	  Abnormal odour of urine

Chromosomal studies	Presence of dysmorphic features or multiple congenital abnormalities
Congenital infection screen Blood viral titres Skull radiography Urine for cytomegalovirus	History of rash/flu-like illness in pregnancy Microcephaly Chorioretinitis Associated deafness Neonatal hepatosplenomegaly
Imaging for brain structural defects Ultrasound scan Magnetic resonance imaging/ computerized tomography scan Electroencephalography	Abnormal head size Neurological signs Skin stigmata (see Fig. 16.7) Seizures (particularly focal)

[a]Because they are potentially treatable conditions, and hence progression of the brain injury can be avoided, the common metabolic disorders and hydrocephalus should also be checked for relatively early in the diagnostic process. Simple and cheap testing of urine for reducing substances, and blood for sugar, ammonia and acid–base status, can provide a useful screening for many of the more common metabolic disorders. Cranial ultrasonography or, in older children when the anterior fontanel is closed, computerized tomography, may be necessary to exclude hydrocephalus

logical sequence. It is not desirable to perform batteries of tests to investigate for everything at the same time. Table 3.4 lists the main investigations in relation to the relevant clinical findings.

Management

This should take the form of a multidisciplinary approach, with involvement of the family as well as the relevant agencies within the health, educational and social services. It is the general practitioner or paediatrician who coordinates all these services and provide the means of continuity, communication and reference for the child and parents.

An initial comprehensive evaluation of a child with mental handicap should be undertaken at a developmental assessment centre. This is carried out over the course of several days by a multidisciplinary team.

Working out and securing the best possible placement for the child with learning difficulty is one of the central tasks of the management process. The community child health services are suitably positioned at the interface between the medical and educational systems, and early referral to the community child health team is crucial. A statement of needs is usually prepared jointly with the educational psychologist and forwarded to the local educational authorities (see Ch. 17).

At the heart of the modern approach to children with mental handicap lies the belief that social prejudice can be as incapacitating for the child and family as the mental handicap itself, and that learning and training at all levels can be best achieved in the context of a stimulating and loving environment.

Based on these beliefs, the concept of normalization is advocated: the mentally handicapped child should be raised in a normal environment, living at home with the family and, whenever possible, making use of ordinary services and schools. In Britain, the 1981 Educational Act promotes integration with 'normal' school children. Institutionalization is no longer advised. Children with mental handicap should be respected as full members of the society; they have the right to live with dignity.

The management of children with mental handicap should be focused on the management of the family, therapeutic measures and support for the child.

Management of the family

This requires a great deal of tact and sensitivity, but from the very beginning openness and trust have to be established. An initial reaction similar to that of bereavement can be expected if the condition has not already been suspected by the parents. It may be necesssary to deal with the feelings of denial, guilt and anger, and these should be given time to resolve. The following steps are crucial in the family management:

- Full explanations regarding the diagnosis, the possible causes and the management should be provided. The limitations in our ability to predict the outcome should be highlighted, without raising unrealistic expectations or unnecessarily painting a gloomy picture.
- Genetic counselling when necessary.
- Parental education about the nature, extent and causes of the handicap and provision of details about the available societies, agencies and support groups. Parents are said to be the best therapists, and many parents will want to participate in the provision of therapeutic and educational measures to their child.
- Financial help, respite care and other measures of support should be made available when required.

Therapeutic measures and support for the child
These should be provided along the following lines:

- Periodic detailed assessment to keep up with the continually changing picture frequently seen in these children, to document strengths as well as weaknesses.
- Intensive training and stimulation in an attempt to overcome deficiencies.
- Strategies to bypass the handicap. This is becoming more feasible with technological progress; computers, word processors with word-initiating or word-completing facilities, and modified calculators can all appreciably improve the level of functioning.
- Treatment of the underlying condition
- Provision of general health care. Lack of judgement may predispose these children to a wide range of accidents and health problems. Communicative difficulties contribute to the delay in diagnosis. In the profoundly handicapped child, there is a higher incidence of constipation, urinary tract infections, recurrent chest infections and reflux oesophagitis.
- Advice regarding education and career. Though the aim should be education in an ordinary school, possibly in a special unit or class within the school, it may be necessary to concede that sometimes the resources of specialized schools will better serve the needs of a child with severe handicap.

Prevention
Prevention of such a common and serious condition as mental handicap requires the orchestrated efforts of multiple agencies and public services. The following is a summary of the main stages at which these efforts should be directed:

- General health education of the public, directed particularly at women of child-bearing age. Risks of drugs, smoking and alcohol should be highlighted.
- Encouragement of the population at risk for inherited disorders (e.g. with a positive family history) to undergo genetic testing with their partners.

- Provision of high standards of antenatal and obstetric care.
- Antenatal screening and detection with a view to in utero intervention (e.g. in utero transfusions, surgery) or, in selected cases, termination of pregnancy.
- Continued refinement and improvement of neonatal care, bearing in mind that although this will improve the outcome for individual babies, the accompanying improvement in overall survival rate may lead to an increase in the total number of babies surviving with significant brain injury.
- Neonatal screening for early detection of certain conditions (e.g. hypothyroidism, phenylketonuria).
- Developmental screening for early detection of delay and early deployment of suitable interventions.

DELAYED WALKING

Walking signifies a new stage of independent mobility for the child. For parents, it is perceived as an important landmark in the child's development, and is awaited with eagerness and anticipation. Many people mistakenly regard early walking as a sign of mental superiority.

The majority of children are expected to have started walking independently by 14 months of age, but the range is wide and probably covers a period between 9 and 18 months of age. A minority of otherwise normal children may not be able to walk independently even at 2 years of age.

Walking, like other developmental skills, is not an all or nothing phenomenon. Children start standing on their own at around 12 months of age, and begin to cruise around furniture and walk with a hand held well before attempting to walk independently. Children who demonstrate these skills are unlikely to have serious pathology as a cause for the delay in independent walking. It is also important to note that before children are able to walk steadily, there is a period of staggering gait with frequent falls and unsteadiness.

Though the four mechanisms of developmental delay should be considered (see above), walking,

like other early gross motor skills, requires little supervised training. Understimulation is an unlikely cause for delayed walking. Similarly, unless its degree is severe, mental handicap per se is an improbable cause of delayed gross motor development.

For the reasons given above, the diagnostic evaluation of the majority of children with delayed walking should focus on the differentiation of two possible mechanisms for the delay: normal variation (see Key diagnosis: normal variation, below) and the presence of a physical/neurological impairment (cerebral palsy (CP), muscular disorders, spinal lesions). Each of these conditions is dealt with in some depth in Chapter 10; here those aspects particularly relevant to delay in walking are described.

Cerebral palsy (see also Chs 10 and 17)

A history of prematurity, difficulties in pregnancy or labour, or a history of severe postnatal illness suggests CP as a possible cause for the delay. Though the characteristic feature of CP is increased muscle tone (see Fig. 10.3), hypotonia can be present in the early years. However, the presence of exaggerated tendon reflexes serves to support the possibility of CP and helps in making the distinction from other causes of hypotonia.

The pattern of delay due to CP is variable. Typically, the gross motor sphere is affected most, but this varies with severity and type of CP. Again, depending on the type and severity of the underlying CP, the gross motor skills may be uniformly delayed or some may be acquired in time while others are delayed. Delayed standing and walking can be the first indication of a problem of development due to CP. This is particularly true of spastic diplegia, a form of CP in which the lower limbs are affected most. When CP arises from a postnatal cause, the resultant pattern of delay in development will reflect the timing of the injury.

Muscular disorders (see also Chs 10 and 16)

These are uncommon but important causes of delayed walking. Here too, gross motor delay may be seen early on, or delayed walking may be the first sign of trouble. Alternatively, these children may present later. Duchenne's muscular dystrophy (see Fig. 16.9), the commonest of the congenital muscular disorders, is frequently first suspected when an otherwise normal boy presents with difficulty in walking upstairs or rising from the sitting or lying position (see Fig. 10.7).

A positive family history, a history of polyhydramnios and the presence of associated abnormalities, such as undescended testicles, suggest a congenital muscular disorder. Hypotonia and weak tendon reflexes are characteristic. Elevated serum creatinine kinase (CK) levels are found from early on in many of these disorders, and is a useful screening tool. Confirmation of the exact diagnosis frequently relies on electromyography, genetic studies and muscle biopsy.

Spinal lesions

Spina bifida (see Fig. 16.10), spinal cord malformations/injuries and deformities of the lower limbs may all be implicated as possible causes for delayed walking. Careful clinical assessment is mandatory, and the use of the relevant imaging techniques may be required.

✳ KEY DIAGNOSIS

Normal variation

Normal variation is a diagnosis of exclusion. The need for, and the extent of, further evaluation and investigations of children presenting with delayed walking should be determined on the basis of the severity of the delay, as well as the presence or absence of clinical data indicating the presence of pathology.

Thus, for mild degrees of delay (18–24 months of age), it is reasonable to adopt an expectant policy provided the history, physical and developmental examinations reveal no other cause for concern. Ascertainment of the serum CK level is a simple and useful test at this stage.

For children older than 2 years who are still unable to walk, normal variation continues to be a possibility. However, the likelihood of the presence of other mechanisms for the delay increases and, even in the absence of other clinical data pointing to pathology, further investigations are warranted. It is important to realize that sometimes the historical data are lacking in children with CP or muscular dystrophy and the physical signs can be subtle; careful evaluation is necessary. Central nervous system imaging, muscle biopsies, electromyography and other tests may be indicated.

In some cases of severe delay in walking, no evidence of pathology can be found in spite of extensive investigation. It may be impossible to resolve the issue as to whether these children have an underlying cause for the delay, or simply represent an extreme of normal variation. In these cases it is reasonable to adopt an attitude of cautious optimism.

Physiotherapy and other measures directed at strengthening various muscle groups, preventing contractures and improving balance and coordination should be employed as appropriate without undue delay for a specific diagnosis.

DELAYED SPEECH

Language is a system of symbols that is utilized in the formation of ideas and concepts and is thus the basis of cognition. Language is also a means of communication with others, i.e. the exchange of concepts and ideas which occurs in the context of social interaction. Language is usually expressed in speech, but it can also be expressed in other ways such as sign language or musical notes.

Speech is the production of words which involves the combination of sounds in a predetermined manner. For words to convey complex concepts and meanings, they themselves have to be combined according to a set of rules: syntax and grammar. The meaning that such combined words convey is referred to as semantics.

A baby begins to communicate using vocal and non-vocal means from birth. The cry, grimace of discomfort, and smile – all can be seen as communicative tools. These, initially, may not be purposeful but simply reflex actions in response to feelings of hunger, discomfort or pleasure. However, as babies learn that they can influence their environment by these actions, through the parents' readiness to respond (a bottle of milk for crying or parents smiling back), they begin to use these tools intentionally. As parents and other care-givers use speech and language more in these communicative episodes, the child's understanding and use of speech and language evolves.

Thus the following factors are crucial for speech and language development:

- Successful social interaction with the environment
- Normal hearing
- Adequate mental functioning to allow understanding and developing of the concepts and ideas
- Normal speech production, which is itself dependent on motor planning and coordination of the complex movements involved, normal articulation and voice production.

Faults at any stage can result in failure of normal speech development. Such faults can arise through one or more of the four mechanisms of delay discussed earlier.

Normal variation

Normal variation, or more specifically delayed maturation, is a common cause of delayed speech. Such children are a heterogeneous group with different patterns of speech delay depending on the step involved. Thus, delayed maturation of mental processing can result in delay in verbal understanding as well as in speech production, while underdevelopment of the motor mechanisms involved can lead to expressive aphasia and immature pronunciation.

Understimulation

This is also a relatively common factor in speech delay. As discussed earlier, successful social interaction with the environment is a prerequisite for the development of communicative skills in general. Furthermore, the child is very much dependent on his or her parents or care-givers for the acquisition of vocabulary and learning language. Television, video and recorded children's stories are far less effective in this respect. Some recent reports implicate the practice of allowing young children to spend long hours in front of the television as a contributory factor in some cases of speech delay.

Mental handicap

Speech and language delay is frequently the first and cardinal manifestation of mental handicap. This is not surprising since learning to talk is one of the most difficult series of skills a child will ever acquire. The finding of a parallel delay in understanding characterizes the delay in speech due to mental handicap.

Autism is a rare and special case related to mental handicap (see Ch. 18). It probably also falls in the domain of failure of social interaction with the environment. Though some ambiguity still surrounds this entity, it is held that the primary defect in autism is a deficit in certain aspects of mental functioning which are necessary for successful social interaction.

Autism is characterized by impairment of verbal and non-verbal communication, as well as failure to engage in imaginative activities or social contact. Autism typically is evident from early childhood. The prognosis is variable but generally must be guarded. Treatment should be undertaken by a team specialized in this area.

Physical/neurological impairment

The presence of a physical or neurological impairment at any point in the system of language development and speech production can lead to speech delay. Such an impairment can affect the input or the output limbs of this system:

- Deafness
- Any impairment in voice production and articulation:
  - Impaired motor function (e.g. cerebral palsy)
  - Structural defects (e.g. cleft palate or tracheostomy)
  - Psychological influences.

Deafness

This is a common underlying cause of speech delay. Even unilateral deafness has been shown to affect children's speech and language. Hearing assessment is a mandatory step in the evaluation of virtually all children with speech and language disorders (see Key diagnosis: hearing loss).

Impairment of motor function/structure

Speech production is dependent on highly coordinated movements of the tongue and lips as well as laryngeal, pharyngeal and facial muscles. Because these same groups of muscles are involved in sucking, swallowing and chewing, a history of difficulties with these activities may be the first clue to a motor impairment affecting these muscles and may forecast problems in speech development. A cleft lip or palate (see Fig. 16.11) interferes with the integrity of the seal required to produce certain sounds.

Psychological influences

Stammering is a disorder of fluency of speech. Though genetic and neurological factors are implicated in its aetiology, the psychological influences are instrumental in the development and persistence of stammering. Many normal children go through a phase of developmental stammering between 2 and 4 years of age. Tolerance and acceptance by the surrounding adults are crucial in allowing this phase to resolve.

Evaluation

In a child presenting with delayed speech, the following steps are crucial:

- The nature of the difficulty should first be ascertained. The social dimension, including the use of other means of communication, should be carefully examined, deafness reliably excluded, mental abilities assessed and speech production evaluated.
- Assessment of other spheres of development should be performed. Global developmental delay suggests mental handicap, while the association of speech delay with gross motor delay suggests cerebral palsy as a possible cause.
- Physical and neurological assessment (history and examination), looking for evidence which may suggest one of the conditions that impair speech. This should include otoscopic examination.
- Early institution of an appropriate speech therapy programme is crucial, whether or not the precise underlying cause of the speech delay has been clarified. Difficulties in speech may become permanent if such an intervention is delayed, even if the underlying mechanism has been dealt with.

✴ KEY DIAGNOSIS

Hearing loss

Hearing is the perception of sounds. There are two main qualities of sound that affect our ability to hear (hearing sensitivity): these are the intensity or loudness of the sound and its pitch or wave frequency. These qualities are utilized in measuring hearing sensitivity, and are expressed in a graphic form as the audiogram (see Fig. 3.5).

The outer and middle ears are structures that facilitate conduction of sound, resulting in more effective and accurate hearing. A lesion affecting the outer or middle ear results in impairment of the conduction of sound through these structures, i.e. conductive hearing loss. However, sound can also be transmitted through the skull bones. The hallmark of conductive hearing loss is that the sensitivity of hearing is reduced for air conduction but is preserved for bone conduction.

The cochlea in the inner ear is the hearing organ proper. It converts sound energy into nerve impulses which are transmitted along the cochlear branch of the eighth nerve to the brain stem. A lesion anywhere in this pathway results in the sensorineural type of hearing loss. The hallmark of this type of hearing loss is that the hearing sensitivity is diminished for both air and bone conduction.

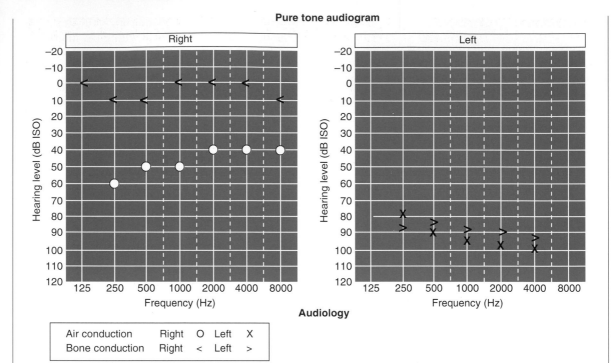

Pure tone audiogram

| Air conduction | Right | O | Left | X |
| Bone conduction | Right | < | Left | > |

Figure 3.5 An audiogram showing right-sided conductive hearing loss. Note the discrepancy between air and bone conduction. There is also left-sided sensory neural hearing loss

The sound impulses are conveyed from the brain stem to the relevant cortical centres for processing. A lesion at this level results in a central type auditory disorder in which the analysis, interpretation and localization of sound are impaired.

Aetiology

Hearing loss of either the conductive or sensorineural varieties (Fig. 3.5) can be congenital or acquired. Table 3.5 illustrates some of the important causes.

Estimates of the prevalence of hearing loss vary according to type and severity; conductive hearing loss due to middle ear effusion is by far the commonest form of deafness in children. It is thought that almost all cases of acute otitis media are followed by a period of conductive deafness due to middle ear effusion. This is usually unilateral and transient, with hearing restored as the effusion resolves, usually within 3 months. It is estimated that 1 in 3 children will experience at least one such episode in the first 5 years of life.

Some of the children with middle ear effusion following otitis media, particularly those with underlying problems predisposing to middle ear infections such as nasal allergy and eustachian tube dysfunction, may develop a chronic form of the disease (chronic serous/secretory otitis media; see Ch. 13) with the accompanying hearing loss taking a chronic course. This usually is of the order of 30 dB across all frequencies (Fig. 3.5), and can be bilateral.

Sensorineural hearing loss is the commonest cause of severe (> 60 dB) bilateral hearing loss in children (Fig. 3.5). It is estimated that 1 in 1000 newborns has severe bilateral sensorineural hearing loss. This figure rises sharply for premature neonates who required intensive care. The autosomal recessive form is the commonest cause of congenital sensorineural hearing loss.

Diagnosis

Children with deafness present in several ways. The mother or health visitor may be concerned

Table 3.5 Classification of hearing loss

Type of hearing loss	Congenital	Acquired
Conductive	Syndromes with ear deformities or those predisposing to recurrent ear infections Example: Pierre Robin syndrome	Recurrent middle ear infections Chronic serous otitis media
Sensorineural	Inherited, isolated or part of a syndrome. Congenital infections, e.g. congenital rubella syndrome Other in utero injuries	Postnatal hypoxic, traumatic or toxic injuries, e.g. gentamicin ototoxicity

Mixed-type hearing loss also occurs. An important example is the spread of infection from the middle to the inner ear

about the baby's poor communication and lack of response, or the school teacher may become worried about the child's behaviour and/or understanding. Some of these children may be suspected of being mentally handicapped or socially maladjusted. Alternatively, the child may present first with a delayed, immature pattern of speech or pronunciation. Obviously, the severity and timing (if acquired) of the deafness also influence the presentation.

Because of its detrimental effect on language development, hearing loss in children should be recognized and the necessary therapeutic measures implemented as early as possible. The lack of specificity of the presenting features means that delays in identifying affected children would be inevitable if the diagnosis depended solely on clinical presentation. To avoid such delay, two strategies are employed:

- Hearing assessment is included as an integral part of all children's surveillance programmes (see below and Ch. 17).
- A high index of suspicion is engendered among primary care physicians and other health professionals. Hearing assessment should be routinely performed following ear infections, meningitis, gentamicin therapy, etc., as well as being part of the process of evaluation of a child with mental handicap, speech delay, behavioural problems, etc., where deafness may be a contributory factor.

Hearing assessment for screening purposes includes history taking as well as the use of the age-appropriate 'clinical' hearing tests. These usually require a degree of cooperation from the child and a certain level of skill and experience from the examiner. Some of these tests, particularly those used at younger ages (see Fig. 13.6), are considered to be crude and of low accuracy (see also Table 3.1).

If there is a reason to strongly suspect hearing loss in a child or if the performance on one of the screening tests raises concern, one of the more objective 'formal' hearing tests should be performed. These are generally more accurate and less dependent on the child's cooperation. They include pure tone audiometry, tympanometry and, particularly when the child's cooperation is unobtainable, electrophysiological measurements. The last generally utilize the measurement of the response of the cochloea, brain stem or the relevant area in the cortex to sound (auditory evoked).

Management

The management of conductive hearing loss due to chronic secretory otitis media is controversial. Surgery is probably still the standard treatment, and involves grommet insertion and/or adenoidectomy. The presence of nasal allergy should be identified and treated (see Ch. 13).

An attempt to determine the underlying cause of sensorineural deafness, whether congenital or acquired, should be made. This includes obtaining a family history, the evaluation of the child and, when appropriate, other family members for the presence of stigmata that may suggest one of the numerous conditions and syndromes of which sensorineural deafness is a feature. Associations of this type of deafness with ocular, skin, renal and cardiac conduction abnormalities are well known. Congenital infections and hypothyroidism should also be excluded. In acquired sensorineural deafness, careful history taking may point to the causative event.

Whether congenital or acquired, sensorineural hearing loss is generally irreversible and not amenable to treatment. The strategy here is to circumvent the handicap by the use of hearing aids. The majority of these children, with appropriate support, will be able to integrate into mainstream education and attend ordinary schools. In some, however, the severity of the hearing defect is such that communication is possible only by means of signing. Cochlear implants and other techniques are indicated for a selected group of deaf children who could not be helped otherwise. The procedure is undertaken only in highly specialized centres.

FURTHER READING

Illingworth R S 1987 The development of the infant and young child: normal and abnormal, 9th edn. Churchill Livingstone, Edinburgh

Illingworth R S 1991 The normal child: some problems of the early years and their treatment, 10th edn. Churchill Livingstone, Edinburgh

CHAPTER 4

Neonatal paediatrics

E. Shinwell

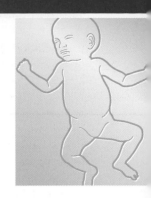

CORE PROBLEMS IN NEONATAL PAEDIATRICS

CORE PROBLEM	KEY DIAGNOSIS	RELATED TOPICS
• Small for gestational age	Placental insufficiency	Congenital infection Hypoglycaemia
• Birth asphyxia	Hypoxic–ischaemic encephalopathy	Resuscitation
• Respiratory distress	(Respiratory distress syndrome)	Pneumonia Meconium aspiration Transient tachypnoea of the newborn (Heart failure)
• Prematurity	Respiratory distress syndrome	Intraventricular haemorrhage Necrotizing enterocolitis Bronchopulmonary dysplasia Retinopathy Apnoea
• Collapse	Sepsis	Congenital heart disease Inborn errors of metabolism Congenital adrenal hyperplasia
• Jaundice	ABO incompatibility	Physiological Rhesus incompatability Breast milk induced

ESSENTIAL BACKGROUND

INTRODUCTION

This chapter provides an overview of the commonest and most important problems seen in the neonatal period. The relevant physiological and anatomical considerations are discussed under the individual diagnostic topic headings. The neonatal examination is outlined in the following section.

ROUTINE EXAMINATION OF THE NEWBORN

The newborn is not simply a small child, and needs to be examined with special considerations in mind. At least two examinations with special content are recommended – the first in the delivery room and the second during the first day of life.

Examination in the delivery room

The first examination of a newborn in the delivery room should assess the immediate cardiorespiratory transition to extrauterine life. In addition, major congenital anomalies or birth injuries need to be ruled out. Relevant information as to high-risk situations which may hinder the newborn's normal transition to extrauterine life should be conveyed prior to the delivery (Table 4.1). The newborn must be closely observed during the first minutes of life. The first few breaths are usually lusty and are followed by irregular breathing and then, after a few minutes,

Table 4.1 **High-risk deliveries**	
High-risk situations	*Common examples*
Evidence of fetal distress	Fetal tachycardia/bradycardia Late decelerations Loss of baseline variability
Suspected chorioamnionitis	Maternal fever Foul-smelling amniotic fluid Cloudy membranes
Delivery problems	Caesarean section Vacuum or forceps delivery Abnormal presentation, e.g. breech Prolapse of cord Multiple pregnancy Antepartum haemorrhage
Prematurity or postmaturity	
Oligo- or polyhydramnios	
Maternal disease	Pre-eclampsia Diabetes
Antenatal fetal diagnoses	Diaphragmatic hernia
Prolonged rupture of membranes	
Meconium-stained amniotic fluid	Intrauterine asphyxia
Maternal opiate administration	

regular respiration is established. The colour changes gradually from dusky blue to pink, and the heart rate should be above 100 beats/min at all times. The tone should be good and the baby responsive to stimulation.

First complete examination

During the first day of life, a complete physical examination should be performed. Ideally, this should take place in a warm, well-lit room, in the presence of the mother (and, preferably, also the father) with the infant naked. This is an opportunity to clearly demonstrate any abnormal findings and allow the parents to ask questions, thus aiding reliable transfer of information and alleviating the parents' anxieties. Also, it is possible to take a family history as required. The examination should include a complete review of all body systems, with a specific focus on identifying any congenital anomalies, such as dislocation of the hip or birth injuries such as a fractured clavicle.

Gestational Age

Weight, length and head circumference should be measured. Assessment of gestational age is usually simple when the infant weighs more than 2500 g and the pregnancy is reported to have lasted at least 37 weeks. If the infant is small, or the reported dating is less than 37 weeks, a formal assessment of gestational age should be made (see Small for gestational age, p. 53).

Inspection

The experienced eye can glean a harvest of information before touching the infant.

Colour

The infant should be pink. However, during the first few days, the hands and feet may have a dusky blue colour (acrocyanosis), resulting from poor peripheral circulation. The face may also be dusky and cyanotic as a result of pressure during birth. The tongue and oral mucosae, however, should be pink/red, which helps to rule out central cyanosis. If it is difficult to distinguish, oxygen saturation by pulse oximetry or arterial Po_2 should be checked.

- Pallor may result from anaemia, hypotension or acidosis. The parents' skin colour should be noted in order to assess baseline colour.
- Plethora may be seen in polycythaemia.
- Jaundice is noted first on the head and progresses down the body.
- Meconium staining of the skin, nails and umbilical cord is seen after meconium has been passed in utero; a common occurrence in postmaturity, with or without fetal distress.

Skin findings

Skin abnormalities are common in the neonate, and most are either transient or of minimal significance.

- Erythema toxicum is a common rash with irregular macular patches, some with a pale centre. Wright's stain of a scraping of a lesion reveals eosinophils. No treatment is required, and the rash fades after 1–4 days.
- Dry, scaly, cracked skin is often seen in postmature infants, but may also occasionally be a sign of ichthyosis, a chronic skin disorder.
- Milia are pinpoint white papules on the nose, cheeks and forehead which contain keratogenous material and which fade after 1–4 weeks.
- Mongolian blue spots are deep-blue pigmented areas most commonly seen on the lower back and buttocks of dark-skinned infants. They usually fade within the first few months of life.
- Breast enlargement is common and transient, and a small amount of milk may be expressed.

Examination by systems/body areas
Head
The scalp should be examined for skin lesions resulting from the process of birth, such as abrasions caused by fetal scalp electrodes or vacuum extraction.

- Caput succedaneum is a diffuse swelling secondary to pressure on the head during delivery which usually clears within a few days.
- Cephalohaematoma is scalp haemorrhage limited by the periosteal boundaries, which may contain a significant amount of blood, and its reabsorption may contribute to jaundice. The haematoma resolves gradually over weeks to months.
- Cranial sutures should be checked for overlapping, excessive width or premature closure.
- The anterior fontanelle varies in size from a fingertip to 5 cm across. Normal tension of the fontanelle (flat with the skull) should be noted. A full or tense fontanelle, when the infant is held at an angle of 45° to the cot, may be seen in hydrocephalus or meningitis and warrants further investigation by cranial ultrasound and clinical evaluation. However, a mildly tense fontanelle, together with a normal cranial

ultrasound examination, can also be a transient benign finding in an otherwise healthy infant. A sunken fontanelle may be seen in dehydration.

Eyes

- The red reflex is a useful check of the transparency of all structures through to the lens. The ophthalmoscope is held approximately 10 cm from the eye, using the +10 diopter lens. A normal red colour should be observed. Cataracts may be seen as black areas or lines.
- The cornea should be noted to be clear. A cloudy cornea may be seen in congenital glaucoma. Leukocoria (white pupil) is seen in congenital cataracts, retinoblastoma and other conditions.
- Small eyes or microphthalmia are seen as an isolated finding and also in various generalized conditions such as congenital rubella and cytomegalovirus infection.
- Subconjunctival haemorrhages are common and transient.
- Conjunctival discharge is seen with infection (often minor, but rarely gonococcal, see Ch. 13), and may also be related to impaired lacrimal drainage as in dacryostenosis.

Nose
Occlusion of the posterior nasal passages (choanal atresia) may be suspected because of respiratory distress in the absence of an obvious pulmonary cause or by noisy breathing (choanal stenosis). The patency of the nares can be checked by occluding the mouth and one nares and holding cotton wool by the other to observe movement. Passing a fine catheter may also confirm patency, but this may cause oedema, worsening conditions such as choanal stenosis. Flaring of the alae nasi is a sign of respiratory distress.

Ears
Low-set ears are a sign found in a number of syndromes and chromosomal anomalies. Skin tags or dimples in the area of the ear may be associated with renal anomalies, but most often are an incidental finding which is of cosmetic significance only.

Mouth

- Clefts of the lips or palate are not uncommon and are of major importance. Cleft palate can be identified either by passing a finger along the palate or on inspection with a tongue depressor and light source.
- A cleft or high-arched palate may be seen as part of the Pierre Robin syndrome, which is characterized by micrognathia (a small, posteriorly displaced mandible), airway compromise and feeding problems.
- Asymmetry of the mouth, which may be a sign of facial nerve palsy, is often more pronounced during crying, and usually resolves spontaneously.
- Natal teeth are an occasional finding, and usually require removal because of the risk of aspiration if loosely attached.
- A large or protruding tongue, macroglossia, can be seen in hypothyroidism and the Beckwith–Weideman syndrome; confirmatory findings should be looked for. In Down's syndrome, the tongue may appear large relative to the disproportionately small mouth.

Neck

- Torticollis is characterized by a sternomastoid mass (often a haematoma) and limitation of neck movement.
- Redundant skin on the back of the neck may be seen in Turner's syndrome (the classical webbed neck appears later (see Fig. 16. 5)) as well as in some other chromosomal disorders including Down's syndrome (see Fig. 16.4).
- Cystic hygroma often presents as a large, soft mass in the posterior triangle of the neck which may even restrict respiration.

Shoulders

Fracture of the clavicle is a common form of birth trauma, particularly when there is difficulty in delivering the shoulders of a large baby. The fracture usually heals spontaneously without intervention within a few weeks. A frequent associated finding is Erb's palsy, which results from damage to the fifth and sixth cervical nerves and is characterized by a limp, adducted arm with an extended elbow, pronated forearm and flexed wrist. Klumpke's paralysis is much rarer and affects the seventh and eighth cervical and first thoracic nerves, causing paralysis of the lower arm and hand.

Cardiovascular and respiratory systems

As the processes of adaptation of the two systems to extrauterine life in the neonate are closely interrelated, it is appropriate to consider the examination of these two systems together.

The infant should be pink, well perfused and have quiet, effortless breathing at a rate which rarely goes above 60 breaths/min. Normal breathing in an infant is often irregular with frequent short pauses. However, apnoeic spells of greater than 20 s duration are pathological, and are often associated with bradycardia and cyanosis. Respiratory distress can present as tachypnoea, grunting, intercostal and subcostal retractions and nasal flaring. Stridor indicates narrowing of the airway, most often at the level of the larynx or trachea (see Ch. 6). The chest should be seen to expand well and symmetrically.

Peripheral pulses must always be checked; they may be bounding in infants with a patent ductus arteriosus, while femoral pulses may be reduced or absent in coarctation of the aorta. If so, blood pressure should be taken in the upper and lower limbs. If all pulses are weak, a low cardiac output state, such as hypoplastic left heart syndrome or septic shock, may exist.

Palpation of the chest has limited value although an occasional precordial thrill may be found. Percussion is useless in the neonate.

Auscultation requires a quiet baby. Try to pacify a crying baby before listening, as no useful information can be obtained otherwise. Air entry should be equal and of good volume. Adventitial sounds, such as crepitations and wheezes, are heard in the first few hours after birth, and clear spontaneously as excessive lung fluid is absorbed. Beyond the first few hours, additional breathing sounds are usually pathological.

The heart rate should mostly be in the range of 120–160 beats/min. However, during crying or physical activity the heart rate may temporarily be faster. Likewise, some healthy infants during sleep may have a pulse as low as 80–90 beats/min. The heart sounds should be clear, and the second sound is heard to be split in 50–75% of babies in the first few days of life. Short, grade 1–2/6 systolic murmurs are often heard transiently during the first 48 h of life. Many murmurs heard in the newborn are innocent, and will disappear within the first few months of life. However, it is often difficult to distinguish on the basis of physical findings alone between innocent and pathological murmurs (see Ch. 7). Thus, if a murmur is loud, long or coarse, heard on two examinations 24 h apart or is associated with abnormal pulses or colour, it should be investigated immediately. It is also important to bear in mind that babies with serious heart disease may have only a soft murmur or no murmur at all. Investigation of a murmur should include blood pressure measurement in the upper and lower limbs, a measure of oxygenation such as pulse oximetry or arterial blood P_{O_2}, electrocardiography, chest radiography and, frequently, echocardiography (some cardiologists question the relative value of the radiograph and electrocardiogram (ECG) when they will see 'all that matters' on the echocardiogram anyway!).

Abdomen

The abdomen should be neither distended as in bowel obstruction nor scaphoid as in diaphragmatic hernia. Check for redness or discharge around the umbilicus, which are signs of omphalitis. Periumbilical hernias are common, and mostly close spontaneously over time. Palpation should be performed when the baby is quiet. In order to relax the recti, it is useful to flex the legs. The liver may be up to 2 cm below the costal margin, and a spleen tip may be felt in a normal baby. The kidneys are not always palpable, but it is important to note an enlarged, hydronephrotic kidney. Abdominal masses are rare but important, and should be checked for by deep palpation.

Genitalia

The genitalia must be checked carefully.

- A degree of phimosis is common. Severe phimosis is rare but is associated with poor urinary stream and warrants urgent evaluation and surgical intervention.
- In hypospadias (see Ch. 16), the urethral meatus is displaced on the underside of the penis between the glans and the base of the shaft. Chordee may be present.
- The presence of both testes in the scrotum should be checked (see Ch. 19). The testes may be undescended, found in the inguinal canal or be retractile, moving from the scrotum to the canal on stimulation.
- A hydrocele is a fluid–filled, transilluminable mass next to the testis (see Fig. 19.5), which usually resolves spontaneously.
- Inguinal hernias are common in premature infants but rare at term.
- In the female genitalia at term, the labia majora cover the labia minora. Skin tags and retention cysts are common and transient. A mucoid or bloody discharge is often seen briefly as an oestrogen-withdrawal phenomenon.
- Ambiguous genitalia may be the only early clue to an underlying endocrine disorder (e.g. congenital adrenal hyperplasia (see Ch. 9)), which can be associated with serious fluid and electrolyte disturbances.

While checking the perineum, it is important to note the patency and position of the anus, which may be imperforate or anteriorly displaced.

Spine

- Neural tube defects such as meningomyelocoele (see Fig. 16.10) are most common in the lumbar region, and are easily recognized as a membrane-covered mass. Occult forms, such as spina bifida, may have an associated swelling, dimple, naevus or tuft of hair on the overlying skin.
- A dermal sinus is a small pit commonly seen in the lumbosacral region, which is usually blind-ending and harmless. However, a small number may communicate with the spinal column and have an associated risk of meningitis; these need to be investigated and repaired.

Limbs

Limb anomalies are common and often require urgent care.

Congenital dislocation of the hip (a more appropriate term is 'developmental dysplasia of the hip') is an important condition to be ruled out as, if missed, permanent damage may result (see Chs 12 and 16). Because at birth the condition is still in its early stages and the pathology is limited to laxity of the hip joint ligaments (unstable hip), clinical detection is dependent on the demonstration of the dislocatability of the hip joint. This is usually achieved by Barlow's manoeuvre, in which the examiner's hands are placed with the middle finger on the greater trochanter, the thumbs on the inner aspect of the thigh and the palms on the knees. The knees and hips should be fully flexed and, with the femur held in slight abduction, downward pressure is applied. A clunk is produced, as the hip is dislocated. The joint relocates spontaneously, when the downward pressure is no longer applied by the examiner. When an unstable hip becomes 'truly dislocated' Ortolani's manoeuvre is used (Fig. 4.1); it aims to relocate the dislocated femoral head in the acetabulum with an attendant 'clunk' felt in the process. The legs are held as above, and then each hip separately should be abducted, and at full abduction, pressure should be applied forwards with the middle finger on the trochanter. A mild click can result from movement of the ligamentum teres, and can be confused with the 'clunk' of dislocation/relocation. If any doubt exists after these procedures, an orthopaedic consultation should be obtained before discharge of the infant.

Club foot or talipes is an important abnormality of the foot (see Ch. 16). In the equinovarus form (see Fig. 16.13) the foot is displaced upwards and laterally and cannot be corrected by mild pressure. This requires orthopaedic correction, but needs to be distinguished from transient positional abnormalities resulting from intrauterine posture.

Other common abnormalities of the limbs include syndactyly, over-riding toes, and flexion deformities of the fingers. Positional abnormalities of the arms are usually neurological in origin.

Neurological examination (see also Ch. 10)

The normal infant lies in a flexed posture, has spontaneous movement and good tone in all four limbs and responds to handling with reflex movement and a good, normally pitched cry. The infant will have good sucking and rooting reflexes. The Moro reflex (see Fig. 3.2) is elicited by pulling the infant's arms so as to raise the head almost off the mattress and then release the arms. In a normal response the arms are then thrown

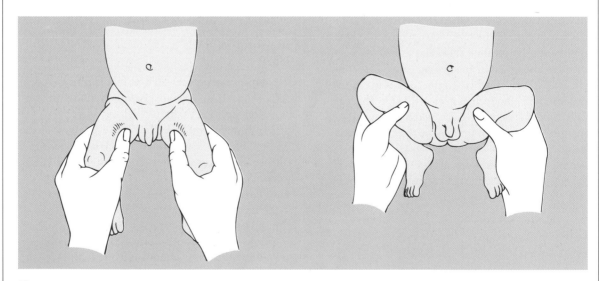

Figure 4.1 Examination for congenital dislocation of the hip (Ortolani's manoeuvre)

out sidewards and then come gradually back towards the midline. Asymmetry may indicate a fractured clavicle, hemiparesis or Erb's palsy. Complete assessment of all the primitive reflexes and behaviour are not part of routine screening.

CORE PROBLEMS

SMALL FOR GESTATIONAL AGE (SGA)

Definitions

In order to discuss the issue of the SGA infant, it is necessary to define a number of concepts:

- Gestational age: the length of the pregnancy from the first day of the last menstrual period to the birth
- Term infant: born between 37 weeks and 1 day and 41 weeks and 6 days of gestation
- Preterm infant: born before 37 completed weeks of gestation
- Post-term infant: born after 42 or more weeks of gestation

- Low birth weight: birth weight less than 2500 g (approximately 6–8% of births)
- Very low birth weight: birth weight less than 1500 g (approximately 1% of births)
- Extremely low birth weight: birth weight less than 1000 g (0.25–0.5% of births)

- Appropriate for gestational age (AGA): birth weight within 2 standard deviations (SD) of the mean for the relevant gestational age
- Small for gestational age (SGA) (or small for dates): birth weight more than 2 SD less than the mean, i.e. less than the 3rd percentile

- Intrauterine growth retardation (IUGR): refers to the in utero condition of an SGA infant, and the terms are often used interchangeably
- Large for gestational age (LGA): birth weight more than 2 SD above the mean.

It is clear from these definitions that an infant born weighing, for example, 1800 g may be classified in different ways, depending on his or her gestational age: preterm AGA, term SGA or preterm SGA. This categorization is important not only for the records but because each definition is associated with a specific morbidity pattern, which may be anticipated and treated accordingly.

Gestational age may be assessed on the basis of both obstetric and neonatal information. The date of the last menstrual period (if regular) and ultrasound dating from early in pregnancy are good indicators of gestational age. In the neonate, scoring systems using a combination of physical and neurologic findings have been developed. The Dubowitz score involves the grading of 'maturity' of 21 physical and neurological features, and the total score correlates with gestational age, with a margin of error usually of ±2 weeks.

IUGR may be caused by maternal placental or fetal disorders (Table 4.2).

✳ KEY DIAGNOSIS

Placental insufficiency

Placental insufficiency is the final common pathway for a number of conditions associated with IUGR. It operates in the later phases of fetal development, through chronic hypoxia and malnutrition, and retards the growth of the body whilst the head tends to be spared, i.e.

Table 4.2 Causes of IUGR	
Maternal/placental	*Fetal*
Placental insufficiency:	Constitutional
Pregnancy-induced hypertension	Congenital infection, e.g. cytomegalovirus infection, rubella
Diabetes	Early fetal toxins, e.g. alcohol, phenytoin, warfarin
Smoking and alcohol	Chromosomal anomaly
Maternal systemic disease	Malformations
Multiple gestation	

asymmetric growth retardation. Conditions such as chromosomal abnormalities or congenital infections tend to affect the fetus early in the pregnancy and are associated with a general reduction in fetal cell number, and result in symmetric growth retardation, i.e. the head and the body are on similar percentiles.

Apart from the difference in body proportions, the clinical manifestations of IUGR are generally the same, irrespective of whether the condition is the result of placental insufficiency or is primarily a fetal disorder.

Clinical features

- SGA infants are at increased risk for perinatal asphyxia, with its associated problems of the meconium aspiration syndrome and persistent pulmonary hypertension. Pulmonary arteries respond to chronic intrauterine hypoxia with medial muscle hypertrophy, which contributes to the pulmonary hypertension.
- Haematological problems such as polycythaemia and hyperviscosity may be secondary to raised erythropoietin levels related to chronic hypoxia. Infants born to mothers with pregnancy-induced hypertension, particularly if treated with hydralazine, often develop leucopenia and thrombocytopenia during the first week of life.
- Diminished glycogen and fat stores raise the risk for hypoglycaemia, which may be severe, requiring high glucose intake for a number of days.
- Reduced subcutaneous fat may predispose the SGA infant to hypothermia.

Management

The management of SGA infants is based on anticipation of the above problems and early intervention. The most common problems are hypoglycaemia and polycythaemia, and these need to be looked for before symptoms appear.

Hypoglycaemia
SGA babies are vulnerable to hypoglycaemia for a number of reasons:

- High energy demands of the brain and heart
- Reduced glycogen deposits in the liver, muscle and heart
- Reduced peripheral glucose utilization/ reduced insulin sensitivity
- Defective lipolysis
- Reduced gluconeogenesis.

Clinical signs of apnoea and convulsions occur only after several hours of hypoglycaemia, by which time irreversible neurological damage will have been done. Hence the need for blood sugar monitoring in SGA infants.

Hypoglycaemia is treated with glucose either by intravenous fluids or by early feeding. Normal glucose intake in a healthy neonate is 4–6 mg/kg/min, but in SGA infants this may reach levels up to 10–15 mg/kg/min during the first few days of life. Occasionally, a central venous line, usually via the umbilical vein, may be required in order to provide the necessary high glucose concentrations.

Polycythaemia
Clinical signs of polycythaemia include respiratory difficulties, lethargy, poor feeding, hypoglycaemia, increased jaundice, convulsions and cerebral or renal vein thrombosis. The management of polycythaemia is a source of much debate. If the venous haematocrit is above 70% and the infant is symptomatic, most neonatologists agree that a partial dilution exchange should be performed in order to reduce the hyperviscosity. However, no consensus exists as to the management when the haematocrit is between 65 and 70% or when the infant is asymptomatic.

Outcome
The outcome of SGA infants is related to the cause of the growth retardation, in particular as regards congenital infections and malformations. Asymmetric SGA infants tend to have a better outcome than symmetric SGA because of the brain-sparing effect. Overall, SGA infants tend to have a poorer growth and developmental outcome than AGA infants at corresponding gestational ages.

PERINATAL ASPHYXIA

The process of birth and adaptation to extrauterine life expose the fetus/newborn to major physiological stress which, in certain cases, may result in injury to body systems and in particular to the developing nervous system. This may lead to major morbidity and mortality in the neonatal period and long-term neurodevelopmental handicap in survivors.

Perinatal asphyxia is the disturbance of normal gas exchange via the placenta or lungs which results in hypoxia, hypercarbia and acidosis. Hypoxic–ischaemic encephalopathy (HIE) is the pathophysiological and clinical picture as it affects the brain, and is commonly seen after perinatal asphyxia (see p. 57).

The *causes of asphyxia* are numerous, and include maternal, fetal, placental and neonatal factors.

- Maternal causes include lung or heart problems, eclampsia, or drugs which may lead to diminished uterine perfusion.
- Fetal factors may include severe anaemia or heart failure, such as in hydrops fetalis.
- The placenta may detach from the uterine wall and present as an acute emergency for both mother and infant.
- The umbilical cord may prolapse into the vagina, and its compression may compromise blood flow to the fetus (abruptio placentae).
- The neonate may not breath effectively if influenced by drugs such as opiates administered to the mother for pain relief.
- If the fetus has been stressed, meconium may be passed before birth. At, shortly before or shortly after birth, the respiratory movements may result in inhalation of particulate meconium into the airways. This may partially or totally occlude airways, resulting in areas of collapse together with areas of hyperexpansion which may seriously compromise respiration.

All of the above-mentioned pathological states (and a few more) can result in defective gas exchange and require prompt intervention in order to prevent widespread tissue damage.

The clinical picture varies in overall severity and, in addition, different organ systems may be affected to a varying degree. The most commonly affected are the central nervous system (see Key diagnosis: hypoxic–ischaemic encephalopathy) and the kidneys. Cardiovascular, pulmonary, haematological, endocrine and metabolic disturbances are also seen.

Resuscitation

In order to perform effective resuscitation, it is helpful to understand the normal responses of the newborn to asphyxia. The initial hypoxia and acidosis lead to a characteristic response with diversion of blood flow to the heart and brain and away from less essential organs, such as the gut, liver, kidneys, muscle and skin. In addition, the pulmonary vasculature responds to hypoxia by vasoconstriction, leading to pulmonary hypertension and right-to-left shunting via the ductus arteriosus and the foramen ovale, thereby worsening the hypoxia. Initially the myocardium will maintain cerebral blood flow, but as the hypoxia and acidosis worsen, the myocardium will fail and cardiac output and blood pressure will fall. Respiration is initially irregular until the infant stops breathing in a period known as 'primary apnoea'. If no resuscitative efforts are undertaken, the infant will begin gasping respirations until finally entering 'secondary apnoea'. Clinically, it is impossible to distinguish primary from secondary apnoea, and thus resuscitation is indicated under all circumstances.

Resuscitative efforts leading to improvement in oxygenation and acidosis will reverse the above pathophysiological process and, if instituted early enough, may prevent organ damage.

Preparation
All high-risk deliveries, as defined in Table 4.1, should be attended by appropriately skilled personnel capable of performing a full resuscitation. Likewise, all necessary equipment should be well maintained and ready for use at all times (Table 4.3).

Use of the Apgar score
The Apgar score is a widely used system for description of the clinical condition of the infant

Table 4.3 Apgar score			
Sign	*0*	*1*	*2*
Heart rate	Absent	<100 beats/min	>100 beats/min
Respiration	Absent	Slow, irregular	Good cry
Colour	Blue or pale	Pink, with blue extremities	Pink
Muscle tone	Limp	Some flexion	Active movement
Reflex irritability	No response	Grimace	Cough or sneeze

shortly after birth (Table 4.3). The score comprises five easily assessed parameters, including heart rate, respiration, colour, muscle tone and reflex irritability. Each item is scored from 0 to 2, giving a range of 0 to 10. A score is assigned at the ages of 1 and 5 min routinely and, if still low, at 10, 15 and 20 min.

The primary purpose of the score is to convey information and not to provide a prognostic assessment. However, Apgar scores which remain below 3 at or beyond 10 min of age are associated with an increased risk of mortality, cerebral palsy and mental retardation in survivors.

Stages of resuscitation

The immediate objectives of resuscitation are establishment of a clear airway, stimulation of breathing and maintenance of body temperature. The baby at birth is wet, and if not dried and warmed under a radiant heat source may begin to lose body heat rapidly. The mouth and nose should be suctioned as necessary in order to open the airway. For the infant who does not breathe spontaneously, stimulation by gentle slapping of the soles of the feet or rubbing the back can be tried first. However, this should be of limited duration and, if there is no response, further measures should be instituted. If there is some respiration, the heart rate is above 100 beats/min but the colour is blue, the infant may improve with oxygen by face mask alone. If there is no or little effective respiration and there is bradycardia of less than 100 beats/min, the infant should be ventilated with a bag and mask. It is important to ensure that the mask has an effective rubber seal

and fits the face well, thereby preventing leak. If after approximately 30 s of effective bagging the heart rate is still low and the colour poor, the infant should be intubated and ventilated via an endotracheal tube. The consideration of when to intubate and how long to ventilate via a mask is influenced by the availability of appropriately skilled personnel.

The vast majority of depressed infants will recover rapidly in response to these manoeuvres. However, a small number of severely asphyxiated infants will require either external cardiac massage or administration of medications, which may include adrenaline, sodium bicarbonate, glucose, naloxone, saline and 5% albumin/saline. The first medication to be considered is adrenaline (1:10 000 – 0.1–0.3 ml/kg) which may be given intratracheally if the infant remains bradycardic and cyanosed despite ventilation via an endotracheal tube with 100% oxygen together with external cardiac massage. If the condition has not improved, venous access should be established. The quickest and simplest method is insertion of a catheter 3–5 cm into the umbilical vein. Adrenaline, sodium bicarbonate, naloxone, glucose and volume expanders may be given by this route.

Special situations in resuscitation

- If the mother received opiates close to the delivery and the infant is depressed after birth, naloxone may be given, often with an almost immediate improvement in the infant's condition. This may be given by puncture of the

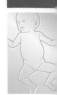

umbilical vein in the cord or via a peripheral vein, and often obviates the need for further resuscitative measures.

- Meconium-stained amniotic fluid poses a significant risk for aspiration, which may be prevented by appropriate care. After the delivery of the head and before the delivery of the shoulders, the nose and pharynx should be suctioned. Following delivery, if the infant is vigorous, crying and pink, observation alone may suffice. However, if the infant is depressed, an endotracheal tube should be inserted and the trachea suctioned. Much debate exists as to whether the thickness of the meconium should influence the care given. No clear answer is available, and some authorities recommend intubation in all cases of thick meconium. Others point out the significant risks which may be associated with intubation (vocal cord trauma, bradycardia, etc.), and suggest a more selective policy as above.

- If a prenatal diagnosis of diaphragmatic hernia is known or the condition is suspected because of respiratory distress together with a scaphoid abdomen, the infant should not be ventilated via a mask as this may distend the intestinal loops in the chest cavity and thus further compromise respiration. Thus, in this situation, the infant should be intubated immediately.

- Hydrops fetalis presents a particularly difficult challenge in the delivery room. The infant may have massive subcutaneous oedema, ascites and pleural and pericardial effusions. If the respiration is extremely compromised in spite of ventilation with high pressures, drainage of fluid from both pleural cavities and from the peritoneum is required as an emergency procedure as part of the resuscitation. In spite of these rather heroic measures, the prognosis is often poor although it is primarily influenced by the underlying diagnosis.

- Shock may result from severe blood loss secondary to conditions such as abruptio placentae (placental separation) or placenta previa. The infant is pale, poorly perfused, tachycardic, tachypnoeic and with low blood pressure. Immediate volume expansion may be achieved by administration of 10–20 ml/kg of saline or 5% albumin saline over 15–20 min. If the situation was anticipated and sufficient time available, O-negative whole blood may be given.

✳ **KEY DIAGNOSIS**

Hypoxic–ischaemic encephalopathy (HIE)

Hypoxia and acidosis cause immediate neuronal damage. In addition, following resuscitation and reperfusion, secondary neuronal damage may take place. This is most marked during the first few hours after birth, but may in some cases continue for many months. The secondary damage is primarily due to apoptosis, the process of programmed cell death. Certain current research approaches, such as hypothermia and magnesium sulphate administration, aim to curtail apoptosis and thereby improve the outcome of infants with HIE.

Clinical features

In mild cases the initial clinical signs are hyperalertness, roving eye movements and hypotonia. More severely affected infants have disturbed consciousness, being either stuporose or even comatose. Seizures are seen before 12 h of age in the majority of seriously affected infants. These may be generalized clonic seizures, but more often are 'subtle'. Subtle seizures include sucking, lip smacking, blank staring or jerky eye movements, irregular random limb movements and apnoeic spells. Disturbances of respiration are commonly seen, and vary from irregular breathing to complete apnoea requiring mechanical ventilation. Severely affected infants show a progressive deterioration of central nervous system function with coma, apnoea and brain stem depression. Brain stem signs include abnormalities of pupillary, oculomotor, caloric and auditory evoked responses.

Diagnosis and investigation

A number of diagnostic modalities are employed in the assessment of HIE. Electroencephalogram

- Immediately following delivery, reflecting the physical and metabolic stress of labour as well as the presence of fetal lung fluid
- Following vigorous physical activity such as after feeding or a prolonged bout of crying.

However, respiratory distress is a cardinal presentation of some of the most common and serious pathological states in neonates (Table 4.4).

The presence of evidence of abnormal ventilatory function (cyanosis, hypoxia, hypercapneoa) without signs of respiratory distress is an important clue to central nervous system depression such as seen due to HIE, or due to drugs given to the baby (e.g. anticonvulsants) or mother (e.g. opiates used for analgesia during labour).

Respiratory disorders

In neonatal practice, respiratory disorders are by far the most common underlying pathology of respiratory distress. The respiratory distress syndrome (RDS; hyaline membrane disease) has traditionally been the single most important condition determining the morbidity and mortality of premature neonates. It also may rarely affect full-term babies in whom certain risk factors are present (e.g. diabetic mothers). Both the incidence and severity of RDS can be favourably altered by the appropriate interventions (administration of steroids to mothers in preterm labour, and prophylactic or rescue treatment of premature babies with surfactant), and in many units these interventions have become standard practices (for further discussion of RDS see p. 61).

Pneumonia (and sepsis)

These are some of the most common and serious conditions underlying respiratory distress in neonates. The infection can be congenital (acquired in utero or intrapartum) or develop postnatally. Prematurity and prolonged rupture of membranes are important predisposing factors.

The clinical manifestations which may include, in addition to signs of respiratory distress, hypotension and thermal instability may ensue soon after birth, and frequently the condition is indistinguishable from RDS. The course can be progressive, in the absence of the appropriate treatment, with rapid deterioration and shock (for a more detailed discussion of neonatal sepsis, see p. 71).

Meconium aspiration

The passage of meconium in utero occurs in response to fetal hypoxia through reflex anal sphincter relaxation. Such response is well developed in post-term babies but is also seen in term and SGA babies. It can rarely occur in

Table 4.4	Causes of respiratory distress in a neonate
Category	*Example*
Respiratory	Respiratory distress syndrome (RDS) Pneumonia Aspiration syndromes including meconium aspiration Pneumothorax Pulmonary hypoplasia, e.g. congenital diaphragmatic hernia (Fig. 4.2) Transient tachypnoea of the newborn (TTN)
Cardiac	Pulmonary oedema and heart failure Right-to-left shunt
Haematological	Anaemias and abnormal haemoglobins
Metabolic	Disorders associated with metabolic acidosis
Neuromuscular	Spinal muscular atrophy Neonatal forms of muscular dystrophy and myasthenia

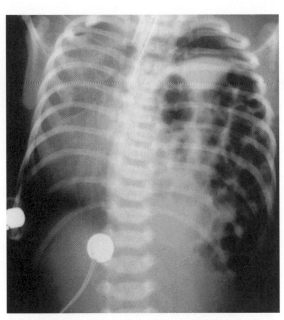

Figure 4.2 Congenital diaphragmatic hernia. A radiograph of a neonate showing tracheal deviation associated with multiple gas-filled bowel loops in the left hemithorax

premature babies in whom the passage of meconium in utero is a clue to certain types of intrauterine infections (e.g. listerosis).

The aspiration of meconium-stained amniotic fluid down the lower bronchial tree largely occurs at birth with the first few breaths. This usually results in mechanical obstruction and chemical irritation of the airways. Secondary infection may complicate the course of this illness and air leak syndromes, including pneumothorax, are other complications to watch out for. Treatment is initially supportive, but the most effective interventions are usually preventative (see resuscitation, p. 55).

Transient tachypnoea of the newborn

In certain cases there is delayed absorption of fetal lung fluid, and signs of mild to moderate respiratory distress persist for 48–72 h of age. Transient tachypnoea of the newborn is impossible to differentiate from other types of respiratory pathology, particularly pneumonia, and these infants are usually managed along

similar lines in the early stages. A short benign course, negative laboratory investigations for infection and rapid resolution of radiological findings (usually limited to prominence of the bronchovascular markings, fluid in the fissures and mild hyperinflation) allow the retrospective diagnosis to be established.

Heart failure

This important cause of respiratory distress is discussed in Chapter 7.

PREMATURITY

Prematurity is a major cause of morbidity and mortality in the newborn. All systems of the body are influenced by being unable to complete the third trimester of gestation within the uterus. The degree of immaturity varies significantly among the different organ systems and among infants of the same gestational age. The following discussion will focus on the major conditions associated with prematurity, although a comprehensive description is beyond the scope of this text.

✳ KEY DIAGNOSIS

Respiratory distress syndrome (RDS)

RDS is a the most common, life-threatening condition affecting premature infants. The primary cause is inadequate surfactant in the alveoli together with structural immaturity. The incidence is inversely related to the length of gestation. RDS is seen in more than three-quarters of infants born before 28 weeks of gestation and in less than 10% after 32 weeks.

Pathophysiology

In order for gas exchange to take place, the infant requires patent airways, thin-walled alveoli and adequate pulmonary circulation. The alveoli are lined by two types of epithelial cells. Type I cells are flat elongated cells which cover most of the alveolar surface, and their thinness is ideally suited to allow gasses to cross to and from the pulmonary capillaries in the interstitium. Type II cells are small, highly specialized, high-energy cells whose main function is the synthesis and secretion of surfactant (together with the absorption of lung fluid at birth). Pulmonary surfactant is a phospholipid–protein complex present mainly on the inner lining of the alveoli. The highly polar phospholipid molecules (the most abundant being dipalmitoyl-phosphatidylcholine) form a monolayer at the air–water interface, markedly lowering surface tension, thus preventing alveolar collapse at end-expiration.

Surfactant production is low throughout gestation until a marked rise is seen between 24 and 34 weeks of gestation with marked individual variation in the timing of surfactant sufficiency. Lack of surfactant at birth results in diffuse alveolar collapse and respiratory distress. Oozing of proteinaceous fluid into the alveoli together with cell debris result in the characteristic histological appearance of hyaline membranes which gave the condition its original name, hyaline membrane disease.

Clinical features

The classical clinical picture of RDS is seen less often since the advent of very early intubation, ventilation and surfactant administration in the early stages of the illness. However, classically, the infant is seen to develop respiratory distress with tachypnoea, grunting, intercostal recessions, nasal flaring and cyanosis when breathing room air. The severity of the respiratory distress worsens over minutes to hours as the existing surfactant pool is metabolized and the alveolar type II cells are incapable of increasing the rate of endogenous synthesis. Chest radiography shows a characteristic homogeneous, reticulogranular pattern over both lung fields. Air bronchograms (Fig. 4.3) show air in the bronchi standing out against a background of atelectatic lung tissue. As the respiratory condition worsens, hypoxia and respiratory acidosis with hypercarbia are seen.

The natural history of RDS is a gradual worsening to a nadir at 2–4 days. Then, if the infant survives, accelerated differentiation of type

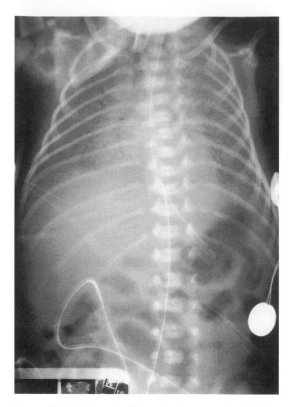

Figure 4.3 A chest radiograph of a premature infant receiving intensive care therapy. There is a reticulogranular pattern (with air bronchograms) in keeping with RDS

II cells results in increased surfactant production with resultant gradual improvement in the clinical condition over the next few days

Treatment

As RDS is a dynamic condition whose severity changes markedly over the first few days of life, continuous monitoring of gas exchange using pulse oximetry and/or transcutaneous Po_2/Pco_2 monitoring together with intermittent blood gas measurements is essential. In addition, heart and respiratory rate, blood pressure and body temperature need to be followed carefully. Serial chest radiographs are useful in following the severity of the disease and also in checking for the appearance of acquired problems such as lobar atelectasis secondary to endotracheal tube misplacement.

The management of RDS varies as to the severity of the clinical condition. Mild cases may do well with supplemental oxygen alone. However, if the infant begins to tire and the oxygen requirement rises or respiratory acidosis (increased CO_2, decreased pH) develops, nasal continuous positive airways pressure (CPAP) may help to stabilize alveoli and improve respiratory status. In many cases, endotracheal intubation and mechanical ventilation are required. This technique is effective in ensuring effective gas exchange, and is an accepted standard of care.

As inadequate surfactant is the primary aetiological factor, it is logical to administer exogenous surfactant in order to improve lung function until endogenous production rises. Surfactant is administered via the endotracheal tube and spreads out over the alveolar surface. In most cases the infant's respiratory condition improves markedly within minutes to hours (Fig. 4.4). Measurements of pulmonary mechanics have shown increased lung volume within minutes and improved compliance within 6–24 h.

Prevention

Prevention of premature labour is crucial, and the value of adequate antenatal care cannot be overemphasized. The likely degree of maturity of the fetal lungs should be taken into account in timing interventions such as caesarean section.

Administration of steroids to pregnant women before term significantly accelerates the maturation process of the fetal lungs. It is currently the standard practice in most centres to administer betamethasone or dexamethasone to women 48–72 h prior to delivery at 32 weeks of gestation or less. Frequently, it is possible to suppress labour activity in women who go into spontaneous premature labour for the 48–72 h necessary to give the required doses of steroids.

The administration of surfactant as a preventative measure is debatable (see Highlights and Hypotheses: a deeper look at surfactant therapy).

There are a number of complications of RDS which although not uniquely associated with RDS can be considered to constitute the 'associated morbidity'. Most important amongst them are chronic lung disease CLD; (bronchopulmonary dysplasia (BPD)), peri-/intraventricular haemorrhage (P-IVH) and necrotizing enterocolitis (NEC)

Bronchopulmonary dysplasia

Even in the era of surfactant therapy and sophisticated ventilators, a significant number of premature infants survive their initial respiratory problems (RDS, recurrent apnoea, etc.), only to develop CLD requiring either ventilation and/or supplemental oxygen for weeks or months.

Aetiology and pathophysiology

The main aetiological factors are prematurity, mechanical ventilation and oxygen therapy. Toxic oxygen free radicals are generated in the presence of high concentrations of administered oxygen in the face of immature oxygen free radical scavenging systems. The accumulated radicals cause widespread cellular damage. Pulmonary oedema, secondary either to excess fluid administration or left-to-right shunting via a patent ductus arteriosus (see below), is a risk factor for BPD. Also, events such as sepsis/pneumonia, pneumothorax (Fig. 4.5) and

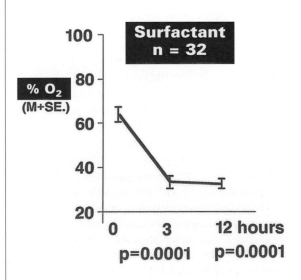

Figure 4.4 The improvement in oxygen requirement in RDS in premature infants immediately after administration of exogenous surfactant

HIGHLIGHTS AND HYPOTHESES

A DEEPER LOOK AT SURFACTANT THERAPY

Surfactant is prepared by two different methods. Natural surfactant is extracted from mammalian lungs (bovine, porcine) and contains >90% polar phospholipids together with small amounts of surfactant proteins B and C. Synthetic surfactants contain phospholipids with or without added emulsifiers and spreading agents. The response to natural surfactants is more rapid than that seen after synthetic surfactant administration. In addition, natural surfactants are associated with a greater reduction in mortality and air leak. Future possible developments include surfactants consisting of synthetic phospholipids together with recombinant surfactant proteins or peptides.

Two different approaches have been employed as to the timing of surfactant administration. In the prophylactic approach, surfactant is administered either in the delivery room or very shortly after birth to all infants at high risk of developing RDS. Studies have mostly viewed infants born at less than 30 weeks of gestation as being at high risk. The main aims of this approach are to optimize even distribution of the surfactant and to minimize lung injury caused by mechanical ventilation of the surfactant-deficient, non-compliant lungs. However, up to 40% of infants born at less than 30 weeks of gestation will not develop RDS and thus the prophylactic approach will result in unwarranted therapy. The second approach, which is termed 'rescue', limits surfactant administration to infants with a clinicoradiographic diagnosis of RDS, who require mechanical ventilation and supplemental oxygen. This approach provides surfactant only to those who need it but involves a delay on average of 2–6 h from birth to treatment. Studies comparing these two approaches have so far been inconclusive as to differences in mortality or major morbidities, and in practice both approaches are employed today. A modification which is gaining support is limitation of prophylactic use to infants born at less than 28 weeks of gestation, thereby targeting the highest-risk infants and minimizing unnecessary administration.

The advent of surfactant replacement therapy, which is now a standard of care for RDS, has dramatically improved outcome. Mortality is significantly reduced, and most residual mortality is related to associated morbidity such as sepsis or intraventricular haemorrhage rather than to the primary respiratory condition. The incidence of air leaks, such as pneumothorax and interstitial emphysema, has been reduced dramatically. The effect on the incidence and severity of other morbidities is as yet unclear. Intraventricular haemorrhage, sepsis, patent ductus arteriosus and necrotizing enterocolitis are probably unchanged. The incidence of bronchopulmonary dysplasia and retinopathy of prematurity is unchanged but their severity seems diminished.

BEYOND CORE

A KINDER, GENTLER APPROACH TO VENTILATION

The delicate, premature lungs are ill prepared to deal with the trauma of mechanical ventilation which may contribute to the development of chronic lung disease (bronchopulmonary dysplasia).

In the search for ways of ventilating babies and causing less barotrauma, two techniques have been proposed. Synchronized or patient-triggered ventilation employs a sensor to detect the start of inspiration and initiate a ventilator breath in time with the spontaneous inspiration. This prevents active expiration against a mechanical breath which may be a contributory factor in the aetiology of pulmonary air leak, such as pneumothorax (Fig. 4.5) or interstitial emphysema. High-frequency ventilation is another technique under investigation. It employs extremely high ventilatory rates of 400–1400 breaths/min with an extremely small tidal volume. Although the exact mechanisms by which gas exchange is effected are not totally clear (possibly facilitated diffusion), this technique has been shown to be useful as a rescue manoeuvre in critically sick infants with conditions such as pulmonary interstitial emphysema.

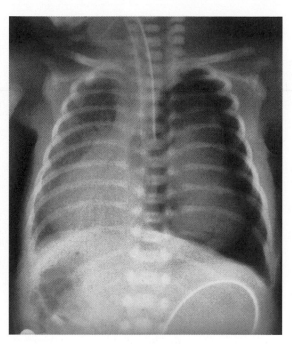

Figure 4.5   A chest radiograph of a ventilated premature infant. There is a right pneumothorax

pulmonary interstitial emphysema which may cause direct lung damage and also result in increased ventilatory and oxygen requirements are aetiological factors.

In the first weeks of life, the primary pathological process is inflammation. Later, diffuse emphysema with areas of collapse and fibrosis are seen. In addition, airway changes are marked with increased mucus production, epithelial metaplasia and increased bronchial smooth muscle, which can cause bronchospasm. Late vascular changes result in pulmonary hypertension.

Clinical findings include worsening of respiratory distress with fine crepitations and occasionally expiratory wheezing. Recurrent flitting atelectasis may be secondary to thick airway secretions. In infants who require prolonged ventilation, thinning of airway cartilage may develop, leading to secondary tracheobronchomalacia.

Treatment and outcome

The treatment of established CLD has many facets. All attempts should be made to minimize the use of supplemental oxygen and mechanical ventilation, without exposing the infant to either hypoxia or respiratory acidosis. For this purpose, continuous monitoring of oxygenation and intermittent blood gas analyses are required. The most widely used and effective therapy is corticosteroids, which have numerous effects including suppression of inflammation, stimulation of antioxidants, enhanced surfactant production and decreased bronchospasm. Intravenous dexamethasone has been shown to improve lung function in the short term, facilitate earlier extubation and also possibly reduce mortality. Steroids may also be administered by inhalation although the effects are not as yet clear. Commonly seen side–effects of steroids include hyperglycaemia, hypertension, gastrointestinal haemorrhage and masking of the signs of infection.

Diuretic therapy has been shown to increase pulmonary compliance in CLD and can help to relieve the excessive work of breathing. In infants with marked bronchospasm, bronchodilators such as β agonists (salbutamol, terbutaline) and methylxanthines (caffeine, theophylline) may be effective.

Nutritional support is of major importance in fostering a full and rapid recovery from CLD. Fluid restriction designed to minimize pulmonary oedema often results in low caloric intake. An additional problem is the high incidence of gastro-oesophageal reflux in infants with CLD. Within these restrictions, efforts must be made to maximize caloric intake, which is closely related to the rate of recovery.

Prevention of pulmonary infection is important as each episode of infection increases the lung damage and slows the rate of repair. Thus, careful nursing technique and appropriate culture-directed antibiotic therapy are recommended where indicated.

In most infants the outcome of CLD is a slow but gradual process of recovery with subsequent normal lung function. CLD-related mortality is probably of the order of 5–10% although reports vary. Long-term follow-up suggests, however, that the most severely affected infants continue to have airway hyper-reactivity, with recurrent admissions due to episodes of wheezing and abnormal pulmonary function between episodes.

Patent ductus arteriosus

During fetal life, blood bypasses the lungs by flowing from the pulmonary artery via the ductus arteriosus into the aorta. Under normal circumstances, the ductus closes within 48 h of birth. In the premature infant, particularly if ventilated for RDS, the immature duct may not close. This may result in a left-to-right shunt via the ductus which leads to pulmonary oedema and cardiac failure, with increased requirements for oxygen and ventilatory support (see Ch. 7).

Peri-/intraventricular haemorrhage

P-IVH is an all too common complication of premature birth and is often associated with significant long-term neurodevelopmental handicap. The incidence in very low birth weight (<1500 g) infants is 10–40% in different reports, with an inverse relationship between the incidence and the gestational age at birth. Most haemorrhages occur during the first 4 days after birth, and most of the remainder are temporally associated with serious illness such as sepsis or pulmonary air leak.

Pathophysiology

The premature brain is particularly vulnerable to injury. In the periventricular area near the foramen of Monro, a structure called the germinal matrix is to be found at 26–34 weeks of gestation, which involutes completely by term. This rich vascular matrix, which consists of a single layer of endothelial cells with no surrounding supportive tissue, is at risk of rupture when exposed to high-risk situations. The cerebral circulation at this early stage of gestation is pressure-passive, i.e. changes in arterial blood pressure result in large swings in cerebral blood flow. Unstable blood pressure is associated with mechanical ventilation (particularly if asynchronous) airway suction and pulmonary air leak. Thus, fluctuations in blood pressure are transmitted to the cerebral circulation, resulting in rupture of the delicate germinal matrix vessels. This subependymal bleeding (grade 1) may spread into the ventricle itself (grade 2). If there is sufficient bleeding, the ventricles may be dilated (grade 3). The term 'grade 4' is used to describe a parenchymal haemorrhagic venous infarction which is usually unilateral and, although usually seen in the presence of significant intraventricular haemorrhage, can occur alone.

Clinical features and investigation

P-IVH can present either as a catastrophic deterioration with hypotension, apnoea, metabolic acidosis and death, or it may follow an intermittent course with cyclical deterioration followed by recovery. However, most cases are silent and are only detected by routine cranial ultrasound screening (Fig. 4.6), which is the preferred method of diagnosis.

The major complication of P-IVH is posthaemorrhagic hydrocephalus, which develops in up to 50% of infants with grade 3 or 4 haemorrhage.

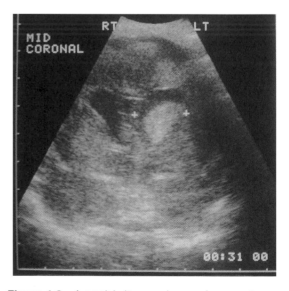

Figure 4.6 A cranial ultrasound scan of a premature baby showing left-sided intraventricular haemorrhage. (Reproduced by courtesy of Dr J. Boyer, St Peter's Hospital, Surrey)

Treatment and outcome

Treatment of P-IVH starts with prevention. As P-IVH is primarily a complication of prematurity, prevention of premature birth is of major importance, with active antenatal care and aggressive use of tocolytic therapy. In addition, prevention of RDS with antenatal corticosteroid administration significantly reduces the incidence and severity of P-IVH. It is important that haemodynamic stability be maintained. Rapid administration of volume expanders or hyperosmolar solutions such as sodium bicarbonate, excessive handling or suctioning should all be avoided. In addition, synchronized ventilation may serve to reduce cerebral blood flow fluctuations, although this has yet to be proven. Management of established haemorrhage is supportive, with administration of blood or other volume expansion as required together with general supportive measures such as ventilation. Posthaemorrhagic hydrocephalus may be managed by repeated lumbar punctures in order to reduce the pressure in the ventricles and thereby hopefully minimize secondary white matter damage. Pharmacological interventions, such as furosemide and acetazolamide, have also been studied. In approximately 50% of cases, a shunt operation will be required, usually ventriculoperitoneal.

The prognosis is primarily related to the grade of the haemorrhage. Grades 1 and 2 are associated with neurodevelopmental delay in up to 20% and mortality in up to 10%. Grades 3 and 4 are associated with up to 80% neurodevelopmental delay and even 50% mortality. The presence of either periventricular haemorrhage or hydrocephalus significantly worsen the prognosis.

Periventricular leucomalacia (PVL)

PVL is necrosis of the periventricular white matter which results from hypoxia and ischaemia. It is seen in 2–20% of very low birth weight infants. During the first week of life, PVL is seen on ultrasound examination as increased echogenicity around the lateral ventricles. As the condition progresses, cysts appear in the echogenic regions with secondary loss of brain tissue. Prematurity, intrauterine growth retardation and chorioamnionitis are recognized risk factors for PVL. Poor prognostic indicators include bilateral as opposed to unilateral cysts, diffuse as opposed to localized cysts, and the presence of subcortical cysts. Cerebral palsy and mental retardation are seen in 60–100% of premature infants with cystic PVL. Those infants in whom periventricular echogenicity does not progress to cyst formation have a lower risk of poor outcome.

Necrotizing enterocolitis

NEC is the most common neonatal surgical emergency, and is characterized by widespread necrosis in the small and large intestine, and leads to significant morbidity and mortality even with modern intensive care. The incidence ranges from 1 to 5% of neonatal intensive care unit admissions, and is highest in the most premature infants. Less than 10% of cases are seen in term infants. Incidence rates vary significantly from centre to centre and from year to year; mortality rates range from 20 to 60% in different reports.

Aetiology and pathogenesis

The pathogenesis of NEC remains unknown in spite of extensive investigation over many years. A number of contributory factors have been identified, although a number of factors which were previously thought to be relevant have subsequently been shown not to be so. Umbilical artery catheters, RDS, thrombocytopenia and anaemia are just a few of those risk factors which have been disproved.

Almost all infants with NEC have received enteral feeding, and a hypothesis has been proposed that hyperosmolar feeds may cause an initial mucosal injury. However, no clear and consistent relationship has been identified in terms of the timing or amounts of feeds which may be detrimental, and it is important to remember that the vast majority of enterally fed premature infants do not develop NEC. Human milk may have a protective effect.

Many cases of NEC, particularly during mini-epidemics, are associated with growth of bacteria (mostly Gram-negative bacilli) or viruses (rotavirus) either from the blood or from the peritoneal cavity. However, it is unclear whether these organisms are of primary or secondary importance as aetiological factors.

Asphyxial events may result in diversion of blood from the splanchnic bed, resulting in relative intestinal hypoxia and/or ischaemia with subsequent reperfusion injury. This may combine with intestinal immaturity to begin the process of diffuse necrosis.

In any individual case of NEC, a combination of the above factors may be active and unfortunately, to date, no specific preventive measure has been identified.

Clinical features

The clinical picture of NEC may vary from a mild transient condition to a fulminant disease with an extremely high risk of mortality. Early signs may be limited to lethargy and gastric residuals (nasogastric aspirates). Later, as the condition progresses, there are bloody stools, poor perfusion, temperature instability, apnoea and bradycardia. Bowel sounds may be absent as ileus develops. Haematological findings include leucocytosis or leucopenia, with left shift and thrombocytopenia. Blood gas analysis may show metabolic acidosis related to hypovolaemia, and both hypoxia and hypercarbia secondary to abdominal distension which may compromise lung excursion. As the disease progresses, third space losses of extravascular fluid within the abdomen may cause hypovolaemia and shock; intestinal perforation then becomes a significant risk. Additional findings in severe cases include oedema and erythema of the abdominal wall.

Investigation

The abdominal radiography may show distended loops and bowel wall oedema. The classic pathognomonic radiography finding is pneumatosis intestinalis, which is the accumulation of intramural gas along the length of the affected bowel (Figs 4.7 and 4.8). Intestinal perforation may be identified by free air in the peritoneal cavity on radiography. As the disease progresses, fluid may accumulate in the peritoneal cavity. Additional signs include a fixed,

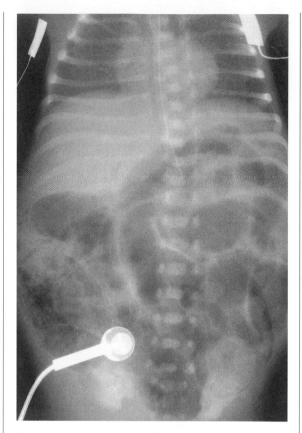

Figure 4.7   An abdominal film from a premature infant requiring intensive support. There are dilated gas-filled loops of small intestine, some of which are paralleled by lines of gas, indicating intramural gas. Some gases are also seen outlining the portal vein: necrotizing enterocolitis (see Fig. 4.8)

distended loop which may be persistent over 1–3 days. This may represent a concealed intestinal perforation which has become sealed off. In some cases, air may be seen in the portal system.

Treatment and outcome

NEC is an acute emergency, and treatment must be started immediately after the suspicion has been raised. Feeding should be stopped, and a nasogastric tube passed to allow bowel decompression by intermittent suction. Cultures of blood, cerebrospinal fluid and urine should be taken, and broad-spectrum antibiotic administration begun. Common combinations include penicillin or ampicillin together with an

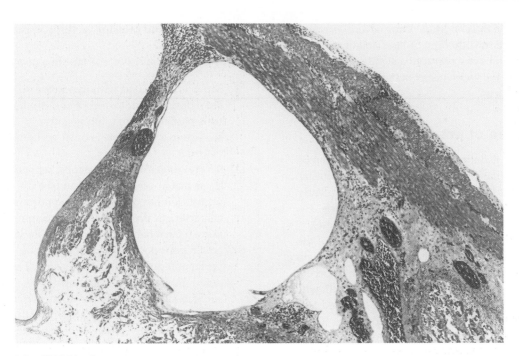

Figure 4.8   NEC histology

aminoglycoside, such as gentamicin or amikacin and metronidazole to provide anaerobic coverage. Fluid replacement should be administered at the maintenance requirements, usually 150–200 ml/kg/day, or occasionally more, and should include a high sodium intake to replace losses into the intra-abdominal third space. Fresh frozen plasma may be incorporated into the fluid regimen as a volume expander and as a source of coagulation factors. Radiographs of the abdomen, including decubitus views, should be taken at frequent intervals in order to detect perforation without undue delay. Blood counts and urea and electrolytes need to be followed carefully. Thrombocytopenia may be treated with platelet transfusions.

Indications for surgical intervention include evidence of perforation, fixed loop and uncontrollable clinical deterioration. At laparotomy, a careful survey of the complete bowel is undertaken to identify the extent of the disease, with the most commonly affected areas being the terminal ileum and the ascending colon, although the whole of the small and large intestines may be affected. The necrotic area is

removed, and a jejunostomy, ileostomy or colostomy is performed.

Late sequelae of NEC include stricture formation and short bowel syndrome. Strictures may develop as a result of fibrosis in affected regions. This may present as intestinal obstruction at 2–8 weeks after the initial event, and usually requires surgical resection although intraluminal dilatation has been used in some cases. Short bowel syndrome is characterized by diarrhoea and malabsorption, and may require prolonged periods of nutritional support either enterally or parenterally.

Retinopathy of prematurity

The immature, incompletely vascularized retina is at high risk of injury. This condition may result in outcomes ranging from normal sight, through refractive disorders to total blindness after retinal detachment. Factors which may contribute to the pathogenesis include prematurity, hyperoxia, shock, asphyxia, vitamin E deficiency, hypothermia and light exposure. Careful regulation of oxygen administration may help to minimize the condition. Once severe disease develops, cryotherapy or laser ablation of the peripheral avascular retina significantly reduces the incidence of subsequent retinal detachment.

Apnoea of prematurity

Apnoea is defined as a pause in respiration of greater than 20 s, and is a common manifestation of prematurity. The apnoeic spell is frequently associated with bradycardia and cyanosis. Two mechanisms contribute to the pathogenesis. Central apnoea results from immaturity of the respiratory centre in the brain stem. Obstructive apnoea results from weakness of the upper airway, in particular the pharyngeal wall, which may collapse during inspiration. A mixed form involving both mechanisms also occurs. The effect of apnoea may result in transient hypoperfusion, hypoxia and ischaemia to organs such as the brain and the gut, and may contribute to the development of periventricular leucomalacia and necrotizing enterocolitis (see above). The differential diagnosis of apnoeic events is extensive, and includes sepsis, intracranial haemorrhage, respiratory disorders, metabolic disturbances and drugs, such as phenobarbitone. Infants of less than 35 weeks of gestation need to be monitored in order that apnoeic spells may be identified and treated and have preventive therapy instituted. Immediate treatment involves gentle stimulation, which in the majority of cases induces respiration. If there is no response, the infant should be ventilated either by bag and mask or, if necessary, via an endotracheal tube. Apnoea of prematurity may be prevented by the administration of methylxanthines such as caffeine or theophylline or ventilatory support, either via nasal CPAP or even with intubation and ventilation. Apnoea of prematurity is a diagnosis of exclusion after other underlying causes have been ruled out and/or treated.

COLLAPSE

Collapse (or shock) is a sudden deterioration in the general condition of the infant, associated with a fall in blood pressure, pallor and poor perfusion.

The common causes of collapse in a neonate are:

1. Sepsis is associated with hypotension, secondary to endotoxaemia and capillary leak, particularly in gram negative septicaemia (this topic is dealt with in detail below).

2. Severe congenital heart lesions, particularly those that are duct dependent (see Ch. 7), such as left hypoplastic heart syndrome. This characteristically presents, in a seemingly normal term baby, at 1–3 days of life with pallor, poor perfusion, poor or absent peripheral pulses and hypotension. The deterioration results from normal spontaneous closure of the ductus arteriosus, which makes the inadequate small left ventricle the only source of blood to the systemic circulation.

3. Inborn errors of metabolism which become manifest shortly after the establishment of enteral feeds and are accompanied by metabolic derangements such as hyperammonaemia, hypoglycaemia and/or acidosis.

4. Endocrine causes, such as the salt-losing form of congenital adrenal hyperplasia, are rare causes of hypotension and will usually be associated with hyperkalaemia, hyponatraemia and metabolic acidosis.

5. Other causes are related to blood loss, tension pneumothorax (see Fig. 4.5), intracranial haemorrhage and reaction to drugs.

Immediate assessment should lead to recognition of the severity of the baby's condition, and guide the physician as to the appropriate resuscitative measures. Further evaluation, after the baby's condition has been stabilized, should involve a detailed history and physical examination, as well as further investigations as necessary.

Immediate management

- Volume expansion with either crystalloid, such as normal saline, or colloid, such as saline albumin, plasma or blood

- Inotropic support with dopamine and/or dobutamine
- Antibiotic cover (see below)
- Ventilatory support
- Correction of metabolic problems such as hypoglycaemia or severe acidosis
- Prostaglandin E_1 infusion may be initiated if closure of the ductus is suspected in order to reopen the duct, at least until a diagnosis is confirmed or ruled out
- Enteral feeding is usually withheld during the acute phase

✳ KEY DIAGNOSIS

Sepsis

Sepsis in the neonate is a common and life-threatening condition, which can present in a multitude of forms and become fulminant in a moment. Even in the age of modern antibiotics, neonatal sepsis results in significant morbidity and mortality.

Incidence

Neonatal sepsis is seen in 1–10 per 1000 live births and in up to 50% of very low birth weight infants. Reported mortality rates vary between 10 and 50%. Meningitis coexists with a significant percentage of cases of sepsis in the neonate, and causes a high mortality rate and significant long-term morbidity.

Risk factors

Factors which are associated with increased risk of sepsis include:

- Maternal bacterial colonization or infection. Organisms such as group B streptococci are commonly found in the cervix and vagina and are a major cause of sepsis (which may be reduced or prevented by intrapartum antibiotics). Numerous other organisms may also be acquired either by ascending infection or by haematogenous spread. Specific infections such as chorioamnionitis and urinary tract infection in the mother add extra risk.

- Prematurity, which is the most powerful independent risk factor. Immaturity of host defences raises the risk of infection markedly in all newborns but in particular in the premature infant. The skin and mucosae are thin and permeable, cellular immunity is inadequate, complement levels are low and IgM and secretory IgA are absent.
- Prolonged rupture of membranes beyond 24 h, which raises the risk of ascending infection.
- Obstetric factors such as instrumental deliveries, fetal scalp electrodes, multiple gestation and need for resuscitation at birth which are associated with increased risk of infection.
- Invasive procedures and multiple broad-spectrum antibiotics, which predispose to infection.

Causative organisms

Sepsis during the first 3 days of life (early sepsis) is generally thought to be related to the birth process, whereas, beyond the fourth day (late sepsis), infection is primarily nosocomial. Accordingly, the causative organisms in early sepsis represent maternal flora whereas the flora of the neonatal unit or the home predominate in late sepsis.

Many studies have reported on the distribution of organisms causing neonatal sepsis, and there is significant variation between reports. In Britain and Europe, early sepsis is mainly caused by group B *streptococci* and Gram-negative bacilli such as *Escherichia coli* and *Klebsiella*. In North America, Group B *streptococci* are found in a much higher incidence, whereas in the Middle East and Eastern Europe, Gram-negative bacilli are predominant. In late sepsis, coagulase-negative *staphylococci* and fungal infections are important.

In addition to varying patterns of organisms, the pattern of antibiotic sensitivities varies between neonatal units and also varies over time within individual units. Thus, in order that appropriate antibiotic cover be administered, it is critical that each unit maintain and regularly review a local database of infections and antibiotic sensitivity patterns.

Clinical features

Signs of sepsis in the neonate are non-specific and the differential diagnosis is extensive. However, as mild initial disease may rapidly progress to severe systemic infection, it is important to maintain a high index of suspicion and begin antibiotic therapy without waiting for culture results. Signs of sepsis include:

- Change in behaviour/neurological state – lethargy, irritability, change in tone, convulsions or bulging fontanelle
- Temperature instability – hypothermia or fever which is unexplained by technical factors such as a malfunctioning incubator
- Respiratory – apnoeic spells or periodic breathing, respiratory distress (tachypnoea, grunting, flaring, retractions), increased oxygen or ventilatory requirement
- Cardiovascular – poor perfusion, hypotension, tachycardia/bradycardia
- Gastrointestinal – poor feeding, vomiting or gastric residuals, diarrhoea, abdominal distension
- Metabolic – unstable glucose homeostasis (hyperglycaemia, hypoglycaemia) or metabolic acidosis
- Skin – rashes, pustules, vesicles, cellulitis or omphalitis
- Hepatic – increased indirect hyperbilirubinaemia, mixed hyperbilirubinaemia

Investigation

Diagnosis of sepsis is difficult in view of the non-specific nature of many of the signs and variation of presentation of the disease. If an appropriately high index of suspicion is maintained, approximately three 'septic work-ups' are usually performed for every one positive blood culture.

Septic work-up routinely includes:

- Full blood count and differential – leucopenia, leucocytosis and shift to the left with abundant immature forms are characteristic.
- Cultures of blood, cerebrospinal fluid and urine.
- Urinalysis, looking for evidence of urinary tract infection.
- Chest and abdominal radiography as indicated.

- Gram stain of fluid from a skin lesion, joint aspirate or other fluid, which may be useful.
- Serum urea, creatinine and electrolytes, for assessment of renal function.
- C-reactive protein, which is used in some centres; its usefulness is limited by the the fact that it usually becomes abnormal in neonatal sepsis 24 h or more after the onset of clinical disease. However, it is a useful tool for following the progress of the disease and its response to therapy.

Treatment

Antibiotic therapy should be initiated as soon as cultures have been taken. As stated above, individual unit policies are based on the antibiotic sensitivity patterns of the local causative organisms. Combinations which are commonly used in early sepsis include penicillin/ampicillin together with an aminoglycoside, such as gentamicin or amikacin. Some centres use a third-generation cephalosporin such as cefotaxime or ceftazidime. (Note that ceftriaxone is contraindicated in the neonate as it dissociates bilirubin from albumin and raises the risk of kernicterus.) In late sepsis, when meningitis is more likely, third-generation cephalosporins and ampicillin are often used.

In special circumstances, such as in the presence of central lines or when the baby's condition does not improve on the usual antibiotic combinations, the addition of other antimicrobial agents is considered. Vancomycin should be included if a diagnosis of staphylococcal infection is made with positive blood cultures or strongly suspected from appropriate clinical findings. Likewise, treatment for fungal infections should usually be reserved until a definite diagnosis is made.

If cultures are negative after 72 h and the infant's clinical condition is acceptable, antibiotic cover may be discontinued. If a specific diagnosis such as pneumonia, in which cultures may be negative, is made, then antibiotic cover may be continued for 7–10 days. In meningitis, cover should be continued for at least 14 days. In sepsis with positive cultures, antibiotic therapy can be tailored to the specific organism.

Supportive therapy in sepsis includes much of the approach described earlier for collapse in general. Experimental, and as yet unproven, approaches to the treatment of sepsis include intravenous immunoglobulins for support of humoral immunity and granulocyte–colony stimulating factor (G–CSF) for stimulation of neutrophil production.

JAUNDICE

Jaundice is very common in the newborn, and is mostly mild and requires no treatment. However, in some infants, it results from serious pathology and, if untreated, can cause serious morbidity and even mortality.

Background

Bilirubin is produced by the breakdown of haem-containing proteins, primarily haemoglobin. In its native form it is lipid-soluble and circulates in plasma primarily bound to albumin. A small amount remains as 'free' bilirubin, and it is this component which, when in gross excess, can cross the blood–brain barrier. This bilirubin causes neuronal damage, leading to the clinical picture of kernicterus, with lethargy, convulsions, opisthotonus and possibly death. Survivors suffer from choreoathetosis, sensorineural deafness and mental retardation.

In the liver, bilirubin is conjugated with glucuronide to produce conjugated or 'direct' bilirubin, which is water-soluble and can be excreted via the bile into the gastrointestinal tract.

Immaturity of the newborn liver results in accumulation of unconjugated bilirubin and physiological jaundice of the neonate. This normally starts by day 2 or 3, reaches a peak between days 3 and 5, and slowly falls off thereafter. Jaundice which begins earlier, or reaches very high and dangerous levels, is termed pathological.

The commonest mechanism of severe, pathological hyperbilirubinaemia is increased haemolysis secondary to blood group incompatibility, either of the rhesus (Rh) or ABO types. In Rh incompatibility, the mother, who is Rh-negative, becomes sensitized by entry of Rh-positive blood into her bloodstream, either at the end of a previous pregnancy or during a miscarriage. The antibodies which she produces against Rh-positive blood can cross the placenta and cause haemolysis in future pregnancies if a fetus is Rh-positive. This may result in severe neonatal hyperbilirubinaemia and anaemia. In the most extreme and often fatal form, intrauterine haemolysis leads to anaemia and generalized oedema, known as hydrops fetalis.

ABO incompatibility is much commoner and milder. The mother is blood group O and the fetus group A or B. Haemolysis results from high levels of anti-A or -B antibodies. Hydrops is not seen, but marked neonatal hyperbilirubinaemia and prolonged anaemia may result. Both ABO and Rh incompatibility cause jaundice, which appears usually on the first day of life.

Another common mechanism of unconjugated hyperbilirubinaemia is breast milk jaundice. Breast-fed infants have a higher incidence and increased severity of jaundice, although this does not reach levels associated with kernicterus. Various mechanisms may coexist, including reduced caloric and fluid intake and exposure to pregnanediol in the milk which inhibits conjugation. Breast milk jaundice is not a contraindication to breast feeding.

Common causes of hyperbilirubinaemia are shown in Table 4.5, and are divided into unconjugated and conjugated types.

Investigation

Jaundice which is visible within the first day of life should be viewed as haemolytic until proven otherwise, and investigated accordingly. Thereafter, investigation of the cause is usually indicated when the bilirubin levels are above those seen in normal physiological jaundice. Much debate has centred in recent years on the question of the bilirubin levels at which to investigate, institute phototherapy or perform an exchange transfusion and recommendations vary.

Standard investigations should include direct and indirect bilirubin levels, a blood count and

Table 4.5   Causes of hyperbilirubinaemia in the newborn

Unconjugated	Conjugated
Physiological	Neonatal hepatitis
increased haemolysis	Intrauterine infection
Rh incompatibility	Cytomegalovirus
ABO incompatibility	Rubella
Glucose-6-phosphate	Toxoplasmosis
dehydrogenase	Biliary tract obstruction
(G6PD) deficiency	Biliary atresia
Spherocytosis	Choledocal cysts
Reabsorption of blood	Parenteral nutrition
Cephalhaematoma	Galactosaemia
Extensive bruising	α_1-Antitrypsin deficiency
Breast milk jaundice	Cystic fibrosis
Hypothyroidism	
Infection (may be mixed)	
Septicaemias,	
Urinary tract infection	
Dehydration	
Deficient glucuronidation	
Crigler–Najjar syndrome	
Gilbert's disease	
Prematurity	

[a] Causes of prolonged neonatal jaundice include all conjugated hyperbilirubinaemias plus breast milk jaundice, hypothyroidism, infection (may be mixed type), the Crigler–Najjar syndrome, prematurity

smear, the mother's and infant's blood group, and an infant Coombs's test. If the parents are of Mediterranean or Middle Eastern origin, or there is a previous family history, glucose-6-phosphate dehydrogenase levels should be checked (see Ch. 11). If the direct bilirubin level is high, liver enzymes should be measured. Persistent or very severe jaundice which is unexplained by the above screening will require more detailed investigation, including thyroid function testing. Sepsis may result in worsening of jaundice, but jaundice is unlikely to be the sole presenting sign of sepsis. Therefore, in an asymptomatic infant, no investigation for infection is usually included in the work-up for jaundice.

Treatment

Phototherapy is the mainstay of therapy. Light in the blue waveband (450 nm) causes conversion of bilirubin in the skin to a stereoisomer which is water-soluble and excretable in the urine. While under the light, the infant is kept almost naked apart from eye patches to prevent retinal damage (and a nappy, perhaps). Heat and fluid loss are important potential problems during therapy. Phototherapy is instituted at bilirubin levels which are well below those which are associated with kernicterus, in order to allow a generous safety margin.

In a small minority of cases, bilirubin levels continue to rise in spite of phototherapy, and exchange transfusion is indicated. Vascular access for the procedure is usually via the umbilical vessels. Gradual exchange in small aliquots of twice the total blood volume produces a significant reduction in bilirubin.

The policy of anticipation, careful monitoring, early phototherapy and exchange transfusion if necessary has made kernicterus a rare event today.

FURTHER READING

Fanaroff A A, Martin R J 1997 Neonatal perinatal medicine. Diseases of the fetus and infant, 6th edn. Mosby, St Louis

Rennie J M, Roberton N R C 1998 Textbook of neonatology, 3rd edn. Churchill Livingstone, Edinburgh

Volpe J J 1995 Neurology of the newborn, 3rd edn. Saunders, Philadelphia

CHAPTER 5

Gastroenterology and nutrition

S. C. Ling   L. T. Weaver

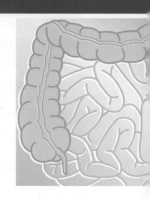

CORE PROBLEMS IN GASTROENTEROLOGY AND NUTRITION

CORE PROBLEM	KEY DIAGNOSIS	RELATED TOPICS
• Acute diarrhoea	Infective gastroenteritis	Haemolytic uraemic syndrome[8]
• Chronic diarrhoea	Toddler diarrhoea	Cow's milk protein enteropathy Coeliac disease Crohn's disease Ulcerative colitis Parasitic infection
• Persistent vomiting	Pyloric stenosis	Gastro-oesophageal reflux Overfeeding
• Constipation	Functional constipation	Hirschsprung's disease
• Recurrent abdominal pain	Functional abdominal pain[18]	Headache[10]
• Jaundice	Hepatitis A infection	Hereditary haemolytic anaemias[11]
• Prolonged neonatal jaundice	Biliary atresia	Neonatal hepatitis
• Failure to thrive	Psychosocial deprivation	
• Nutrition	Infant feeding	Breast feeding Formula feeding Weaning
	Healthy eating beyond infancy	

Where the primary location of a topic is in another chapter, this is indicated by a superscript

ESSENTIAL BACKGROUND

INTRODUCTION

Digestion and absorption of nutrients requires the integration of gastrointestinal, pancreatic and hepatic functions (Table 5.1). This complex process generates substrates needed to support growth, and to maintain the structure of the body and its metabolism.

The developing intestine

The embryonic gastrointestinal tract is formed within 3 weeks of conception, and by 12 weeks

Table 5.1   Function and malfunction in the digestive tract

Function	Malfunction	Effects of malfunction
Motility	Uncoordinated swallowing	Aspiration
	Retrograde flow at the gastro-oesophageal junction	Gastro-oesophageal reflux
	Uncoordinated small intestinal motility	Pseudo-obstruction
	Rectal/internal anal sphincter incoordination	Constipation
Secretion, digestion and absorption	Impaired pancreatic secretion	Maldigestion and malabsorption (e.g. cystic fibrosis)
	Absent or reduced disaccharidase	Maldigestion and malabsorption (e.g. postenteritis syndrome)
Defence	Reduced tolerance of foreign protein	Inflammation (e.g. cow's milk protein enteropathy, coeliac disease)
	Pathogens overcoming gastrointestinal immune system	Gastroenteritis or systemic infection

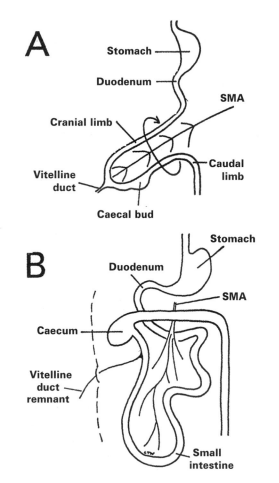

Figure 5.1   Fetal gut rotation during development (SMA = superior mesenteric artery)

gestation the midgut (small intestine and proximal colon) has returned to the abdominal cavity, rotating into the normal position found in the adult (Fig. 5.1). Villi appear during the subsequent 10 weeks, and the gastrointestinal secretory processes develop during the second trimester of fetal life. The stomach secretes hydrochloric acid, intrinsic factor and pepsin, with small intestinal lactase activity at 25% of childhood levels. However, even at term, pancreatic lipase secretion is only 10% of adult levels, although lingual and gastric lipases contribute to lipolysis.

By the end of the second trimester of pregnancy, the fetal gut is structurally complete, lies in its mature anatomical position within the abdomen, and has secretory and absorptive activity. Gastrointestinal motility, however, remains immature. The fetus swallows amniotic fluid containing small amounts of protein, including trophic factors such as epidermal growth factor which may stimulate gut development. Gastric antral motility, transit of fluid through the small intestine, and immature peristalsis occur in the third trimester, but mature migrating motor complexes develop nearer term.

The mucosal defence system of the neonatal intestine is immature. T and B cells, macrophages and dendritic cells accumulate in the intestinal tract and mechanisms for their coordinated

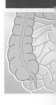

ENTEROCYTE TURNOVER AND FUNCTION

Although functionally still immature at birth, the microscopic appearance of the small intestinal mucosa is similar to that of the older child and adult. The mucosal surface is covered with villi, which project into the lumen and substantially increase the surface area for absorption. At the base of the villi are the crypts of Lieberkühn, which secrete mucus, water and electrolytes and are the origin of rapidly dividing undifferentiated cells which migrate on to the villi. Here they mature into enterocytes with a well-developed brush border containing the enzymes and transporters necessary for absorption of nutrients, water and electrolytes. Digestive enzymes within the brush border membrane include: disaccharidases (lactase and sucrase–isomaltase), enterokinase, peptidases and glucoamylase. As the cells reach the villous tip they degenerate and drop off into the lumen. The whole cycle takes 4–6 days. This rapid turnover explains the susceptibility of the small intestine mucosa to toxic insult (e.g. infection, chemotherapy, radiation) and its ability to recover quickly from such insults.

function develop during the second trimester of pregnancy. Secretory immunoglobulin (IgA) in breast milk acts at the intestinal mucosal surface and other protective factors, such as lactoferrin and lysozyme, defend against ingested microorganisms. Maternal lymphocytes in breast milk contribute to passive cell-mediated immunity of the neonate.

The choice of feeds during the first months of life must take into account the immaturity and continuing development of the gastrointestinal tract and other organs. Human milk is the ideal feed because, in addition to providing all the nutrients necessary for the infant, it contains digestive enzymes and immune and other protective factors but little in the way of antigenic protein.

THE FATE OF FOOD

Seeing, smelling, or thinking about food stimulates salivary, gastric and pancreatic secretion, and biliary flow. Foods are chewed and mixed with saliva in the mouth where they are formed into boluses ready for swallowing.

Motility

Swallowing begins the movement of food along the intestinal tract, and involves the integrated activities of the muscles of the oral cavity, pharynx and oesophagus, coordinated with muscles regulating breathing. Swallowing can be initiated voluntarily but, once initiated, proceeds as an involuntary reflex which is coordinated centrally. Both central neurological disease and acute respiratory disease (the latter mainly in infancy) can result in incoordination of swallowing and aspiration of food. Gastric emptying is regulated by the composition of food: fat and hyperosmolar foods delay it. In the small intestine, integration of contractions that mix lumenal contents, and peristalsis (contraction and relaxation moving lumenal contents distally from one region to the next) is controlled by enteric neural, endocrine and paracrine mechanisms. Retrograde flow is largely prevented by the lower oesophageal sphincter and the anatomy of the gastro-oesophageal junction, by the pyloric sphincter, and by the ileocaecal valve. Small intestinal motility thus propels, liquefies, and mixes food with intestinal secretions. In the colon, peristalsis is less frequent, slowing the progression of its contents and enabling absorption of water and electrolytes. Defaecation is initiated by involuntary relaxation of the internal anal sphincter in response to faeces dilating the rectum and by voluntary relaxation of the external anal sphincter.

Secretion

Gastric mucosal cells secrete hydrochloric acid, pepsinogen, intrinsic factor and mucus. Acid secretion by parietal cells, which is stimulated by gastrin, cholinergic nerves and histamine, converts pepsinogen to pepsin (a protease) and maintains a hostile environment for microorganisms. Excess acid secretion is prevented by somatostatin (which inhibits gastrin and acid release) and negative neural and hormonal feedback from the duodenum. Intrinsic factor, secreted by parietal cells, combines with vitamin B_{12} in the gastric lumen, enabling absorption of this complex by a specific carrier mechanism in the terminal ileum.

Acid, fats and amino acids in the small intestine promote vagal activity and release of secretin and cholecystokinin (CCK). The pancreas secretes bicarbonate and water in response to secretin, and digestive enzymes (lipase, amylase and proteases) following stimulation by CCK and cholinergic nerves. CCK also induces gallbladder contraction and expulsion of bile into the duodenum. Bile acids are reabsorbed in the ileum and recycled by the liver via the enterohepatic circulation.

Digestion and absorption

Saliva, gastric juice, bile, pancreatic and small intestinal brush border secretions contain digestive enzymes, as does breast milk, which act to break down macronutrients (fat, carbohydrate and protein) into fatty acids, monoglycerides, monosaccharides, amino acids, and oligopeptides that are then absorbed (Table 5.2).

Lipases hydrolyse dietary triglyceride to fatty acids and monoglycerides, which combine with bile salts to form micelles to facilitate their absorption. Complex carbohydrate is digested by amylase in the intestinal lumen, and the resulting disaccharides and oligosaccharides are hydrolysed to monosaccharides by the small intestinal brush border enzymes. These sugars are then absorbed by active, facilitated and passive transport mechanisms across the enterocyte.

Protein digestion requires activation of inactive precursors of enzymes. Pancreatic trypsinogen is activated in the intestinal lumen to trypsin by enterokinase, and trypsin then converts other pancreatic proteases to their active forms. This process prevents autodigestion. Amino acids, di- and tripeptides are absorbed by specific carrier mechanisms. Vitamins and minerals are absorbed largely in the small intestine. Most water-soluble vitamins are absorbed passively, except for vitamins C, B_1, B_{12} (with intrinsic factor), and folic acid which are absorbed by active mechanisms. Fat-soluble vitamins (A, D, E and K) are solubilized within bile salt micelles to facilitate absorption. Calcium absorption is by an active, vitamin D-dependent process, responsive to circulating calcium levels. Dietary haem iron is absorbed intact, but inorganic iron absorption depends upon the carrier protein transferrin.

Water absorption occurs principally in the small intestine (see Beyond Core: small intestine fluid absorption), but also in the colon, where the liquid ileal effluent is dehydrated and compacted to formed stool. Within the colon, bacteria ferment carbohydrate, including lactose in infants and starch in older children, forming short-chain

Table 5.2	Digestive enzymes	
Macronutrient	*Principal digestive enzymes*	*Main products of digestion*
Triglyceride	Lipase (lingual, gastric, pancreatic, breast milk)	Fatty acids, monoglycerides
Carbohydrate	Amylase (salivary and pancreatic) Disaccharidases	Disaccharides, oligosaccharides Monosaccharides
Protein	Pepsin, trypsin, chymotrypsin, elastase, carboxypeptidases	Amino acids, dipeptides, tripeptides

fatty acids which can be absorbed and used as an energy source.

Defence

Defence against ingested microorganisms and antigenic proteins is provided by the immune system and by other mechanisms within the gastrointestinal tract. Although immature in the neonate, these mechanisms are augmented by the protective factors present in breast milk (see Beyond Core: antimicrobial factors in breast milk).

Gastric acid, pepsin, pancreatic proteases, peptidases and lipases create a hostile environment for microorganisms in the upper gastrointestinal tract and degrade antigens. Mucus inhibits microbial replication and denies microorganisms access to the mucosal cell surface, where they might damage the glycocalyx (resulting, for example, in lactase deficiency in gastroenteritis) or bind to receptors (e.g. enteropathogenic *Escherichia coli*). Likewise, enterotoxin binding to receptors is reduced by mucus (e.g. cholera toxin). If epithelial damage occurs in the intestine, a proliferative enterocyte response maintains mucosal integrity.

Gastrointestinal-associated lymphoid tissue (GALT) is found diffusely within the epithelium mucosa and submucosa throughout the gastrointestinal tract, and in aggregates (Peyer's patches) in the small intestine. IgA is secreted into the intestinal lumen, where it binds antigen and prevents bacterial and viral colonization and injury to the mucosa. Unlike other immunoglobulin classes, IgA does not participate in many proinflammatory and cytotoxic responses; this is important given the wealth of mostly harmless antigens encountered in the gastrointestinal tract.

M cells overlying Peyer's patches 'sample' lumenal antigens by endocytosis and process them for presentation to closely associated underlying lymphoid tissue. CD8+ cytotoxic T cells predominate in mucosal lymphoid tissue (including intra-epithelial lymphocytes), and CD4+ T helper cells in the submucosa. In health, antigen delivered to these cells will result in either the production of secretory IgA, or to 'oral tolerance' whereby a more generalized immune reaction is avoided. Only rarely do gastrointestinal lumenal antigens precipitate a systemic immune response. Products of the GALT are therefore secreted into the gastrointestinal lumen, and are also transported in the systemic circulation. In lactating mothers, plasma cells migrate to the breast from Peyer's patches in the gut ('the enteromammary circulation') where antibodies and T cells pass into the milk, providing early passive humoral and cell-mediated immunity to the infant.

HISTORY TAKING, PHYSICAL EXAMINATION AND INVESTIGATION

History

Poor appetite, diet and growth

Normal growth depends on adequate nutrition throughout childhood, which in turn requires an intact and functioning gastrointestinal tract, pancreas and liver. Poor growth may result from:

- Inadequate diet (e.g. too many sugary drinks diminishing other nutrient intake)
- Inability to swallow (e.g. the bulbar palsy of spastic quadriplegia)
- Inadequate digestion or absorption (e.g. cystic fibrosis)
- Inability to utilize absorbed nutrients (e.g. chronic liver failure)
- Excessive energy requirement (e.g. chronic infections)
- Excessive gastrointestinal losses (e.g. diarrhoea and vomiting).

A well-taken history should detect which of these is likely, and whether the primary problem is gastrointestinal or lies elsewhere. Direct questioning will obtain a record of the frequency and quantity of foods taken, from which nutrient intake can be calculated using food tables.

Vomiting

The importance and severity of vomiting varies across a spectrum, ranging from possetting (regurgitation of small volumes of feed with no weight loss) to vomiting associated with, for instance, signs of blood loss and oesophagitis in severe gastro-oesophageal reflux. The sudden onset of forceful vomiting is likely to be pathological. Bilious vomiting, with abdominal distension and pain, suggests obstruction below the level of the ampulla of Vater. Frequency of vomiting will help determine the risk of dehydration. It is important to remember that in young children vomiting is a non-specific response and may result from a wide range of causes.

Pain
Babies cannot say when they are in pain but the nature of their cry may suggest it. Parents are experts at distinguishing different cries, but it should be remembered that a 'colicky' baby may appear very distressed whilst having no serious pathology. Recurrent central abdominal pain (greater than three episodes in 3 months) in children is common and usually no organic cause is found; the decision to investigate depends on the history and examination. Abdominal pain localized away from the umbilicus is more likely to be associated with underlying pathology than is periumbilical pain. Some organic disease presents insidiously with pain (e.g. Crohn's disease), and a period of follow-up and growth assessment may be required before a diagnosis can be made or reassurance given (see p. 90).

Disordered bowel habit – diarrhoea and constipation
The frequency, size and consistency of children's stools must be recorded. Normal bowel habit in childhood ranges from three times a day to once every 3 days, but is more frequent in young infants. Delayed passage of the first meconium stool for more than 24 h after birth is suggestive of Hirschsprung's disease.

Diarrhoea is the passage of frequent, runny or watery stools. The duration and frequency of the diarrhoea should be recorded as an indication of severity. In constipated children, small, hard stools, soiling, or overflow diarrhoea may be present. Pieces of undigested food, mucus or slime in the stool are a feature of toddler diarrhoea. The frequency of bowel motions must be placed in the context of the child's growth; normal growth makes pathology less likely.

Comprehensive history
Many gastrointestinal diseases are associated with abnormalities in other systems, e.g. recurrent respiratory infections in cystic fibrosis, eczema in cow's milk protein enteropathy, or anaemia in coeliac disease. It is essential to take a full paediatric history, including the past medical history, family history, infectious disease contacts, and recent foreign travel.

Examination
General inspection
Nutritional status, dysmorphism, pallor or jaundice can be assessed on general inspection. Body weight and height should be measured and plotted on appropriate growth centile charts. Certain skin rashes and hair quality may suggest nutrient deficiencies.

Hands and arms
Examination of the nails may reveal: leukonychia in hypoalbuminaemia; koilonychia in iron deficiency; or clubbing in cystic fibrosis and chronic gastrointestinal diseases. Pulse, respiratory rate and blood pressure should always be measured.

Face
The conjunctivae may appear anaemic, or the sclerae jaundiced.

Oral cavity
Examine the oral cavity carefully, especially for: angular stomatitis in iron or riboflavin deficiency; glossitis in iron or B vitamin deficiency; oral ulceration in inflammatory bowel disease; and dental caries.

Abdomen
Gaining a child's cooperation to palpate the abdomen is one of the challenges of paediatrics;

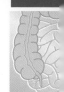

the child will form an opinion of you based on your communication with his or her parents and your approach to examination. Expose the abdomen completely and inspect it, noting distension, movement with respiration, and evidence of previous surgery. Ask if the tummy is sore, and start palpation away from a painful area. Talk reassuringly to the child. Asking questions about familiar things such as school, family, favourite toys can help gain the child's confidence. In the younger child, a useful strategy is to pretend that you are feeling what he or she had for breakfast. A child exaggerating or feigning pain will often be distracted by conversation and 'forget' to wince. Feel for masses and organs. The spleen in infants is superficial, and enlarges from the left hypochondrium towards the left iliac fossa. The liver may be palpable in young children up to 2 cm below the right costal margin in the midclavicular line. Feel in the epigastrium for an enlarged left lobe of the liver. Percuss for the upper edge of the liver. Auscultate the abdomen, listening for the presence and quality of bowel sounds.

Examine the hernial orifices, genitalia (including whether the testes are in the scrotum or inguinal canal) and perianal area. Although it is sometimes argued that rectal examination has adverse psychological effects, it is important to perform when indicated. With full explanation the procedure should not be traumatic and often reveals valuable information (e.g. narrowed segment in Hirschsprung's disease, bloody stool or masses not palpable abdominally) missed by general physical examination or investigations. Rectal examination is not performed routinely in children, and when indicated should be undertaken by an experienced paediatrician.

Other systems

The assessment of the gastrointestinal system should always be set within a comprehensive examination of the child, because findings in other systems may provide essential clues to gastrointestinal disease. For example, evidence of chronic respiratory illness suggests cystic fibrosis, and arthritis of the knee or ankle may be associated with inflammatory bowel disease.

Investigation

Imaging

Ultrasound scanning provides images of organs and anatomical lesions, such as pyloric sphincter hypertrophy in pyloric stenosis, a dilated biliary tree in extrahepatic biliary obstruction, hepatic parenchymal abnormalities in cirrhosis or periportal biliary abnormality in cystic fibrosis. Doppler ultrasound can be used to measure blood flow in, for example, the portal and hepatic veins, which may indicate the presence of early liver disease and portal hypertension with varices. It avoids the radiation associated with radiographic studies but does not provide information about the morphology of the intestinal mucosa.

Barium meal or barium enema is used to provide images of the intestinal mucosa (e.g. in suspected inflammatory bowel disease), of strictures and dilatations, and of gut rotation (e.g. in malrotation). Barium swallow may reveal a hiatus hernia or oesophageal varices but is not ideal for the diagnosis of gastro-oesophageal reflux.

Radio-isotope scans are increasingly used in paediatric practice. A technetium-labelled white blood cell scan can detect inflammation and is used in the assessment of inflammatory bowel disease. Labelled pertechnetate has an affinity for gastric parietal cells and is used to detect the presence of a Meckel's diverticulum.

Endoscopy

The mucosa of the oesophagus, stomach and duodenum can be directly visualized by upper gastrointestinal endoscopy and that of the rectum, colon, caecum and terminal ileum by colonoscopy. Indications include suspected oesophagitis, duodenal ulcer, haematemesis, rectal bleeding and inflammatory bowel disease. Children require either heavy sedation or general anaesthesia for these procedures. Multiple mucosal biopsies can be taken and are essential for the diagnosis of some disorders, such as Crohn's disease.

Oesophageal pH monitoring

In suspected gastro-oesophageal reflux, a 24 h trace of pH can be obtained by passing a pH probe through the nose and into the lower oesophagus. The severity of acid reflux is measured from the duration of recordings of less than pH 4 and the number of episodes of acid reflux.

Small bowel biopsy

The classical technique for obtaining jejunal mucosal biopsies is the Watson or Crosby capsule, passed under radiographic screening in a sedated child to beyond the duodenal–jejunal flexure. More recently, this approach has been superceded by the use of endoscopy to obtain multiple biopsies from the duodenum. Biopsies are essential for the formal diagnosis of coeliac disease and may be useful in detecting other small bowel enteropathies.

Tests of absorption and pancreatic function

In suspected malabsorption, faeces should be collected for measurement of fat content. Direct microscopy, after staining with Sudan red, provides a subjective impression of the number of fat globules present. Alternatively, a 3 day fat balance study, measuring fat intake (by dietary assessment) and fat output (by a 3 day faecal fat collection), will detect normal fat absorption (>90% of ingested fat is absorbed) or malabsorption (<90% absorption). A 3 day fat balance study will indirectly measure pancreatic lipase activity, but assumes normal hepatobiliary and intestinal mucosal function for accurate interpretation. Pancreatic insufficiency is suggested by reduced faecal chymotrypsin.

If carbohydrate malabsorption is suspected, the presence of reducing sugars (e.g. undigested lactose) in the faeces can be measured using faecal fluid and a Clinitest tablet. This must be performed immediately after the stool is passed.

Breath tests

Breath tests rely upon the principle that a product of the metabolism of an oral substrate may be excreted and measured in the breath. For example, lactose is usually completely absorbed in the small intestine, but any reaching the colon is fermented by bacteria, generating hydrogen, which is absorbed and then excreted in breath. In children with lactase deficiency, ingestion of lactose is followed by a significant rise in breath hydrogen when the sugar reaches the large bowel. Another important breath test uses carbon-13-labelled urea to detect colonization with *Helicobacter pylori* (see Beyond core: peptic ulcer and *Helicobacter pylori*).

Liver function

Serum alanine transaminase, aspartate transaminase and γ-glutamyl transferase are used as measures of hepatocyte damage, and levels are

---

BEYOND CORE

ASSESSMENT OF SMALL INTESTINAL AND PANCREATIC FUNCTION

Small intestinal function

The xylose absorption test involves giving this sugar by mouth followed by measurement of its concentration in the blood 1 h later. The lactulose: mannitol test involves measurement of the ratio of these two sugars in a timed urine collection after an oral load.

Pancreatic function

Direct measurement of pancreatic exocrine function is performed by duodenal intubation and aspiration of secretions following intravenous injection of secretin and CCK. This test is invasive and not frequently undertaken in children. The stable isotope-labelled mixed triglyceride breath test is more specific for pancreatic lipase function but less widely performed. It requires access to an isotope ratio mass spectrometer, which is not available in all hospital laboratories.

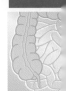

raised many times above the upper limit of normal in diffuse inflammatory liver diseases, such as hepatitis A. Levels may remain normal or only marginally elevated in patchy liver disease. Transaminases may also be elevated in muscle disorders or haemolytic anaemia.

Serum alkaline phosphatase levels are elevated most markedly in disorders involving biliary obstruction. Circulating levels may also be raised in parenchymal liver disease. Serum alkaline phosphatase levels are generally higher in growing children than in adults, reflecting the higher level of bone-derived alkaline phosphatase, which is a different isoenzyme to that derived from liver. Individual isoenzymes must be measured if there is doubt as to the cause of an elevated serum alkaline phosphatase level.

Serum bilirubin is used as a measure of hepatic excretory function (as well as haemolysis), and serum albumin and prothrombin time measure liver synthetic function. Serum albumin levels are diminished in a variety of other conditions (e.g. nephrotic syndrome), and should be interpreted with care.

CORE PROBLEMS

ACUTE DIARRHOEA

As with vomiting, the passage of frequent and loose stools is a non-specific response seen in a wide range of childhood illnesses including meningitis, pneumonia, urinary tract infection and otitis media. The presence of associated features specific to those entities may point to the correct diagnosis. Occasionally, dehydration may overshadow other clinical signs and therefore failure to achieve the expected degree of improvement after rehydration should prompt a careful reassessment of the working diagnosis. Acute diarrhoea is usually the most prominent feature of a short-lived, self-limiting illness caused by gastrointestinal infection. It remains one of the commonest diseases of childhood throughout the world and a major cause of early mortality in developing countries, leading to about 4 million deaths in childhood each year. Although less common and usually milder in developed countries, gastroenteritis continues to account for a significant proportion of hospital admissions and a few deaths.

Infective gastroenteritis

Pathogenesis
Childhood gastroenteritis in the developed world is caused by viruses in 50–70% of cases, bacteria in 15%, parasites in 1%, and no pathogen is identified in the remainder (Table 5.3). The commonest cause of infective gastroenteritis is rotavirus, occurring with a peak incidence in the winter, often accompanied by respiratory symptoms and occasionally a non-specific rash. Rotavirus selectively invades and damages mature enterocytes at the tips of the villi, causing shortening of the small intestinal villi and leaving predominantly crypt-like cells which have little disaccharidase activity or fluid absorptive capacity (see Beyond Core: enterocyte turnover and function); the colon is unaffected. Diarrhoea caused by rotavirus is thus caused by a combination of malabsorption and fluid loss as a result of the damaged epithelium. Adenovirus acts in a similar way. However, the mechanism of action of *Vibrio cholerae* and enterotoxin-producing *E. coli* is somewhat different: toxins produced by these orgnisms stimulate active fluid secretion by the crypt cells.

Clinical features
Acute diarrhoea with vomiting suggests gastroenteritis. However, vomiting may precede diarrhoea and increases the risk of dehydration. Associated respiratory symptoms commonly occur in viral gastroenteritis, while blood or mucus in the stool suggest an invasive, bacterial or parasitic enteritis (or inflammatory bowel disease). The risk of gastroenteritis is higher in formula-fed infants and decreased by breast feeding. It is therefore important to record the type of feeds that the infant is taking and, if bottle fed, to enquire how the feeds are made up, stored and how often they are reheated. Other useful

Table 5.3   Causes and pathogenic mechanisms of acute infective diarrhoea in UK children[a]

Organism	Pathogenic mechanism
Rotavirus	Infection and damage to small intestinal enterocytes
Adenovirus	Infection and damage to small intestinal enterocytes
Campylobacter jejuni	Invasion of terminal ileum and colon
Escherichia coli	Invasion (enteroinvasive), toxin production (enterotoxigenic, enteropathogenic, enterohaemorrhagic)
Salmonella enteritidis	Invasion of terminal ileum and colon
Shigella species	Invasion and production of entero- and cytotoxin in the terminal ileum and colon
Cryptosporidium	Infection of enterocytes in small and large intestine
Giardia intestinalis	Unknown mechanism in small intestine

[a] Age under 3 years and lack of blood and mucus in the stool favour a viral aetiology. However, a similar picture may be seen with enterotoxin-producing *E. coli*

information that helps to determine the microbiological cause includes contact with other cases of gastroenteritis, recent diet and foreign travel.

General examination may reveal signs of dehydration (Table 5.4). Whilst the abdomen may be slightly distended and mildly tender, it should feel soft, with no palpable masses. Bowel sounds are usually active. Variation from these findings should raise a suspicion of other pathology, including acute intestinal obstruction, intussusception, or appendicitis. A non-specific erythematous rash, and evidence of upper airway infection support a diagnosis of viral gastroenteritis. Infective gastroenteritis may progress to chronic diarrhoea, which is discussed below.

In a child with vomiting, but little or no diarrhoea, alternative diagnoses should be considered (Table 5.5). A clean catch or suprapubic aspirate of urine should be obtained to exclude urinary tract infection.

Investigation

Stool samples should be examined for the presence of viruses (by electron microscopy or antigen detection), bacteria (following culture) and parasites (by microscopy). When there are signs of severe dehydration, plasma urea and

Table 5.4   Signs of dehydration

	Fluid deficit (%)	Signs
Mild dehydration	<5	Dry oral mucosa Thirst
Moderate dehydration	5–10	Loss of skin turgor Tachycardia Sunken eyes/anterior fontanelle
Severe dehydration	>10	Cool periphery Tachycardia Hypotension Oliguria Unconsciousness

Table 5.5   Causes of acute vomiting with little or no diarrhoea

Diagnosis	Clinical features	Investigations
Gastroenteritis	Diarrhoea, respiratory symptoms, contact history	Stool for virology and bacteriology
Urinary tract infection	Pyrexia, dysuria	Urine for microscopy and culture Full blood count (neutrophilia) Plasma urea, electrolytes and creatinine
Intussusception	Abdominal distension, pallor, pain, bloody stools (late)	Abdominal ultrasound Gastrografin or air enema
Hepatitis A	None, or jaundice	Liver function tests Hepatitis serology
Malrotation with volvulus	Abdominal distension, pain	Abdominal radiography
Cyclical vomiting	Previous history	None

electrolyte levels should be measured. Hypernatraemic dehydration is now rare in developed countries but still occasionally occurs. It requires careful attention to the rate and composition of fluid replacement; too rapid fluid replacement or the use of hypotonic solutions may provoke a sudden shift of fluid into the intracellular compartment of the brain, causing cerebral oedema, raised intracranial pressure and, possibly, seizures. More commonly, the plasma sodium level is normal or low. Potassium may be lost in vomit and stool, resulting in hypokalaemia, and the plasma urea level may be elevated.

Treatment

The treatment of gastroenteritis aims to correct and prevent dehydration, and to minimize the further spread of the pathogen. Mothers who breast feed their infants should be supported to continue throughout an episode of gastroenteritis. Children with little or no dehydration must maintain their fluid intake. Children with moderate dehydration should be encouraged to drink oral rehydration solution (ORS) (see Beyond Core: oral rehydration solution and fluid absorption). The volume to be consumed should be calculated by adding an estimate of the fluid deficit, calculated from the degree of dehydration, to the normal maintenance requirement and an allowance for ongoing losses. Using this figure, small but frequent volumes should be given to the child to reduce the likelihood of further vomiting. ORS can usually be taken orally, but sometimes a nasogastric tube is necessary. Severely dehydrated children, and those who are moderately dehydrated and continue to vomit, may require intravenous fluids. Dehydrated children in shock require restoration of the circulating volume with a plasma expander or isotonic saline but their total intravenous fluid requirement is also calculated from the sum of their normal requirement, the estimated fluid deficit and any ongoing losses.

Antibiotics should not be used to treat viral gastroenteritis, and most episodes of bacterial gastroenteritis are self-limiting. Cholera, *Shigella* dysentery, *Salmonella* infection in infants less than 3 months, *Clostridium difficile* infection, and any enteric infection causing septicaemia require antibiotic treatment; the choice of drug depends on local patterns of resistance. *Giardia intestinalis* and *Entamoeba histolytica* infections are usually treated with oral metronidazole.

Complications of gastroenteritis include lactose intolerance, manifest by persisting diarrhoea testing positive for reducing sugars. A breast-fed child with transient lactose intolerance rarely needs to stop breast feeding. If bottle fed, such children may require 4–12 weeks on a lactose-free formula milk (e.g. Wysoy, Enfamil). Cow's milk protein intolerance may follow gastroenteritis, and is managed with a cow's milk protein-free diet.

BEYOND CORE

ORAL REHYDRATION SOLUTION AND FLUID ABSORPTION

Oral rehydration solution

An understanding of the physiology of fluid absorption in the small intestine (see below and Fig. 5.2) led to the development of oral rehydration solution (ORS) in the 1960s. Use of ORS in the developing world has saved millions of lives through the treatment and prevention of dehydration.

In the UK, ORS contains three essential ingredients: water, sodium (50 mmol/l) and glucose (111 mmol/l). In the developing world the sodium concentration is higher (90 mmol/l), and complex carbohydrate from cereals such as rice or wheat is used in the place of glucose. These solutions may reduce stool output as well as replace lost fluid.

Small intestinal fluid absorption

Fluid absorption in the small intestine is driven by the osmotic gradients set up by sodium cotransported with organic solutes (amino acids and glucose). These cotransporters (symports) are located in the apical brush border membrane of the villous epithelium (Fig. 5.2). Both sodium and solute must bind to the cotransporter protein before it undergoes the conformational change which permits sodium to enter the cell via the sodium gradient established by the sodium pump. Sodium is then pumped out of the cell at the basolateral membrane by the sodium pump, which uses ATP as its energy source, thus maintaining the gradient for further sodium absorption. Water moves passively via paracellular pathways.

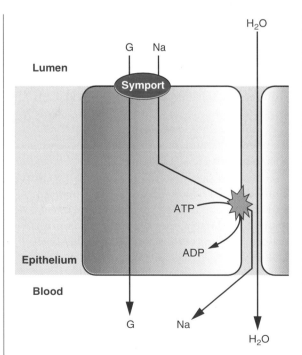

Figure 5.2 Mechanism of action of ORS; cotransport of sodium (Na) and glucose (G) by the villous epithelium drives water absorption (see Beyond Core: oral rehydration solution and fluid absorption)

CHRONIC DIARRHOEA

Chronic diarrhoea is arbitrarily defined as diarrhoea of greater than 14 days duration. Age and characteristic clinical features (Tables 5.6 and 5.7) may point to the likely diagnosis. Thus, the onset of diarrhoea due to cow's milk protein enteropathy is usually in early infancy and may be associated with vomiting, whereas coeliac disease presents later in the first or second year of life after exposure to gluten-containing foods and is associated with abdominal distension and wasting. Toddler diarrhoea is a likely diagnosis in a thriving preschool child with chronic diarrhoea containing undigested food particles. Inflammatory bowel disease presents first in late childhood or adolescence with chronic diarrhoea and abdominal pain; bloody stools suggest colonic involvement. A history of recurrent respiratory infections should prompt investigation for cystic fibrosis (see Ch. 6); the diagnosis is usually made in the first year of life, but mild phenotypes may present later.

In all cases, body weight and height should be plotted on appropriate growth centile charts. Other features to seek on examination are listed

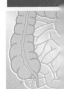

Table 5.6 Causes and mechanisms of chronic diarrhoea

Mechanism	Disease	Characteristic features of stool
Unknown	Toddler diarrhoea	Undigested pieces of food
Maldigestion	Liver disease (disordered secretion of bile) Cystic fibrosis (pancreatic insufficiency) Disaccharidase deficiency (lactase, sucrase-isomaltase)	Steatorrhoea Steatorrhoea, reduced faecal chymotrypsin Watery, acidic stools, positive for reducing sugars
Malabsorption	Coeliac disease Crohn's disease Cow's milk protein enteropathy Parasitic infection (e.g. *Giardia intestinalis*)	Steatorrhoea (may be constipated) May contain blood (20–30%) May be positive for occult blood Organism seen on microscopy
Excess losses	Inflammatory bowel disease (ulcerative colitis or Crohn's disease)	Often contains blood

Table 5.7 Signs to look for in chronic diarrhoea

Sign	Significance
Finger clubbing	Cystic fibrosis, inflammatory bowel disease
Leukonychia	Hypoalbuminaemia
Mouth ulcers	Inflammatory bowel disease
Uveitis	Inflammatory bowel disease
Harrison's sulci	Cystic fibrosis
Abdominal distension	Coeliac disease
Distended abdominal veins	Portal hypertension
Hepatosplenomegaly	Liver disease, portal hypertension
Right iliac fossa mass ± tenderness	Crohn's disease
Left iliac fossa tenderness	Colitis (Crohn's disease, ulcerative, infective)
Nappy rash	Malabsorption (disaccharidase deficiency)
Perianal skin tags, fissures, abscesses	Crohn's disease
Arthritis (especially of the knee or ankle)	Inflammatory bowel disease

in Table 5.7. In addition, children with chronic diarrhoea are at risk of developing specific nutrient deficiencies and signs of these may be present, such as pallor, koilonychia and angular stomatitis in iron deficiency. Children with chronic diarrhoea who fail to thrive require full investigation. This may include imaging, endoscopy and mucosal biopsy, but examination of the stool and blood tests will usually be undertaken first.

Maldigestion and malabsorption are suggested by increased fat in the stool (on microscopy or, more accurately, by a 3 day fat balance study) or reducing sugars in the stool (in disaccharidase deficiency). Stool microscopy may reveal infection with *Giardia intestinalis* or other enteropathogens;

three specimens should be tested. Pancreatic insufficiency is suggested by reduced faecal chymotrypsin.

Blood tests may not lead to a diagnosis in chronic diarrhoea but may detect secondary nutrient deficiencies and, if abnormal, suggest the need for further investigation. Iron deficiency (low serum iron and ferritin levels) suggests malabsorption of iron, or chronic intestinal bleeding (e.g. inflammatory bowel disease or cow's milk protein enteropathy). Elevated serum alanine aminotransferase and aspartate aminotransferase together with reduced serum albumin levels indicate the need to investigate further for liver disease or inflammatory bowel disease (in which iron deficiency may also be present). Coeliac disease is suggested by positive serum anti-gliadin, anti-endomysium and anti-reticulin IgA antibodies.

✱ KEY DIAGNOSIS

Toddler diarrhoea

Clinical features
A child of 2–5 years with chronic diarrhoea and few other symptoms (perhaps occasional abdominal pain or vomiting), with no abnormalities on examination and normal growth, is likely to have toddler diarrhoea. The child's diet may be low in fat and high in carbohydrate. The stool may contain undigested food particles and mucus, but not blood, and the clinical picture is of an irritable, hyperactive bowel. The aetiology of toddler diarrhoea is unclear, but rapid intestinal transit may play a part. There may be a family history of functional bowel disease (e.g. irritable bowel syndrome).

Treatment
The management of toddler diarrhoea centres on reassuring the parents that their child will grow out of the problem, usually by school age, and is digesting and absorbing food properly, even though bits appear in the stool. Slowing intestinal motility by increasing dietary bulk with bran or methylcellulose may improve symptoms, in some cases a fat supplement (such as a long-chain triglyceride emulsion) may reduce stool frequency (colonic motility is reduced by fat in the small bowel: the 'ileal brake').

Cow's milk protein enteropathy (CMPE)

Clinical features
CMPE usually presents in infancy and may follow gastroenteritis. In addition to chronic diarrhoea, the clinical picture may include vomiting, and iron deficiency anaemia secondary to occult blood loss is often present. Eczema occurs in some children with CMPE, but usually persists following exclusion of cow's milk, suggesting a multifactorial aetiology for this component of the disorder. No single laboratory test can diagnose the disease; specific circulating IgE against cow's milk protein lacks sensitivity and specificity.

Investigation
Diagnosis relies on the resolution of symptoms with a cow's milk-free diet, and the recurrence of symptoms on challenge with cow's milk. Multiple small bowel mucosal biopsies often show patchy subtotal villous atrophy.

Treatment
One-third of children with cow's milk protein intolerance also react to soya protein, and therefore a soya-free milk may need to be used as treatment. Casein hydrolysate milks (e.g. Pregestimil) or elemental formulae (e.g. Neocate) are suitable alternatives but are expensive and have an unpleasant taste. In those children with persisting cow's milk protein intolerance, weaning foods should also be free of cow's milk. Rechallenge with cow's milk 12–18 months later (or sooner in those with postenteritis enteropathy) shows that the majority of affected children have outgrown their intolerance.

Coeliac disease

Clinical features
Intolerance to gliadin (a fraction of the gluten protein of wheat, rye and barley) causes the small bowel enteropathy of coeliac disease. Genetically susceptible individuals exposed to this environmental trigger are thought to develop coeliac disease by an immune-mediated mechanism. It presents after exposure to gluten-containing foods, sometimes following a latent

period that may extend to late childhood or adulthood. Under 2 years of age, children with coeliac disease usually have prominent symptoms and signs such as diarrhoea, abdominal distension and wasting; presentation later in childhood is more insidious, with failure to thrive and iron deficiency anaemia often the only features. Over 80% of children have chronic diarrhoea at diagnosis, and some of the remainder have constipation. Irritability, pallor and lassitude are common accompanying symptoms.

Investigation

Diagnosis relies on the demonstration of typical histological changes in a small bowel mucosal biopsy (Fig. 5.3), with a subsequent clinical response to a gluten-free diet. However, if the child is less than 2 years old at biopsy, or if the

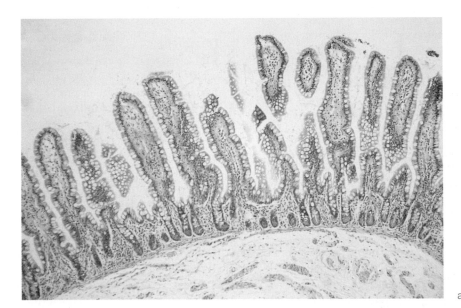

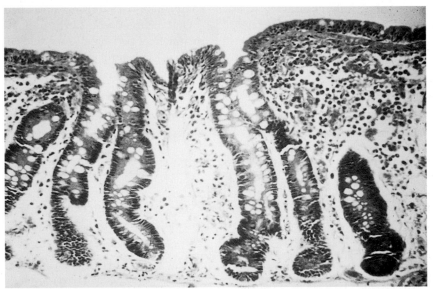

Figure 5.3 Small bowel biopsy histology. **a** In a normal child. **b** In coeliac disease showing total villous atrophy and crypt hyperplasia

clinical presentation or histological findings are atypical, the diagnosis should be confirmed by later dietary challenge followed by repeat biopsies. Positive serum antigliadin and anti-endomysial IgA antibodies are usually found in coeliac disease (provided the child is not IgA deficient), and indicate which children should be biopsied, but are not sufficiently sensitive or specific to make a definite diagnosis.

Treatment

Management involves life-long adherence to a gluten-free diet. This requires parental awareness of food ingredients and proper labelling by food manufacturers. The guidance of a paediatric dietician is essential. There is a small risk of gastrointestinal malignancy in coeliac disease in adult life, especially small bowel lymphoma, which is reduced by dietary compliance.

Crohn's disease

Clinical features and investigation

Crohn's disease is an inflammatory bowel disease of unknown aetiology. Its presentation is usually insidious, with abdominal pain, loose stools (bloody in 20–30%) and poor growth. Other gastrointestinal presenting features include perianal discomfort (fissures, abscesses, skin tags), oral symptoms (owing to thickened buccal mucosa and lips, or recurrent mouth ulcers). Extra-intestinal symptoms (arthritis, uveitis, fever,

erythema nodosum) also occur. It can affect all regions of the gut from the mouth to the anus, and is characterized by 'skip lesions' (regions of affected bowel separated by regions of normal bowel). The terminal ileum is frequently involved and can be biopsied at endoscopy. Inflammation causes typical endoscopic and microscopic appearances (Table 5.8), on which the diagnosis is based. The natural history is one of remissions and relapses.

Treatment

Mild acute relapses can be managed with oral 5-amino salicylic acid (5-ASA) preparations, such as olsalazine. More severe or prolonged relapses require suppression of inflammation with oral corticosteroids or liquid enteral nutrition. The side-effects of corticosteroid therapy include growth inhibition, which may exacerbate growth-retardation due to the primary disease. Treatment with a liquid enteral diet is as effective as corticosteroids, has few side-effects, and maintains better nutrition and growth during treatment compared with corticosteroids. However, the child must stop eating all food while drinking 1.5–2.0 litres of liquid formula for 6–8 weeks; a nasogastric tube is usually required (owing to the poor taste of the formula), and compliance, not suprisingly, may be poor.

Oral metronidazole can be useful in the treatment of perianal disease, and corticosteroid enemas can control proctitis. 5-ASA preparations may help to prevent relapse in Crohn's disease.

Table 5.8	Disease pattern in inflammatory bowel diseases	
	Crohn's disease	*Ulcerative colitis*
Distribution	Mouth to anus (ileocaecal region most common),'skip lesions'	Large bowel, continuous from rectum proximally
Endoscopic appearances	Inflammation, 'snail track' ulcers, 'cobblestone' mucosa	Inflammation, ulcers
Mucosal histology	Non-caseating granulomata, chronic inflammatory cell infiltrate	Chronic inflammatory cell infiltrate, mucus depletion, crypt abscesses
Other pathology	Transmural inflammation, strictures, fissures, fistulae	Inflammation limited by muscularis mucosae

Ulcerative colitis

Clinical features

Ulcerative colitis affects the large bowel from the rectum proximally, and bloody diarrhoea occurs in 80% of cases. Although usually easily distinguished from Crohn's disease (Table 5.8), it also follows a course of relapses and remissions with extra-intestinal manifestations. Acute colonic dilatation ('toxic megacolon') and necrosis occasionally accompany severe exacerbations and may require emergency colectomy.

Treatment

Management of acute relapses relies on 5-ASA preparations, systemic corticosteroids and corticosteroid enemas. An elemental diet is ineffective in ulcerative colitis. Long-term administration of 5-ASA preparations reduces the risk of relapse. The prevalence of large bowel cancer in ulcerative colitis rises rapidly from 10 years after diagnosis, when a decision must be taken between repeated colonoscopic screening or prophylactic colectomy.

Parasitic infection

The most common intestinal parasitic infection of children in the UK is *Giardia intestinalis*. This is transmitted by the faecal–oral route, and the microorganism multiplies in the small intestine, where it adheres to the mucosa, and can cause malabsorption and diarrhoea. It may be acquired from contaminated food or water and therefore may affect other members of the family. Diagnosis is made by microscopic examination of stools; 75% sensitivity is achieved by examining three stools. Sensitivity is further improved by microscopy of a small bowel mucosal biopsy, which can show subtotal villous atrophy and the microorganisms adjacent to the mucosa. Treatment with metronidazole will eradicate the organism, and family members should be screened and treated to avoid reinfection.

PERSISTENT VOMITING

Projectile vomiting after feeds in a 4–6 week old infant who is failing to thrive and hungry again immediately after vomiting suggests pyloric stenosis. Effortless, small vomits, frequent 'poseting' and waterbrash suggest gastro-oesophageal reflux. Calculation of the daily amount of feed taken by a baby may suggest overfeeding, and is often seen in those who are overweight for their age. Diarrhoea usually accompanies vomiting in gastroenteritis. It is important to remember that vomiting is a common non-specific sign of systemic illness, including infection.

General examination will reveal the extent of dehydration (see Table 5.4), and nutritional status, and may suggest systemic illness. If the infant appears systemically unwell, investigation to identify septicaemia, urinary tract infection, neurological disease, metabolic disease or other systemic illness is indicated. Specific investigations are undertaken according to the working diagnosis. Although barium swallow is often used to diagnose gastro-oesophageal reflux, oesophageal pH monitoring is the preferred investigation (see p. 82). Abdominal examination of a baby with suspected pyloric stenosis should be performed during a feed (see below).

✱ KEY DIAGNOSIS

Pyloric stenosis

Pathogenesis

The pyloric sphincter is formed from an expanded band of circular muscle that controls the emptying of the gastric contents into the duodenum. Occasionally this sphincter undergoes significant hypertrophy following birth and causes obstruction to the gastric outlet. The cause is unknown, but inheritance is polygenic; boys are four times more commonly affected than girls, first-born children more than subsequent siblings, and there may be a family history, especially in the mother.

Persistent vomiting of gastric contents leads to loss of hydrochloric acid and retention of bicarbonate. In the kidney, potassium is preferentially secreted in exchange for hydrogen, and is lost in the urine. Thus, hypokalaemic, hypochloraemic, alkalotic dehydration develops.

PEPTIC ULCER AND *HELICOBACTER PYLORI*

Peptic ulcer

Peptic ulcer disease is uncommon in childhood. Diagnosis is by upper gastrointestinal endoscopy when a gastric or duodenal ulcer may be visualized. Over 90% of duodenal ulcers are found within the duodenal bulb. Gastric antral biopsies should be taken to identify gastritis caused by *H. pylori* (present in over 90% of children with duodenal ulcer – see below). Gastric ulcers may occur following corticosteroid treatment, acute stress (e.g. burns) and treatment with non-steroidal antiinflammatory drugs (NSAIDs).

Helicobacter pylori

H. pylori causes the majority of duodenal ulcers that are not related to medication (e.g. NSAIDs), and has a role in the aetiology of gastric ulcer and gastric cancer. It is often acquired in childhood, and 50% of 50 year olds in Scotland are infected. Early colonization is highest in poor social circumstances and overcrowded housing.

H. pylori colonizes the gastric antrum, where it lives in the mucus overlying the epithelium. The majority of colonized individuals are asymptomatic, but for reasons relating to the host and/or the bacteria, some develop excessive gastric acid secretion that predisposes them to duodenal ulceration.

Diagnosis of *H. pylori* is made at endoscopy by histology and urease test of an antral mucosal biopsy. The urease test relies upon the bacteria's ability to convert urea to ammonia, which turns a coloured marker from yellow to red. The non-invasive ^{13}C-urea breath test which can be used to assess response to treatment also relies on the presence of bacterial urease in the stomach, which generates $^{13}CO_2$ when [^{13}C]urea is given orally. The $^{13}CO_2$ expired in the breath can be measured by isotope ratio mass spectrometry. Carbon-13 is a stable, non-radioactive isotope of carbon, and is therefore safe for use in children.

Treatment of *H. pylori* requires triple therapy for 1–2 weeks, with metronidazole, omeprazole (proton pump inhibitor) and either amoxycillin or clarithromycin. The omeprazole can be given for longer. Resolution of ulcers and symptoms follows eradication of the bacteria. Failed treatment may be due to non-compliance or to bacterial resistance.

H. pylori has not been shown to cause gastro-oesophageal reflux, oesophagitis or non-ulcer dyspepsia. Finding *H. pylori* in children with chronic abdominal pain and no evidence of gastric or duodenal ulceration raises an unresolved therapeutic dilemma. Treatment of such children risks drug side-effects and the generation of drug resistance with little evidence of symptomatic benefit. However, there is an unquantified risk of gastric cancer associated with *H. pylori* colonization.

---

abdomen, and rectal examination may reveal an empty rectum followed, on removal of the finger, by a spurt of liquid faeces.

Functional constipation

Clinical features

Constipation will often have been present for many months before medical advice is sought.

There may be no clear history of its onset but sometimes the parents will remember an episode of pain from an anal fissure, or of dehydration associated with a transient illness. There follows a pattern of infrequent passage of small amounts of hard or pasty stool, with occasional large and painful stools. Soiling can occur and may be exacerbated by overflow diarrhoea which can confuse the diagnosis. Intermittent attempts at treatment with short courses of laxatives may have been undertaken.

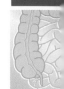

Functional constipation may follow a transient illness or overzealous attempts at early toilet training. Retained stool becomes more difficult to pass, and an anal fissure causes pain on defaecation, reinforcing the child's reluctance to defaecate. Chronic distension reduces the rectum's sensitivity and thereby the urge to evacuate is lost. Soiling then follows, because the child can neither empty the rectum fully nor prevent faecal loss from overflow.

Treatment

Management begins with an explanation of the mechanism of constipation, the rationale for treatment, and its likely duration. A successful outcome relies on good parental understanding and compliance to treatment, which is aimed firstly at emptying the large bowel of the impacted hard stool and secondly at rehabilitating large bowel function. Impaction is usually relieved by large doses of stool softener, such as lactulose, sometimes followed by stimulant laxatives. In severe impaction, enemas may be required over a 2–3 day period, followed thereafter by oral therapy. The child should be encouraged to drink large volumes of fluid during this phase of treatment. Only rarely is manual disimpaction under general anaesthetic required.

Rehabilitation of large bowel function begins once disimpaction is complete and often lasts more than a year. The stool must be kept soft and bulky with a stool softener such as lactulose, and large bowel motility is encouraged with a stimulant laxative such as senna. No further therapy is usually required once appropriate doses of these medicines are reached. Recognition of behavioural disturbance, including encopresis (see Ch. 18), is important. It is sometimes difficult to determine whether behavioural problems are primary or secondary to constipation. Successful treatment of constipation will often be accompanied by spontaneous improvement in behaviour, but the help of a child psychologist may be required.

Hirschsprung's disease

Pathogenesis and clinical features

During fetal development, ganglion cells migrate from the neural crest distally down the gastrointestinal tract towards the anus, where they are involved in the control of motility. Failure of migration results in a section of aganglionic, narrow and immotile bowel, manifest clinically as Hirschsprung's disease. A baby who did not pass meconium within 48 h of birth (unless born prematurely), or whose parents date the onset of constipation to the time of birth, raises the possibility of a congenital abnormality such as Hirschsprung's disease. Although the child with Hirschsprung's disease frequently presents shortly after birth, presentation may be later in childhood, especially if only a small area of bowel is affected ('short segment Hirschsprung's disease'). Soiling is uncommon when Hirschsprung's disease presents in older children with constipation. Rarely the child may present with gross abdominal distension and enterocolitis.

Investigation and treatment

A contrast enema may suggest Hirschsprung's disease (Fig. 5.5) but a suction rectal biopsy of the full thickness of the mucosa showing the absence of ganglion cells is required for diagnosis. Treatment is surgical, using one of several procedures that involve excision of the aganglionic bowel and anastomosis to the rectal stump. Sometimes a defunctioning colostomy is required before anastomosis at a second operation.

RECURRENT ABDOMINAL PAIN

Recurrent abdominal pain is defined as pain recurring for more than 3 months affecting normal activity. If no underlying pathology is found, the term 'functional abdominal pain' is used.

It is essential to take a detailed history from children with recurrent abdominal pain in order to avoid unnecessary investigations of those with no underlying pathology. Functional abdominal pain is usually peri-umbilical and often worse in the morning, whereas pain localized away from the umbilicus, nocturnal pain, persistent diarrhoea, bloody stools, or urinary symptoms suggest an alternative diagnosis.

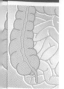

(see Ch. 11), infection and defects in bilirubin glucuronidation. Breast milk-induced jaundice is a common cause of prolonged unconjugated hyperbilirubinaemia. This is a harmless condition, and neither for diagnosis nor for its treatment should stopping breast feeding be advocated (see Ch. 4). The Crigler–Najjar syndrome, of which there are two variants of differing severity, is a rare condition due to complete absence (type 1) or low (type 2) UDP–bilirubin–glucuronyltransferase activity. Type 1 presents as a severe unconjugated hyperbilirubinaemia in the newborn period while type 2 may present in later childhood.

Immediate investigations should include urine and blood cultures to identify bacterial infection, a coagulation screen to identify a prolonged prothrombin time, a full blood count and reticulocyte count if haemolytic anaemia is suspected, and a urine Clinitest analysis for reducing sugars in galactosaemia. Further investigations are undertaken as appropriate for the differential diagnosis (see Table 4.5).

✳ KEY DIAGNOSIS

Biliary atresia

Extrahepatic biliary atresia is a rare condition (1 per 14 000 live births) of uncertain aetiology but accounts for 25–30% of infants with cholestatic jaundice. Its importance lies in the need to differentiate affected infants from those with other causes of jaundice as early as possible in life because the effectiveness of surgical treatment declines markedly after 8 weeks of age. Diagnosis can be difficult and lengthy, and investigation must therefore begin as soon as evidence of cholestasis is found. Jaundice may be noted soon after birth but is commonly delayed until 2–3 weeks of age.

In extrahepatic biliary atresia, bile cannot enter the duodenum because of sclerotic obstruction to the common bile duct, the hepatic duct, or the right and left hepatic ducts at the porta hepatis.

Investigation

In an infant with biliary atresia, conjugated hyperbilirubinaemia and raised serum transaminase and γ-glutamyl transferase levels will be present, and a coagulopathy may coexist. Abdominal ultrasonography will reveal an enlarged liver, may show splenomegaly and portal vein abnormalities in portal hypertension, and will usually exclude other structural causes of conjugated jaundice such as a choledochal cyst. Failure of ultrasound identification of the gallbladder and other parts of the extrahepatic biliary tree in a jaundiced infant before a feed is common in biliary atresia. The patency of the extrahepatic biliary system may be investigated by radio-isotope scan using ^{99m}Tc-DISIDA, which is taken up by the liver and secreted in bile. If the diagnosis of biliary atresia remains likely following these investigations, then a percutaneous liver biopsy should be performed. Characteristic pathological findings include bile duct proliferation, polymorphonuclear infiltration and histological cholestasis. Operative cholangiography is a confirmatory diagnostic test performed at laparotomy, when contrast infused directly into the proximal bile duct fails to appear in the duodenum.

Treatment

The treatment of biliary atresia is by hepatoportoenterostomy, in which the porta hepatis is dissected and the liver surface cut back to fashion an area through which bile may drain, and a Roux-en-Y loop of small bowel is anastomosed to the prepared liver surface.

Approximately 20–40% of operations will be unsuccessful in establishing bile drainage, or will later fail. In these infants, liver transplantation may eventually be required. Some treated infants will suffer progressive hepatic fibrosis and portal hypertension, and their survival will also ultimately depend on transplantation.

Neonatal hepatitis

Following the diagnostic process outlined above, 30–35% of cholestatic infants will be left with a diagnosis of neonatal hepatitis. The number of these infants has progressively fallen over recent decades, due to the identification of more specific diagnoses. They can be grouped into those with a

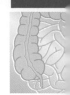

family history (presumably due to genetically determined disease) and sporadic cases. Management is aimed at optimizing nutritional support, supplementation of fat-soluble vitamins A, D, E and K, and attention to other complications of chronic liver failure such as pruritus.

FAILURE TO THRIVE

Failure to thrive describes the infant or child who does not gain weight or height at the expected rate for his or her age. It is a common association with many chronic illnesses and therefore requires comprehensive assessment. Its recognition relies upon serial measurements of height and weight which should be plotted on appropriate growth charts. The recognition that some chronic diseases, such as cystic fibrosis, inflammatory bowel disease and chronic urinary tract infection may present in this way may lead to their early diagnosis.

There are many causes of failure to thrive, but assessment should focus on the three main reasons why affected children may not grow properly. Firstly, they may not be eating enough of the right food; secondly, they may not be digesting or absorbing the food; and thirdly, their energy requirement may exceed their energy intake because of the demands of chronic disease.

A dietary assessment should be undertaken by a paediatric dietician, who will calculate nutrient intakes relative to the recommended requirements. A history of symptoms referable to the gastrointestinal tract should be sought, such as vomiting, abdominal pain, and frequent, loose or smelly stools. Other chronic diseases may be apparent from the history, such as recurrent respiratory infections in cystic fibrosis, or recurrent urinary symptoms in renal disease. A social history may point towards the cause; a single parent of several children living in inadequate accommodation, with a chaotic lifestyle and part-time work at antisocial hours may struggle to provide adequate food at appropriate times to the youngest child.

Health care workers should plot the body height and weight of the child on appropriate centile charts as an assessment of nutritional status. General examination may provide further evidence of the cause of failure to thrive, and signs of specific nutrient deficiencies. Measurement of parental height and weight, plotted on appropriate charts, may show a discrepancy between the actual and expected size of the child. An impression should be formed of how well the child is cared for.

Specific investigations are indicated by abnormalities found on clinical examination. If no such diagnostic features are identified, a child

Table 5.9 Initial investigation of failure to thrive		
Sample	Investigation	Significance of abnormality
Blood	Full blood count differential	Sepsis, anaemia, inflammation, immune deficiency
	Urea and electrolytes, creatinine, calcium, phosphate, bicarbonate	Renal dysfunction, metabolic disease
	Liver function tests, albumin	Liver disease, malabsorption, protein loss (urinary or gastrointestinal)
	Immunoglobulins	Immune deficiency
	Anti-gliadin, anti-endomysial IgA	Coeliac disease
Urine	Microscopy and culture	Urinary tract infection
	Urinalysis (protein and blood)	Renal disease
Stool	Microscopy (3 specimens)	Parasitic infection (e.g. G. intestinalis)
	Culture and virology	Intestinal infection
	Fat globules (3 specimens)	Malabsorption
	Chymotrypsin (3 specimens)	Pancreatic insufficiency
Sweat	Electrolytes	Cystic fibrosis

with failure to thrive should have a number of basic investigations (Table 5.9).

Psychosocial deprivation

Inadequate nutrition may result when a parent lacks the time, money, knowledge or emotional attachment required to feed their child. Associated inadequate stimulation of the child results in psychosocial failure to thrive, with poor growth and development. Clues to the diagnosis are found in the history and by observing the child and parent(s). Investigations should exclude other diagnoses and may reveal signs of inadequate nutrition, such as iron deficiency anaemia.

The diagnosis requires careful and full explanation to the parent(s). Admission to hospital for assessment of the child's feeding, or for a period of supervised nasogastric feeding, may help to confirm the diagnosis. The child may feed ravenously, or be anorexic due to undernutrition or previous unpleasant experience of feeding. On provision of adequate feeds, through a nasogastric tube if necessary, rapid catch-up growth will occur.

Management is multidisciplinary, and specific contributory problems within the social background that are amenable to change should be identified. Discussion with the child's general practitioner and health visitor is essential and involvement of a social worker may be indicated. Recurring failure to thrive at home following hospital admissions indicates more complex and severe problems, and a case conference should be organized to discuss possible solutions with the parents. If no improvement occurs in spite of maximal social support, persisting psychosocial failure to thrive may be an indication for transfer of the child into foster care.

NUTRITION

Infant feeding

During infancy, food must provide for basal metabolism, physical activity, and growth. The newborn doubles in weight in 3 months and, by 2 years, has half his or her eventual adult height. The choice of food for the infant is important because digestive system function is incompletely developed at birth, and continues to mature during the first months of life.

Breast feeding

The ideal food for the human infant is human milk, a complex mixture of nutrients and of immunological and other bioactive substances which confer protection against bacterial and viral infections, and thereby help adaptation to life outside the womb. The composition of human milk changes both during the course of lactation and during a single feed. At the beginning of each feed the fat content is low but later doubles in concentration so that the most energy-dense milk is secreted at the end of the feed.

Colostrum is secreted by the breast during the first few days of lactation. It has about ten times more protein (around 100 g/L) than milk later in lactation, mostly in the form of 'protective proteins', especially secretory IgA and lactoferrin (which competes with bacteria for iron, thereby reducing their viability). There are many other protective factors in human milk (see Beyond Core: antimicrobial factors in breast milk). Nutrients in human milk are more readily absorbed than those in formula milk; for example, although the iron content of human milk is low, it is well absorbed. In addition, human milk contains digestive enzymes, such as lipase, which augments fat digestion at a time when pancreatic lipase activity is relatively low.

Establishing and continuing breast feeding requires help and advice in the first few days to master the technique, and support thereafter when problems arise. Milk production is regulated by circulating prolactin, which increases following each breast feed; frequent suckling therefore results in greater milk production, whilst some drugs (such as bromocriptine and contraceptive agents) and maternal stress may inhibit secretion. During each feed, oxytocin is released from the anterior pituitary and causes myoepithelial cell contraction in the breast alveoli,

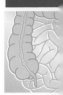

which in turn expels milk from the breast. This 'let-down reflex' is essential for successful breast feeding, but may be disturbed by maternal stress. Mothers who seem to have an 'insufficient milk supply' are often feeding too infrequently to maintain adequate prolactin stimulation, or are stressed by pain, illness, fear of failing to breast feed, or by their partner's, family's or friend's apparent disapproval of breast feeding. Milk production and let-down are improved by frequent feeding and removal of the source of stress.

An infant that does not 'latch-on' properly to the breast will receive inadequate milk and will want to feed more often; sore and cracked nipples may develop in the mother. Helping the mother and infant to breast feed successfully avoids many of the problems associated with breast feeding and prevents early resort to bottle feeding.

Breast-fed babies feed frequently and the mother needs to be available at all times. It may be difficult for a breast-feeding mother to return to work unless her employer has made provision for this (e.g. crèche facilities and flexible 'breast-feeding breaks'). The introduction of bottle feeds to allow the mother to spend longer away from the baby may be successful but may accelerate cessation of breast feeding through the baby's confusion about which way to suck.

Formula feeding

Approved infant formulas are manufactured from various sources (usually cow's milk and vegetable materials) and provide a safe alternative to human milk, although they lack enzymes and immunological and bioactive substances. 'Follow-on formulas' containing more protein, iron and calcium are available for infants from 6 months of age. However, infectious disease is more common in formula-fed than breast-fed infants, especially of the gastrointestinal tract and respiratory system. Neurodevelopment may be superior in breast-fed infants, although evidence for long-term advantage is less certain.

Formula feeds must be prepared and stored according to the printed guidelines. Water must be boiled and put in a sterilized bottle; the appropriate amount of formula powder must be added using the scoop provided, one scoop per fluid ounce (30 ml) of water; after shaking, the bottle must be stored in the fridge until needed; the feed must be given using a sterile teat, rewarmed only once. Milk not taken by the infant should be discarded. In the developing world, the difficulty of performing this routine without introducing contamination, and the value to the baby of the anti-infective factors in breast milk in protecting against enteropathogens, dictate that breast feeding must be the method of choice.

BEYOND CORE

ANTIMICROBIAL FACTORS IN BREAST MILK

Factor	Mechanism of action
Immunoglobulin A	Protects intestinal epithelium from luminal antigens
Lactoferrin	Competes with bacteria for iron
Lysosyme	Antibacterial enzyme lyses cell walls
Bifidus factor	Stimulates lactobacilli in colon
Macrophages	Engulf bacteria
Lymphocytes	Secrete immunoglobulins and lymphokines
Protease inhibitors	Inhibit digestion of bioactive proteins in milk
Complement	Assists bacterial lysis
Interferon	Antiviral agent
Oligosaccharides	Inhibitors of bacterial adhesion to epithelium
Vitamin B_{12} and folate-binding proteins	Compete with bacteria for these vitamins
Anti-staphylococcal factor	Lipid with anti-staphylococcal action

Weaning

At 4–6 months of age, non-milk foods should be introduced into the diet to replenish iron stores which will have become depleted, chewing needs to be developed and milk alone is insufficient to meet the growing nutritional requirements of the infant. Solids are introduced gradually, initially in smooth, pureed form, then gradually increasing their lumpiness as the infant learns to tolerate the changing texture and taste of the food. Non-wheat cereals, fruit, vegetables and potatoes are all suitable first weaning foods. Between 6 and 9 months of age, meat, fish, all cereals, pulses, and eggs can be introduced. No salt should be added to home-prepared foods and only enough sugar should be used to make sour fruits palatable. Breast or formula milk feeding should continue, but if milk intake is poor, vitamin A and D supplements should be provided. Whole ('doorstep') cow's milk should not be introduced into the diet until the age of 1 year.

Healthy eating beyond infancy

During childhood, food should change from the energy-dense diet of the infant, which provides around 50% of energy as fat, to that of the adult, where around 35% of energy should be derived from fat. This change occurs largely in the toddler years. Many toddlers are fussy and difficult with meals, but a varied intake of solid foods should be maintained as far as possible along with approximately 500 ml of milk per day. Full fat milk can be used from 1 to 2 years, and semi-skimmed from 2 to 5 years of age. Care should be taken with fluids. Many toddlers begin to substitute easily assimilated liquids for solid food which requires chewing and the use of cutlery. Dental 'bottle caries' are a result of continual ingestion of sweetened liquids from a teated bottle. After the first year of life, all drinks taken during the day should be given with a cup.

After the age of 5 years, the diet can change towards that advised for adults. Fibre intake should be increased with generous consumption of fruits, vegetables and high-fibre cereals such as wholemeal bread, pasta and breakfast cereals. Efforts should be made to moderate saturated fat intake by the use of skimmed or semi-skimmed milk, low-fat or polyunsaturated spreads, low-fat dairy products and fish, poultry and lean meats. The intake of non-milk extrinsic sugars between meals should be avoided because of its association with dental caries. A reduction in energy intake from a lowering of fat intake should be compensated for by a commensurate increase in starch intake. Fibre is also an increasingly important component of diet with advancing age; not only does it help to maintain healthy colonic function but it also protects against many adult diseases, including obesity, cardiovascular disease and diabetes mellitus.

Many teenagers adopt a 'grazing' eating pattern, consuming snack foods and 'fast food' meals. Their diets may be low in various nutrients, in particular iron, calcium, thiamine and riboflavin. Energy intake averages 90% of estimated average requirement, which may reflect the sedentary lifestyles of many children. Vegetarianism is increasing, and encompasses a range of dietary cultures. 'Vegetarian' diets which include some animal foods such as milk, cheese or eggs usually achieve adequate nutrient intakes. Teenagers who elect to follow a vegan regimen should take supplements of vitamin B_{12}, calcium, vitamin D, iron and zinc. Avoidance of specific foods on religious or cult grounds may result in severe nutrient deficiencies unless the dietary regimen has been based on long-established traditional practices.

FURTHER READING

Walker W A, Durie P R, Hamilton J R, Walker-Smith J A, Watkins J B, eds 1996 Pediatric gastrointestinal disease: pathophysiology, diagnosis, management, 2nd edn. Mosby, St Louis

The respiratory system

P. J. Helms

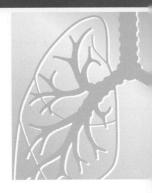

ESSENTIAL BACKGROUND

INTRODUCTION

Respiratory disorders are the most common clinical problems presenting in primary care and in hospital practice. Whereas the prevalence of symptomatic lower respiratory tract illnesses is similar throughout the world, mortality and morbidity vary greatly. In the third world, symptomatic respiratory infections are the single largest identifiable cause of death, and are often due to bacterial agents such as *Streptococcus pneumoniae*, *Haemophilus influenzae* and *Mycobacterium tuberculosis*. By way of contrast, morbidity and mortality are low in the developed world, where the vast majority of symptomatic respiratory infections are due to common respiratory viruses such as respiratory syncytial virus, parainfluenza viruses and the ubiquitous rhinoviruses.

A remarkable feature of the pattern of respiratory illness in industrialized countries is the so-called 'asthma epidemic' with reported prevalences more than trebling in the same communities over the past 30 years (Fig. 6.1). Symptomatic respiratory disorders are most common in young preschool children, which is both a consequence of the relative immaturity of the host defence mechanisms and anatomical development. Lung development is not complete until approximately 3 years of age (see p. 104), and

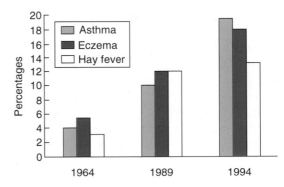

Figure 6.1 Increase in childhood asthma and atopic disease (Aberdeen City, 1964–1994)

growth in size and physiological development continue until full adult stature has been achieved. Consequently, respiratory disease in early childhood may cause significant morbidity in adult life (see Highlights and Hypotheses: Early influences on later health in Ch. 1).

With the increasing success of neonatal intensive care in recent years, increasing numbers of babies exposed to long-term oxygen therapy and intermittent positive pressure ventilation are surviving (see Ch. 4) and producing a population of children with chronic obstructive lung disease of prematurity. These children, together with those suffering from cystic fibrosis, very severe (steroid-dependent) asthma and a heterogeneous group of relatively uncommon lung disorders (e.g. lung hypoplasia, ciliary dyskinesia, fibrosing alveolitis) will require lifelong medical management.

ANATOMY, PHYSIOLOGY AND NORMAL VALUES

Growth and development of the lungs

The lung consists functionally of two zones: conducting, principally the airways, and gas-exchanging, principally the alveoli. Anatomical (Fig. 6.2) and functional development of the gas-exchanging zone of the lung are the major factors determining viability of the preterm infant. The lungs first develop as an outpouching of the primitive foregut at approximately 4 weeks of gestational age and, following a process of repeated branching, the full complement of conducting airways (16 generations) is present by 16 weeks. At around 20 weeks of gestation, primitive alveoli (saccules) begin to develop, and the epithelium begins to synthesize the complex phospholipid, surfactant, which is responsible for lowering the surface tension of the alveolar lining postnatally, thus preventing alveolar collapse at low lung volumes (see Ch. 4).

At birth, approximately half the adult number of alveoli are present, with most of the additional alveoli being added by the age of about 3 years. It is therefore in intrauterine life and early childhood that significant disturbance to this ordered sequence of development can result in serious consequences for the developing lung and subsequent respiratory health. The most dramatic example of such maldevelopment in utero occurs as a consequence of diaphragmatic hernia in which the small intestine and liver are displaced into the thorax and compress the lung, rendering it hypoplastic. Another more subtle but significant

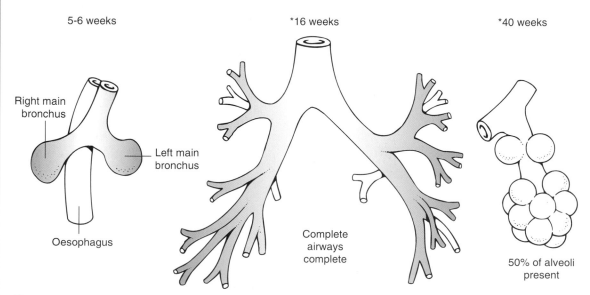

Figure 6.2   Lung development from 5–6 weeks post-conception to full term

influence on lung growth and development in utero is maternal smoking, which has been shown to be associated with increased respiratory symptoms and decreased baseline airway function in early life.

The volume at which the lung operates is a function principally of the outward recoil of the chest wall and diaphragm on the one hand, and the surface tension of the fluid lining the inner surface of the alveoli, on the other. Infants and preschool children are at a particular disadvantage in terms of the mechanics of the respiratory system due to the fact that the chest wall in early life is exceptionally soft and compliant, and thus offers relatively poor support to the lung. Thus, not only is some of the work of breathing wasted on distortion of the elastic thoracic cage but also the lung operates much closer to its residual volume (volume at the end of a complete expiration) than in older children and adults. For this reason, the lung of the infant and young child copes poorly with the additional burden of airway obstruction due to mucous hypersecretion and mucosal oedema associated with lower respiratory infections, with the result that basal areas of the lung collapse. This results in shunting of blood through poorly aerated parts of the lung and a lowered arterial oxygen tension – a common feature of severe lower respiratory infections such as bronchiolitis.

Anatomical immaturity also contributes to the pattern of upper respiratory tract symptoms in young children. The infant and very young child has a large cranial vault but a very underdeveloped facial skeleton relative to the mature adult. Indeed, frontal sinuses are difficult to visualize radiologically until the age of 5 or 6 years. The close apposition of the anterior pharyngeal wall to the posterior-pharyngeal wall, together with hypertrophy of tonsillar and adenoidal tissue and the small cross-sectional area of the larynx in early childhood, results in a susceptibility to obstruction in association with intercurrent, mainly viral, infections. Any further narrowing of this crowded space due to infection results in a further increase in the resistance to air flow, particularly during inspiration (since the extra-thoracic airways are normally narrowed

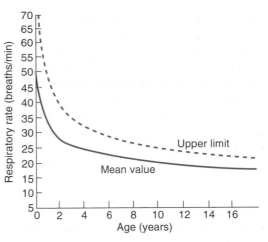

Figure 6.3 Change in baseline respiratory rate with age

during the inspiratory phase of the cycle). This in turn necessitates an increase in the force of contraction of the inspiratory muscles to generate a more negative pressure in order to overcome the increased resistance and to maintain an adequate airflow. However, the resulting increased gradient between the intrapleural and atmospheric pressure encourages collapse of the extra-thoracic airways, and thus may exacerbate the obstruction. These features largely explain the marked inspiratory stridor often heard in young children with symptomatic upper respiratory tract infections and the whoop which accompanies inspiration after a coughing spasm in children with pertussis. A further consequence of the overcrowding of the pharyngeal space and hypertrophy of lymphatic tissue in this region is that eustachian tube drainage is impaired, predisposing to the development of otitis media which is common in children (see Ch. 13).

The respiratory rate, which is high in infancy, falls progressively, to reach adult levels by the age of 3 years (Fig. 6.3).

HISTORY AND EXAMINATION

History taking

A full pregnancy and perinatal history is a prerequisite for formulating an adequate differential diagnosis. Congenital lung disorders, such as lung hypoplasia due to diaphragmatic hernia or oligohydramnios, and acquired disorders, such as the respiratory distress syndrome, may have long-term effects on lung growth and function. Low birth weight is a known risk factor for recurrent wheezing episodes in early childhood and, if ventilatory support is required in the newborn period, may result in damage to the developing lung (chronic obstructive lung disease of prematurity or bronchopulmonary dysplasia) (see Ch. 4).

Asthma and atopic disease are extremely common, and a positive family history favours such a diagnosis. Approximately 40% of children with one atopic parent will also develop atopy, including asthma and if both parents are atopic, approximately 60% of their offspring will be at risk. Further enquiry can establish whether the problem is one of recurrent episodes of breathlessness on exertion or exposure to domestic pets; both are suggestive of atopic asthma.

Recurrent respiratory infections with production of sputum, particularly if associated with failure to thrive and gastrointestinal disturbance, would suggest the possibility of cystic fibrosis.

Passive smoke exposure, particularly maternal exposure in pregnancy, is a well-established risk factor for recurrent wheezing in early childhood. If such a history is elicited there may be the opportunity for health education, although it has to be recognized that the success rate, in terms of cessation of smoking, is low. Often convincing the parents not to smoke in the presence of their children is the most that can be achieved.

Physical examination

As in all paediatric assessments, the differential diagnosis will be established largely on the basis of a careful history and observation; the physical examination is mainly confirmatory. In acute lower respiratory disease there are a number of signs which provide an indication of severity of disease and are termed collectively 'respiratory distress'. These are: nasal flaring, grunting, raised respiratory rate (see Fig. 6.3), use of accessory muscles, and recession (suprasternal, costal, intercostal, subcostal). In the presence of

significant airway obstruction, or parenchymal lung disease where there is significant shunting of blood through poorly aerated lung (see p. 105) there may be associated central cyanosis. Clubbing is difficult to elicit in children under 1 year of age unless it is very severe.

There are a number of different types of chest deformity found in childhood, some of which have specific aetiological significance: Harrison's sulcus, pectus carinatum (pigeon chest), pectus excavatum (funnel chest) and hyperinflation (barrel chest). The term 'Harrison's sulcus', named after its first British observer, refers to a fixed groove in the lower rib cage at the site of insertion of the diaphragm. It is most commonly associated with severe asthma of early onset during the period of greatest compliance of the chest wall in infancy and early childhood. Pectus carinatum is another form of chest deformity associated with asthma in which the long-term effect of the respiratory muscles is to force the sternum forward; it may coexist with Harrison's sulcus. Pectus excavatum (funnel chest) is usually an incidental finding and is not usually of direct significance to the respiratory system; the exception is in children with severe obstructive sleep apnoea, where it may be a prominent feature in association with the daytime somnolence and repeated night awakenings.

Hyperinflation as a result of air trapping is a chronic feature of cystic fibrosis, and is seen acutely in asthma and bronchiolitis. Evidence of hyperinflation can be inferred from the shape of the chest. In children from the age of 3 years, the lateral diameter should be approximately one and a half to twice the antero-posterior diameter. In infants, the chest wall is more circular in shape, and antero-posterior to lateral dimensions are not as helpful in this regard. However, in the infant and young child, depression of the diaphragm will result in downward displacement of the liver extending beyond the usual 1–2 cm below the right costal margin. Absence of cardiac dullness on percussion, after confirmation that the heart is in the usual position by locating the apex beat, is evidence for significant hyperinflation – with the lingula extending over the anterior border of the heart.

Deviation of the trachea points to the possibility of a collapsed lung on that side or a pneumothorax or large space-occupying cyst on the contralateral side. Percussion and ausculation of the chest should allow clear differentiation between these two. In the infant, the breath sounds appear to the uninitiated to be bronchial in nature. This is because of the relatively short distance between the conducting airways and the chest wall as alveolarization is not yet complete (see Fig. 6.2). Infants and young school age children are often found to have fine crackles in association with asthma, and infants with acute bronchiolitis often have showers of fine crackles over all lung areas, which could be misinterpreted as evidence for left ventricular failure. Wheeze, which is a polyphonic sound in expiration, has to be differentiated from stridor, which is monophonic and predominantly inspiratory in timing.

INVESTIGATION

Imaging

Radiological assessment in infants and young children shows what appears to be an enlarged heart as a consequence of the relative

underdevelopment of the lung at this stage, an appearance which is emphasized by the use of antero-posterior films rather than the traditional postero-anterior films used in older children and adults. The uses of computerized tomography include assessment of congenital anomalies (e.g. sequestered lobe) and determining the extent and localization of bronchiectasis (Fig. 6.4).

Respiratory function assessment

Classical spirometric measurements, including forced vital capacity (FVC), can be achieved reproducibly in children as young as 5 years of age but more typically after the age of 7 years. Peak expiratory flow rates (PEFR) are valuable in monitoring of response to therapy in asthma and can be used in children as young as 4 years, but performance is more consistent above 5 years. In infants and young children, specialized measurements can be performed in research laboratories, but these are not widely available or used in routine clinical practice. As would be expected, all lung function measurements are

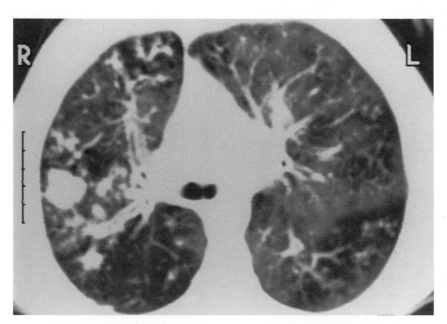

Figure 6.4   A computerized tomography scan of the thorax in a child with cystic fibrosis showing bilateral dilated thick-walled bronchi in keeping with the diagnosis of bronchiectasis

closely related to stature (Fig. 6.5), which explains approximately 70% of the changes with increasing child age.

Although airway development is complete in the mid-trimester of pregnancy and alveolar development is virtually complete by the age of 3 years, growth in body dimensions (including the rib cage) and the stretch that this imposes on the underlying lung, results in a significant growth in size without a significant increase in new lung units. The growth in respiratory function, the brief plateau in early adult life and the subsequent decline with ageing, highlight the importance of achieving the full potential of lung development in early childhood. Failure to reach full genetic potential will result in the early expression of respiratory symptoms associated with ageing. The effects of smoking over a whole lifespan are considerable and significantly increase the rate of normal ageing; hence the need to prevent the habit in childhood and adolescence.

Measurement of arterial gas tensions and pH are essential in the objective assessment of those at risk of respiratory failure and those on ventilatory support. Less invasive techniques,

such as transcutaneous oxygen and carbon dioxide estimation and pulse oximetry, are useful adjuncts, with the latter technique now a routine part of clinical assessment and monitoring.

Bronchoscopy

Although use of the rigid bronchoscope invariably requires ventilation under general anaesthesia, it remains the technique of choice for the removal of foreign bodies because of its wide calibre.

Flexible bronchoscopy can be performed under sedation, and has the additional advantage of providing access to the upper lobes and distal bronchi.

Indications for bronchoscopy
- Infants with persistent stridor (to exclude causes other than laryngomalacia)
- Persistent wheeze and/or recurrent pneumonia (to exclude anatomical abnormalities and the possibility of a foreign body)
- Atelectasis or obstructive hyperinflation not responding to antibiotics and physiotherapy (for aspiration of mucous plugs/thick secretions)

Bronchoscopy also offers an opportunity to obtain lavage specimens for microbiology and cytology studies. Other, much less common indications, include bronchial biopsy for the diagnosis of chronic granulomatous diseases (e.g. sarcoid) and transbronchial biopsy for infiltrative lung disorders.

CORE PROBLEMS

UPPER RESPIRATORY TRACT INFECTION

This is the single largest cause of morbidity in children of all ages. In young preschool children and infants it is a common reason for urgent paediatric referral and can, on occasion, mimic signs of meningitis with irritability and neck stiffness. The majority of upper respiratory tract infections are viral in origin, and antibiotics are rarely indicated, although pressure to prescribe

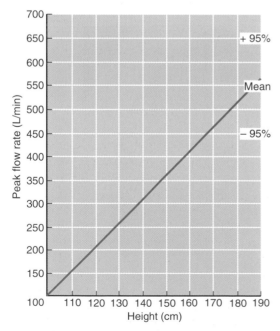

Figure 6.5 Peak flow in relation to height

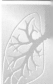

them may be difficult to resist as a consequence of combined parental and doctor anxiety.

Acute pharyngitis

Pharyngeal and tonsillar inflammation (pharyngotonsillitis) associated with coryza is particularly common in infants and preschool children, in whom up to six symptomatic infections per year are the norm. Nasal discharge and obstruction can cause feeding difficulties in infancy. Examination of the throat often reveals an infected red posterior pharynx but no exudates over the tonsils. Dull or pink ear drums are often seen and, together with a low-grade pyrexia (up to 38.5°C), are often incorrectly interpreted as evidence for bacterial otitis media and the need for antibiotics (see Ch. 13).

Cervical lymph nodes are often palpable. Tonsillitis (see Fig. 13.8) with exudates, cervical lymphadenopathy (particularly if painful, anterior and unilateral) and high fever may be due to streptococcal infection. Scarlet fever is a particular form of streptococcal disease (see Ch. 14), while acute glomerulonephritis and rheumatic fever are potential post-streptococcal sequelae (see Chs 8 and 12). Exudates and palatal haemorrhages may suggest glandular fever, a diagnosis which becomes more common in school age children and adolescents.

Investigation

In the presence of features described above, it is rarely necessary to perform further investigations apart from careful observation. If the infant is feeding well, has good peripheral perfusion, is responsive and handles normally, further investigations are rarely required. In the presence of a high fever, above 38.5°C, and if tonsillar exudates are present, a throat swab, full blood count and ASO titre may be appropriate in order to identify possible streptococcal infection for which penicillin will be required. Blood cultures should be considered in children who are systemically unwell with a disproportionate degree of toxicity.

Treatment

Treatment is largely symptomatic for coryzal symptoms, with paracetamol in appropriate dosages for temperature reduction together with removal of clothing, particularly in young children who are at risk of rapid rises of temperature and associated febrile convulsions (see Ch. 10). Antibiotics are rarely required, even in the presence of pink tympanic membranes, as the majority of infections are viral. Antibiotics in themselves can cause problems, and it has been shown that the use of broad-spectrum antibiotics for upper respiratory tract infections has a higher associated morbidity than if antipyretics are given alone. This is true particularly in young infants in whom the commonly used broad-spectrum penicillins not only alter the normal bacterial flora of the upper respiratory tract but also alter the gut flora, resulting in colonization by candida and diarrhoea. Furthermore, penicillins are commonly implicated in the aetiology of skin rashes. Nevertheless, children who have obvious tonsillar exudates, have marked changes of otitis media (Ch. 13) with cherry red rather than pink ear drums, with or without perforation, and who are toxic (temperature above 38.5°C) merit antibiotic treatment even though there is no conclusive evidence that clinical resolution will be hastened. Infants and children in this category are a small minority of those presenting with upper respiratory tract symptoms.

WHEEZE

Wheezing is a common feature of respiratory disease in infants and young children; this may reflect the smaller diameter of the airways at this age, so that any further narrowing of the airway will be sufficient to cause turbulence in the air flow and results in wheezing. The oedema and exudation which accompany inflammation of the airways, whether due to infections, viral or bacterial, or irritation such as that due to passive smoking, are thus more likely to be associated with wheezing than later on in life. Furthermore, at this age there is less smooth muscle in the peripheral airways and more mucus producing

characteristically episodic, associated with virus infections interspersed with long symptom-free intervals. Episodic nocturnal cough in the preschool child, even in the absence of wheeze, may indicate asthma. Children of school age are more likely to have chronic symptoms, such as exercise-induced asthma, sleep disturbance and seasonal exacerbations, as well as virus-associated episodes. Other school children may have unremitting symptoms despite therapy (Fig. 6.6).

In addition to viral infections, environmental factors such as passive smoking may trigger wheeze in infancy. Food allergy is a recognized but less common trigger of wheeze in infants. As the child grows older, inhaled allergens and exercise play an increasingly important role and emotional disturbance can exacerbate symptoms.

The long-term pattern and severity of asthma are best assessed by home monitoring. This is achieved by means of a daily record card in which

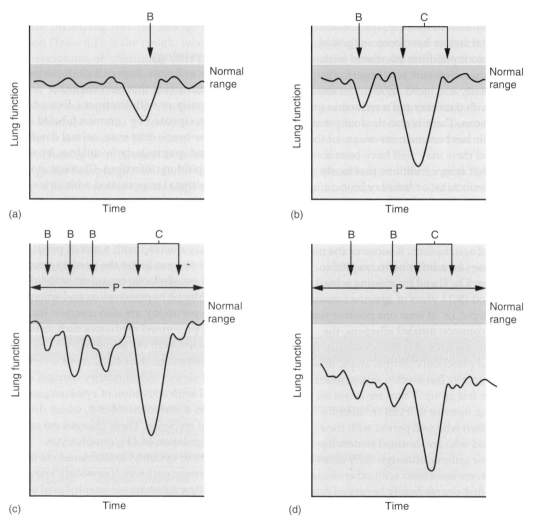

Figure 6.6 The pattern of a patient's asthma largely dictates the drug treatment they should receive. This figure shows the basis for the use of bronchodilators (B), corticosteroids (C) and long-term prophylactic agents (P) in each of the four patterns of asthma: **a** mild episodic symptoms; **b** episodic with intercurrent symptoms; **c** chronic intercurrent and episodic symptoms fully reversible at times; **d** chronic intercurrent and episodic symptoms which never resolve completely

symptoms (particularly important is the degree of night disturbance), peak flow and use of bronchodilators are recorded.

In acute severe asthma, the most important physical signs are extreme dyspnoea, manifest by the degree of difficulty in speaking and use of accessory muscles, and cyanosis, which indicates a very severe degree of airways obstruction. Loudness of wheezing does not correlate reliably with severity but the finding of a 'silent' chest on auscultation indicates critically severe asthma.

Investigation

Chest radiography is indicated at the initial acute presentation and may show, in addition to hyperinflation, evidence of coexisting infection and scattered areas of collapse due to mucus plugging of small airways. Subsequently, chest radiography may be omitted, unless there are features suggestive of bacterial pneumonia, pneumothorax or if the response to seemingly adequate therapy is poor. In young preschool children, assessment is largely clinical. Older children should be encouraged to perform PEFR measurements and this can be used to monitor response to treatment (see Fig. 6.6). Although no substitute for a careful history, skin prick tests may be useful in older children (over 6 years of age), as positivity to common inhaled allergens will confirm the atopic diagnosis and may identify important allergens which could be targets for exposure reduction. Enquiry as to parental smoking habits should also be included in the assessment. Oxygen saturation monitoring is essential in acute severe asthma, and blood gas measurements may be needed (see below).

Treatment

Nationally and internationally agreed guidelines have been produced in recent years including the 1995 British Asthma Guidelines (Fig. 6.7). The mainstay of symptomatic treatment remains bronchodilator therapy with β_2 agonists administered by the inhaled route. Young children and infants who are unable to accept nebulizers or masks attached to spacer devices may require oral treatment but this is less effective. Infants and

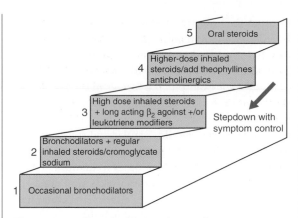

Figure 6.7   Stepwise approach to asthma management

very young children under the age of 2 years are difficult to treat and many of the established treatments that work well in older children and adults are ineffective. Short courses of systemic steroids are effective in treating acute episodes but their long-term use can cause growth failure; thus they should only be used for a small minority of severely affected individuals with frequent interval symptoms and severe acute episodes.

Long-term or prophylactic treatment is required for children who are using more than two or three bronchodilator treatments a week. The British Asthma Guidelines suggest the optional use of cromoglycate as the first prophylactic treatment, followed by inhaled steroids. Nevertheless, it is accepted practice to use inhaled steroids as first-line prophylaxis. The latter should be stepped down as control is achieved. It is important to educate children and their parents in the appropriate use of their medication and to ensure that they know the difference between asthma relievers (β_2 agonists) and preventers (cromoglycate or steroids). It is also important to identify the appropriate delivery device for the child's age and ability. In general, aerosol devices with spacers are used in infants and young children of preschool age, with a face mask rather than a mouthpiece for those too young to use the latter. Older children can usually use dry powder devices, which have the advantage of delivering a higher concentration of drug to the lungs than pressurized aerosols. Second-generation antihistamines and the newly introduced leukotriene-modifying agents may also have a role in clearly defined settings – for example, the former in the atopic infant and the latter as a steroid-sparing treatment.

In the acutely ill child, regular and frequent assessment (including pulse oximetry and arterial blood gases) is required in order to identify impending respiratory failure which may need ventilatory support. In acute attacks, hypoxaemia is an important feature and all nebulized treatments should be delivered with oxygen as the driving gas.

Emergency treatment of acute severe asthma includes: oxygen, nebulized β_2 agonist (initially as frequently as every 30–60 min); rarely, subcutaneous or intravenous β_2 agonist if nebulizer therapy is either unavailable or ineffective; intravenous aminophylline infusion if the patient is unresponsive to β_2 agonist therapy (omit the loading dose if patient has previously had a slow-release theophylline preparation); and intravenous hydrocortisone. Rarely, ventilatory support may be necessary.

Bronchiolitis

In younger children, an increased respiratory rate with costal/subcostal recession and difficulty in feeding are features which are also seen in acute viral bronchiolitis. The latter condition is mostly (70%) due to the respiratory syncytial virus (RSV), and affects each new cohort of newborn infants as they pass through their first winter, the majority presenting between 2 and 4 months of age. Although approximately half of the children admitted to hospital with bronchiolitis persist with wheezing for at least 6 months after discharge, the relationship between this condition and later wheeze and asthma is controversial. Studies have suggested that this group is over-represented in the symptomatic wheezing population in mid-childhood. It is not clear whether this is due to a predisposed host or to a triggering of the allergic IgE-mediated response

associated with the primary RSV infection. A strong family history of asthma or other manifestations of atopy may help prognostically.

In the majority of cases, bronchiolitis results in a mild illness which manifests as a 'heavy cold' associated with some increase in the respiratory rate and a slightly noisy breathing. Reassurance, observation and attention to fluid intake are all that is required, and these children can be managed at home. On the other hand, some cases of bronchiolitis may be severe enough (Fig. 6.8) to precipitate respiratory failure and warrant Intensive Therapy Unit admission and ventilation. Dehydration and secondary bacterial infection are major complications. Severe forms of the illness are more likely in the presence of other pathology such as bronchopulmonary dysplasia, significant congenital heart disease or immunodeficiency. Inhaled ribavirin (tribavirin), an antiviral drug active against RSV, may be beneficial in these cases.

The distinction between acute bronchiolitis and an initial attack of asthma may be very difficult. An onset before 6 months of age favours the

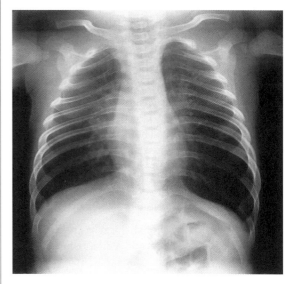

Figure 6.8 A radiograph of an infant showing bilateral hilar enlargement with relatively clear lung fields. On examination, however, the baby had marked respiratory distress (tachypnoea and intercostal indrawing) and widespread high-pitched crackles

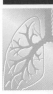

diagnosis of bronchiolitis, while asthma is more likely if there are other features of atopy (family history, coexisting eczema). Second attacks of bronchiolitis are unusual but, as noted above, the illness can be followed by a period of several months of increased reactivity of the airways. This may be manifested mainly as recurrent cough but occasionally also as wheeze and respiratory distress in response to various triggers including other viral infections.

STRIDOR

Stridor is a clinical term used to describe harsh breathing sounds due to obstruction of extrathoracic airways anywhere between the pharynx and upper trachea, and is most commonly heard during inspiration, usually being audible without the use of a stethoscope. Extrathoracic airway obstruction can be congenital or acquired. The common causes of stridor include laryngomalacia, inhaled foreign body, and croup. Laryngomalacia ('floppy larynx') presents soon after birth as mild chronic stridor and usually requires no special investigations unless another, more serious, congenital anomaly is suspected. Stridor due to inhaled foreign body has a characteristically sudden onset and occurs without preceding upper respiratory symptoms, unlike croup. Most causes of acquired extrathoracic obstruction are acute (Fig. 6.9).

Subglottic stenosis is the most common form of iatrogenic chronic stridor and is the result of the long-term intubation required for ventilation of the preterm infant with lung disease (see Ch. 4).

Tonsillar hypertrophy, subglottic stenosis and laryngomalacia are important causes of upper airway obstruction but their course, unlike croup, is chronic.

Certain forms of acute tonsillitis and pharyngeal infections may be associated with significant acute upper airway obstruction but, since no laryngeal or paralaryngeal structures are usually involved, the clinical picture is distinct from that of croup.

✱ KEY DIAGNOSIS

Viral croup

Croup is a symptom complex comprising stridor, barking cough and respiratory distress due to upper airway obstruction. Viral croup, which is far and away the most common form of croup, involves infection of the larynx, trachea and bronchi, hence its full name – acute laryngotracheobronchitis – which describes the site and extent of the infection. It predominates in infants and young preschool children; parainfluenza viruses are the usual infecting agent. It is important to distinguish this common, distressing, but rarely life-threatening disease

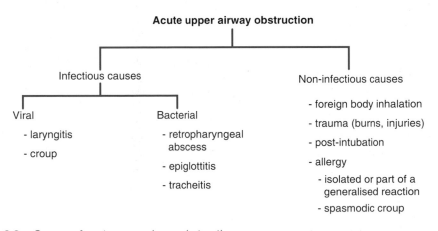

Figure 6.9 Causes of acute upper airway obstruction

from the very severe illness associated with *H. influenzae*: epiglottitis (see Epiglottitis and bacterial tracheitis below). Young children are particularly prone to croup because of their relatively crowded upper airway tract (see p. 105). This may be further exacerbated by reduced cartilaginous support around the larynx (laryngomalacia), resulting in collapse of the larynx during each inspiration.

Clinical features

The harsh tracheal breath sounds are usually audible as the cot is approached. Characteristically, the predominant sound is monophonic, but there may be associated wheeze (polyphonic) if there is bronchial involvement. Another characteristic feature of croup is the deep tracheal cough said to be reminiscent of a barking sea lion. The infant may be distressed but is usually well perfused and otherwise looks well. As in other cases of respiratory distress in children, a prominent feature is subcostal and costal recession; indeed, in severe cases there may also be marked sternal recession due to the negative intrathoracic pressure generated by the diaphragm as it attempts to overcome the severe inspiratory obstruction. As the site of the obstruction is extrathoracic, the stridor will be particularly prominent during the inspiration when the soft tissues of the airway collapse.

Acute episodes of croup usually resolve within 2–3 days and have no long-term sequelae. Episodes of recurrent croup are often described as 'spasmodic croup', and can be part of the clinical presentation of asthma; as such they may respond to asthma therapies.

Investigation

The diagnosis is based on the clinical features, and on no account should the throat be examined since this manoeuvre may precipitate respiratory obstruction. Radiography of the chest and neck is indicated if an inhaled foreign body is suspected (e.g. sudden onset of stridor in the absence of preceding coryzal symptoms). Severe cases of viral croup may present a picture indistinguishable

from that of epiglottitis and should be managed along similar lines (see below).

Children and infants with a prolonged history, particularly those who first present in early infancy, should have congenital abnormalities considered and may require further elective investigations. These include direct microlaryngoscopy in order to visualize endotracheal pathology, together with a lateral barium swallow to exclude extratracheal compression such as a vascular ring.

Treatment

Treatment is essentially supportive unless, of course, endotracheal intubation is required. Antibiotics are only indicated for epiglottitis and/or bacterial tracheitis. It is common practice to increase the humidity of the inspired air with steam or water mist as this appears to give symptomatic benefit. For the child who does not require hospital admission, humidification can be achieved by boiling kettles in the same room as the child or by taking the child into the bathroom and filling the bath or sink with hot water (taking care not to leave the child unattended). Pyrexia should be treated with paracetamol and, where there is obvious respiratory distress, steroids may be given in order to reduce the severity of symptoms and speed recovery. Intramuscular dexamethasone is the most effective, followed by oral dexamethasone or prednisolone. Nebulized steroids are more expensive and are no more effective.

Epiglottitis and bacterial tracheitis

Due to the efficacy of the programme of immunization against *Haemophilus* type b (Hib), epiglottitis is now a rare condition. Unlike croup, in which the onset is typically insidious and the child systemically well, epiglottitis is characteristically of sudden onset and the child is toxic and unwell – classically leaning forwards and drooling in order to avoid the exquisite pain of swallowing.

A toxic child with a temperature above 38.5°C may have bacterial tracheitis. If the intrathoracic

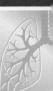

trachea is involved there may be an expiratory component to the stridor due to the tendency of the lower trachea to collapse during forced expiration.

In cases of suspected epiglottitis/bacterial tracheitis or very severe croup, the child should not be left unattended, and a senior member of staff experienced in intubation should be involved. If required, intubation should be performed under anaesthesia, and tracheostomy/cricoidotomy sets should be available in case of intubation failure. The priority is to assess the severity of the obstruction before pursuing any further investigations. After stabilization, blood cultures should be undertaken before antibiotic treatment is initiated.

Inhaled foreign body

The sudden onset of cough, with no prodromal upper respiratory tract symptoms and clinical signs such as stridor, unilateral wheezing or diminished breath sounds, is strong supporting evidence for the diagnosis of inhaled foreign body. The initial symptoms may be followed by apparent resolution and then recurrence. A chest radiograph may be required to exclude unilateral gas trapping or lobar collapse. Inspiratory and expiratory chest radiography and/or screening of the chest demonstrate mediastinal movement away from the area of the impacted foreign body as air cannot escape from the affected part of the lung during expiration (the so-called 'ball valve' effect). Treatment is by bronchoscopic removal. In cases where the diagnosis has been missed or the treatment inadequate, complications invariably arise, with recurrent chest infections, persistent respiratory symptoms and bronchiectasis.

COUGH

Cough as an isolated respiratory symptom is a common reason for medical consultation. It is often considered as part of the asthma syndrome, but increasing evidence points to a different natural history for cough and its poor response to symptomatic or prophylactic asthma medications. Epidemiological evidence has also shown that when presenting alone, cough is rarely the first sign of asthma. Cough can be the presentation of a wide range of respiratory problems ranging from a mild upper respiratory tract infection to life-threatening pneumonia. As a symptom this can be distressing for the child and the parents, and is usually worse, or more noticeable, at night. Grandparents and great grandparents who remember tuberculosis as a serious and common problem consider cough to have a greater significance and hence cause for concern.

The deep tracheal bark often occurring in winter months in very young children is virtually diagnostic for croup (see p. 115) and will usually be associated with inspiratory stridor following prodromal upper respiratory tract symptoms. Cough associated with asthma often has a wheezy component whereas a dry irritating cough associated with significant pyrexia would suggest a lobar pneumonia. A loose productive cough is characteristic of cystic fibrosis in its later stages, and is often seen during the resolution of an acute asthmatic episode when, together with the purulent-looking sputum (due to heavy eosinophilic infiltration), it may be erroneously interpreted as being due to secondary bacterial infection. Paroxysmal cough in an infant or young child associated with vomiting may be due to the severe respiratory illness of whooping cough. Cough may also be the first presentation of an inhaled foreign body in an inquisitive toddler, classically between the ages of 10 months to 3 years.

Treatment of cough, not associated with asthma, lower respiratory tract infection (e.g. pneumonia, or inhaled foreign body) is supportive. Irritating cough, particularly at night, may be helped by proprietary antihistamines, but their effect is likely to be modulated through their sedative rather than antitussive action. Although antibiotics are often demanded by parents and the pressure to resist their prescription can be difficult, they are only indicated where there is evidence of likely lower respiratory tract bacterial infection.

✳ KEY DIAGNOSIS

Pertussis (whooping cough)

Whooping cough can be a particularly serious illness in infancy. It is highly contagious, with infectivity rates approaching 100% among exposed susceptible children, and can be associated with significant morbidity and mortality. Before the introduction of specific immunization, pertussis was the cause of substantial morbidity in the child population, with over 150 000 notifications annually in the UK. During the early 1950s, this high attack rate fell to extremely low levels, but in the 1970s it rose again after widespread publicity surrounding rare cases of encephalopathy possibly linked to pertussis immunization. The excess mortality of approximately 40 deaths per year associated with this period of decreased immunization uptake in the UK emphasized the need to protect this most vulnerable infant group.

Clinical features and investigation

The illness first presents with upper respiratory tract symptoms of a watery nose or discharge followed after 1–2 weeks by severe and persistent paroxysmal coughing. Coughing episodes may be associated with cyanosis, and on completion of the episode a loud inspiratory whoop is often heard.

Vomiting is frequently associated with coughing paroxysms which can be of such severity that subconjunctival haemorrhages and facial petechiae may be seen as a result of the rise in venous pressure. Surprisingly few respiratory symptoms or signs are found in-between coughing episodes unless secondary infection develops (a recognized complication). In small infants, recurrent apnoea is a major complication. Rarely, a diffuse encephalopathy develops. The responsible organism, *Bordetella pertussis*, is difficult to isolate, and is only identified in affected individuals if cough swabs or pernasal swabs are taken during the early phase of the illness. The illness has a long course, and takes up to 3 months to resolve. During this time, feeding can be problematic and the effects on the parents, quite apart from the child, quite trying.

Treatment

The treatment of established whooping cough is not curative. There is some evidence that erythromycin may modify the illness if given during the coryzal stage. The other goal of antibiotic treatment is to shorten the infectivity period. However, the mainstay of management is supportive. Reassurance of the family and observation at home with special attention to fluid intake is appropriate for the mildest cases. Admission to hospital may be necessary for monitoring, airway suctioning and supplemental oxygen to overcome the severe hypoxia which may accompany the cough spasms or apnoea. Nasogastric tube feeding or intravenous fluid therapy may be required. Hospital admission may also provide much needed respite to the family.

✳ KEY DIAGNOSIS

Cystic fibrosis

Cystic fibrosis is the commonest lethal inherited disorder in Caucasian populations; the majority of children presenting before the age of 2 years. The carrier rate of this recessively inherited condition is approximately 1 in 20 but the overall incidence is slightly less than expected at 1 in 2000. The risk to carrier couples of having an affected child is, however, 1 in 4. Presentation is usually with recurrent lower respiratory tract infections and is often, but not always, associated with loose, offensive and bulky stools. Meconium ileus in the newborn, although accounting for less than 10% of cases, is important because it presents acutely with intestinal obstruction and requires urgent surgical intervention. Differential diagnosis includes conditions which are individually rare: immune deficiency, ciliary dyskinesia, or the even rarer Kartagener's syndrome (chronic sinusitis with dextrocardia and immotile cilia leading to chronic sinus and pulmonary infection). A common mistake is to assume that the presenting chronic respiratory symptoms are due to asthma. Initial findings on chest radiography are hyperinflation and peribronchial infiltrates which become larger and more extensive with disease progression (Fig. 6.10). These changes are invariably associated with the development of

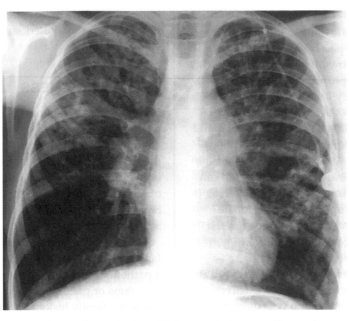

Figure 6.10 A chest radiograph showing an implantable Portocath, increased lung volumes, tramlining, and changes in keeping with bronchiectasis in a child with cystic fibrosis

bronchiectasis (damaged and dilated intermediate bronchi; see Fig. 6.4).

Pathophysiology

Although reference to a disease characterized by salty sweat goes back as far as the Middle Ages, it was not until 1989 that the gene encoding the faulty protein responsible for cystic fibrosis was finally cloned. The commonest mutation, accounting for over 70% of all cases in patients of northern European origin, is a 3 base-pair deletion at position 508 coding for a phenylalanine residue. These patients are referred to as being homozygous for the ΔF508 mutation. The abnormal protein, the cystic fibrosis transmembrane conductance regulator (CFTR), is ubiquitously expressed in epithelia, although its main pathological impact is in the lungs and gastrointestinal (including biliary tract) and reproductive systems. CFTR is a chloride channel, but it also has the ability to regulate other chloride channels and sodium channels. Since fluid transport is regulated by the balance between the opposing osmotic forces generated by Cl^- (secretory) and Na^+ (absorptive) ion

transport, it can be appreciated that an abnormality of CFTR may have wide-ranging effects. In the lung, the organ which finally determines survival in cystic fibrosis, abnormal fluid transport affects both the amount and composition of the fluid secreted into the airways. The result is plugging of small airways with viscid mucus and impaired lung epithelial defence mechanisms and hence the predisposition to chronic bacterial infection which is characteristic of cystic fibrosis.

Investigation

Diagnosis is by estimation of electrolytes in sweat – the so-called 'sweat test'. The abnormality of the chloride channel characteristic of cystic fibrosis results in high sweat levels of chloride and sodium (see above). The prevalence of the main mutations varies between different population groups and can be used to confirm the diagnosis. Genotyping can also be used for antenatal screening. Although there are several hundred different mutations resulting in the abnormal chloride channel, 80% are attributable to five mutations, and the rest are 'private' (i.e. restricted to a particular family).

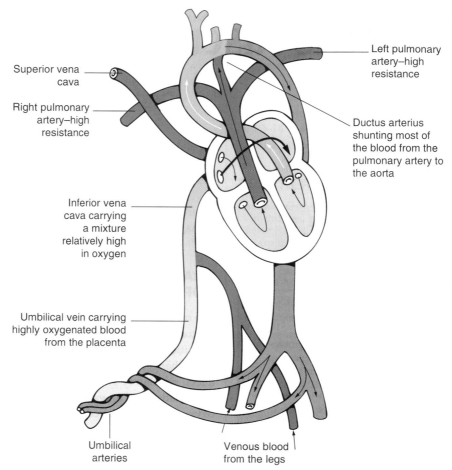

Superior vena cava

Right pulmonary artery–high resistance

Inferior vena cava carrying a mixture relatively high in oxygen

Umbilical vein carrying highly oxygenated blood from the placenta

Left pulmonary artery–high resistance

Ductus arterius shunting most of the blood from the pulmonary artery to the aorta

Umbilical arteries

Venous blood from the legs

Figure 7.1 Fetal circulation

and, via the umbilical artery, the placenta (Figs 7.1 and 7.2).

The major properties of fetal circulation are:

- An unexpanded vascular bed in liquid-filled lungs with high pulmonary vascular resistance and consequently high pulmonary artery pressure.
- Presence of a run-off through the umbilical arteries which contributes to the significantly lower systemic vascular resistance.
- Considerable right-to-left shunting at two levels: at the atrial level (through the foramen ovale, where blood is channelled to the left atrium) and at the level of ductus arteriosus. Here, the factor that governs the flow in the right-to-left direction is the pressure gradient.

Physiological changes at birth

With the interruption of the umbilical flow (which occurs as a result of spasm even if the umbilical cord is not divided) there is a sudden increase in the systemic vascular resistance. Since placental gas exchange is no longer taking place there is also a rapid rise in P_{CO_2} and a drop in P_{O_2} and pH. These and other factors (tactile and thermal) stimulate the respiratory centre and, with the first breath and expansion of the lungs, a rapid and considerable decrease in the pulmonary vascular resistance occurs with a corresponding increase in the pulmonary blood flow. The increased pulmonary venous return to the left atrium raises the left atrial pressure and closes the flap-like valve of the foramen ovale, resulting in cessation of the large right-to-left shunt. The consequent

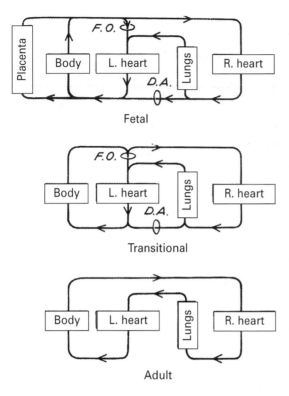

Figure 7.2 Schematic transition of fetal to adult circulation

Table 7.1 Changes in pulse rate and blood pressure with age[a]		
Age (years)	Pulse rate (beats/min)	Blood pressure (mmHg)
Newborn	125	75/55
1	120	85/55
6	100	95/60
10	90	100/70

[a]These values are for boys; they are slightly lower for girls

increase in the Po_2 results in closure of the ductus arteriosus. Complete functional closure of the foramen ovale and ductus arteriosus is not instantaneous, and the circulation during this time can be said to be in a transitional phase (Fig. 7.2).

Anatomical closure of foramen ovale and ductus arteriosus occurs over several days, and thus the early newborn period is characterized by the ease with which those adaptive changes can be reversed back to the transitional state. During this period, the pulmonary vessels are very sensitive to hypoxia and hypercapnia, to which they react by constriction, raising the pulmonary artery pressure and predisposing to the right-to-left shunting. Hypoxia and acidosis may also result in the reopening of the ductus arteriosus. In premature babies, closure of the ductus arteriosus may be delayed.

The process of physical change and physiological adaptation is not limited to the dramatic events at birth. The cardiovascular system continues to grow and develop in the same way as other organ systems in the child. The heart rate and blood pressure also change with age (Table 7.1), emphasizing the need to interpret the values of the heart rate and blood pressure in relation to the age of the child.

Aetiology and haemodynamic principles

Cardiovascular disorders can be congenital or acquired. With the improvement in social and economic circumstances in the developed world and also with the widespread use of antibiotic treatment for streptococcal throat infections, rheumatic fever has become rare (see Ch. 12). Consequently, acquired cardiac valvular lesions have become far less common, and children with congenital heart disease form the largest group seen at a paediatric cardiac clinic. Nevertheless, the cardiovascular system can be involved in a wide range of acquired pathology such as bacterial and viral infections, connective tissue and vasculitic disorders.

Congenital heart disease may be isolated or associated with other congenital abnormalities, possibly as a part of a syndrome. Chromosomal disorders, most notably Down's syndrome, are frequently associated with cardiac abnormalities. Another group of conditions associated with congenital heart are the congenital infections, the most important of which is the congenital rubella syndrome. A history of a flu-like illness with rash and lymphoadenopathy during pregnancy may be significant.

Some inheritable disorders are known to include cardiac abnormalities. Marfan's syndrome is an example. Some of the cardiomyopathies are also thought to be hereditary. Recently, great interest has been generated by the concept of the congenital nature and fetal origins of adult cardiovascular diseases such as hypertension and ischaemic heart disease (see Barker's hypothesis, Ch. 1, and Fig. 1.4).

Congenital heart disease is subdivided into two categories: those with cyanosis (cyanotic) and those without cyanosis (acyanotic). The incidence of all congenital heart disease is estimated at 1% of live births. By far the commonest abnormality is the ventricular septal defect (VSD). Tetralogy of Fallot is the commonest cyanotic congenital heart disease.

Acyanotic cardiac disorders

Most congenital heart lesions belong to this group, and the following are relatively common:

Conditions with left-to-right shunt
Ventricular septal defect (VSD)
Atrial septal defect (ASD)
Patent ductus arteriosus (PDA)

Conditions with obstructive lesions
Coarctation of the aorta
Aortic stenosis
Pulmonary stenosis

Combined lesions also occur. The haemodynamics are then complex and reflect the interaction of the underlying lesions.

It is important to appreciate that although the lesions in both left-to-right shunt and obstructive disorders are congenital in nature, they evolve and may change in severity with age. This is a function of growth and development that continues throughout childhood. As these lesions may change in severity, their management may require revision and hence it is important to keep even those children with initially mild cardiac lesions under surveillance. Fortunately, in the majority of cases, the tendency is for the lesion to become less severe with age. This is particularly true of the VSD, the commonest congenital cardiac lesion (>30% of all lesions), which is

discussed in some detail later. Reference to the other conditions will be made where relevant and in the appropriate depth and context (for an outline of the more important conditions see Beyond Core: scanning more defects 1 – other acyanotic defects (see p. 134)).

Conditions with left-to-right shunt
A spectrum of severity exists for each of these conditions. At one end, small defects leading to small-volume shunts result in little or no symptoms. They may, however, produce loud murmurs, as in the classic case of a small VSD.

At the other end of the spectrum, large defects lead to large-volume shunts, resulting in significant haemodynamic disturbances and hence are symptomatic. In the presence of a large-volume left-to-right shunt, blood is diverted from left to right as a function of the higher pressure on the left. This means that the pulmonary circulation has to cope with an increased volume of blood, and pulmonary plethora results. This clinically may present with increased frequency of chest infections and decreased exercise tolerance. In more severe cases frank heart failure results. Overt heart failure presents as dyspnoea, further limitation of tolerance for physical activity and increased sweating. Cyanosis from pulmonary oedema and cold extremities from poor peripheral perfusion are also symptoms of severe cardiac failure. In infants, a characteristic feeding cycle may be seen (see p. 140). Children in a compensated state may be tipped into heart failure by intercurrent chest infections.

If the pulmonary circulation is chronically overloaded by a left-to-right shunt, irreversible damage occurs to the pulmonary vasculature, leading to increased pulmonary vascular resistance and pulmonary hypertension. Consequently the pressure in the right side of the heart increases, and when it becomes higher than on the left, the shunt reverses and cyanosis ensues. This state of affairs, Eisenmenger's syndrome, is a serious and incurable condition. The approach to children with large left-to-right shunts is governed by the need to avoid the development of pulmonary hypertension, and should include monitoring for the signs of early changes in the pulmonary circulation.

Conditions with obstructive lesions
The clinical manifestations here also depend on the severity and mild cases are asymptomatic. In severe aortic stenosis the left ventricular output is restricted, while in coarctation, flow to the lower half of the body is compromised (see Beyond core: scanning more defects 1 – other acyanotic defects (see p. 134)). In pulmonary stenosis, right ventricular output is restricted.

Cyanotic heart disorders

The haemodynamic feature which leads to cyanosis in this group of conditions is the right-to-left shunt. The existence of such a shunt is usually governed by the presence of structural abnormalities that result in elevation of pressure within the pulmonary circulation to a level above that in the systemic circulation. This pressure gradient represents the driving force for right-to-left flow. Shunting usually occurs through an associated defect that involves a communication between the two sides of the heart (e.g. VSD, PDA).

As a consequence of the shunt, deoxygenated blood mixes with oxygenated blood designated for systemic supply. When the overall amount of deoxygenated haemoglobin in this systemic blood reaches a certain level, cyanosis occurs. As this 'mixing' occurs via a communication between the pulmonary and systemic circulations that bypasses the lungs, cyanosis persists even if the oxygen concentration in the inspired air is increased to 100%. This is the basis of the hyperoxia test, which is a useful way of distinguishing cyanosis caused by a right-to-left shunt from that due to respiratory disorders in which raising the inspired oxygen raises the arterial oxygen saturation.

It may be difficult to recognize mild degrees of cyanosis in babies, in whom it may be regarded simply as deep colouring. The cyanosis may be mild at rest but worsens with physical activity or crying. In certain uncorrected congenital heart disorders, babies with mild cyanosis may have episodes of sudden increase in the cyanosis and irritability. These are called hypercyanotic or blue

spells. The habit of 'squatting' is also seen in children with untreated cyanotic heart disease (see p. 136).

Many combinations of cardiac structural abnormalities belong to the group of cyanotic congenital heart disorders. Some of these are quite complex and rare. In the next section, only tetralogy of Fallot is discussed, but it will serve to exemplify the basic haemodynamic and pathophysiological principles which are to a variable extent shared by most other cyanotic cardiac conditions. A brief description of transposition of the aorta and pulmonary artery is provided in Beyond core: scanning more defects 2 – transposition of the great arteries.

HISTORY, EXAMINATION AND INVESTIGATION

History taking

Parents of children with possible cardiac disease usually have high levels of anxiety, and sensitivity in dealing with these families is essential.

The vast majority of children evaluated for suspected cardiovascular disease are asymptomatic. The suspicion of possible cardiovascular disease may have arisen because of a murmur discovered in the course of a physical examination conducted for some other purpose (screening or during an illness, etc.). The majority of the children will prove to have innocent (non-organic) murmurs. Even in the minority who prove to have an organic murmur, this is usually a small VSD of no haemodynamic significance, giving rise to no symptoms. Children with large septal defects and other serious cardiovascular pathologies may be symptomatic.

In general the symptomatology in children with cardiovascular disorders is usually related to:

- Left-to-right shunt
- Heart failure
- Right-to-left shunt
- Inadequacy of cardiac output in obstructive lesions (rare)
- Associated abnormalities, syndromes, etc.

Large left-to-right shunts result in pulmonary plethora, which may present with increased frequency of chest infections and limitation of tolerance of physical activity. This may progress to overt heart failure, which manifests itself as dyspnoea, further limitation of the tolerance of physical activity and increased sweating. Heart failure may also be caused by obstructive lesions. Cyanosis (see Fig. 16.4) is the cardinal manifestation of right-to-left shunt.

The symptoms of the individual lesions are discussed under the relevant headings.

Physical examination

Common omissions in physical examination of the cardiovascular system in children are:

- Looking for signs of respiratory distress
- Checking the femoral pulses
- Noting the quality and splitting of the second heart sound
- Measuring the blood pressure (occasionally four-limb blood pressure)
- Palpating for hepatomegaly
- Looking for dysmorphic features and other associations.

Inspection
Nutritional state, colour and signs of respiratory distress should be noted. Specific signs to look for are: bulging of the precordium as a sign of cardiac hypertrophy, surgical scars as a clue to previous cardiac surgery, and clubbing of fingers. One should look also for dysmorphic features and associated abnormalities.

Palpation
Feeling the precordium provides useful information about the site and character of the apical beat, the presence of any thrills, right or left ventricular heaves or the presence of an active precordium (a sign of a hyperdynamic circulation, classically seen in babies with patent ductus arteriosus).

Feeling the pulses is an important part of the cardiovascular examination. In neonates and infants, absent or weak femoral pulses are the classical signs of coarctation of the aorta. Radiofemoral delay is another cardinal sign of this condition which can be checked for in older children with slower heart rates. Full pulses are a

sign of hyperdynamic circulation. Feeling the pulses is also crucial in the evaluation of the peripheral circulation and state of hydration; thready pulses are characteristic of a shocked state, severe dehydration and bleeding.

Hepatomegaly is as significant a sign of heart failure in a child as ankle oedema in an adult, and palpating the abdomen is an integral part of the cardiovascular system examination in children. Splenomegaly also ensues in long-standing heart failure; pitting oedema is uncommon.

Auscultation
The objectives of this examination technique are to:

- Appreciate the quality of the heart sounds
- Detect additional sounds including murmurs
- Note the presence or absence of pulmonary oedema.

It is important that each of these objectives be pursued in a systematic manner. The detection of one abnormal sign should not overshadow the value of pursuing the systematic examination for the possible presence of other signs.

Heart sounds are usually loud in children. This reflects the thin chest wall. Obese children may, however, have 'quiet' heart sounds. Splitting of the second heart sound is normally accentuated during inspiration as the negative intrathoracic pressure increases flow to the right side of the heart, thus delaying pulmonary valve closure.

Cardiac murmurs are classified as systolic or diastolic, and systolic murmurs are further qualified as pansystolic and ejection systolic. Diastolic murmurs are described as early or mid-diastolic. Such characterization is not easy in children who have relatively fast heart rates and whose cooperation cannot be guaranteed. It is also helpful to define cardiac murmurs in children in terms of their location, radiation and, when possible, quality of sound.

Murmurs best heard at the lower sternal edge are likely to represent VSD. Rarely an atrioventricular valve lesion may be the source. These murmurs are low pitched and are better appreciated using the bell of the stethoscope.

Murmurs heard at the base of the heart (adjacent to the upper part of the sternum;

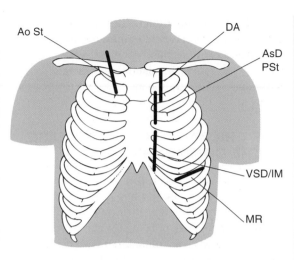

Figure 7.3 Diagrammatic representation of the precordium showing the usual sites at which the murmur of the most common acyanotic lesions are heard. IM, innocent murmur; DA, ductus arteriosus; AoSt, aortic stenosis; PSt, pulmonary stenosis; MR, mitral regurgitation

Fig. 7.3) are high pitched and are better heard using the diaphragm of the stethoscope. These murmurs usually arise from aortic or pulmonary valve lesions. Murmurs arising from aortic valve lesions tend to radiate to the neck; those from pulmonary valve lesions tend to be transmitted to the back. In coarctation of the aorta, the murmur radiates to both the neck and back.

A murmur that is musical or vibratory in nature, heard at the lower sternal edge, tends to be functional or innocent, although a small VSD can sometimes mimic this quality (see Innocent murmurs, p. 132).

Pulmonary oedema is a serious manifestation of advanced heart failure. Fine crepitations at the base of the lungs are an important sign (located posteriorly in children spending most of the time in supine position). This finding is usually accompanied by other signs of respiratory distress and heart failure.

Blood pressure measurement
Measuring the blood pressure is an integral part of the evaluation of the cardiovascular system in children, and it is important to use the appropriate size cuff, usually two-thirds of the length of the arm.

BEYOND CORE

FINE TUNING TO HEART SOUNDS

Normal splitting of the second heart sound is strong evidence against the presence of a range of conditions including tetralogy of Fallot, and severe pulmonary stenosis (atresia). Fixed splitting of the second heart sound (no change during the inspiration/expiration cycle) is the classic sign of an ASD.

Sinus arrhythmia is prominent in children, and is by far the commonest cause of an irregular heart beat or irregularity on the electrocardiogram (ECG). This physiological 'arrhythmia' is characterized by increase of the heart rate on inspiration followed by a decrease on expiration. Apart from murmurs, other added sounds include clicks (noises made by the opening of abnormal valves) and a pericardial rub (an important sign of pericarditis; a condition that is usually caused by viral infections or involvement of the pericardium in connective tissue disorders).

In heart failure, a prominent third heart sound together with the usual tachycardia generates a three-component effect known as gallop rhythm.

There are certain difficulties with the technique of auscultation in children not seen in adults. Two considerations have to be kept in mind. Firstly, one is likely to encounter fast heart rates, particularly in neonates and infants (rates of 150 beats/min or more are not unusual). At high rates, it becomes difficult to distinguish the first from the second heart sound, let alone additional sounds and murmurs. Secondly, high respiratory rates are the norm in infants and small children. In a tachypnoeic baby, a respiratory rate of 100–120 beats/min is not unusual, and differentiating the short whiffing noise of inspiration and expiration from a murmur can be difficult. As a general rule, it is worth investing some time in trying to get in tune with the fast heart rhythm and rapid breathing, before concentrating on any specific signs.

Blood pressure varies with age (Table 7.1), and it also varies among healthy children of the same age. Like many other anthropological parameters, the use of centile charts is necessary for the correct interpretation of the values obtained. Measurement of blood pressure on all four limbs is necessary in children presenting with a murmur or with heart failure. It is also necessary in all hypertensive children, as coarctation of the aorta is an important cause of such presentations in this age group.

Investigation

Some congenital heart defects may be diagnosed antenatally by ultrasound scanning.

Chest radiography provides useful information about the size and shape of the heart and the vascularity of the lungs: cardiomegaly is the typical finding in heart failure, while a boot-shaped heart is what is classically seen in tetralogy of Fallot (Fig. 7.4). Right-to-left shunts are associated with a decrease in the vascularity of the lung fields (oligaemia), while left-to-right shunts are associated with an increase in lung vascular markings (plethora, see Fig. 7.5).

The ECG is helpful in evaluating chamber hypertrophy and rhythm disturbances. Echocardiography is a non-invasive technique that frequently allows a specific diagnosis to be established. This is particularly true of the modern echo machines with added facilities, such as Doppler echocardiography.

Cardiac catheterization, usually as part of preoperative preparation, outlines the exact anatomical relationships, and may be the only way to establish a diagnosis in certain situations.

THE CHILD WITH HEART DISEASE IN THE COMMUNITY

The presence of heart disease in a child usually generates levels of anxiety in parents and teachers which is higher than the situation merits. Such children run the risk of being overprotected.

In the vast majority of children with heart disease, no alteration in life-style is required and no restriction of activity is necessary. These children should be allowed to lead normal lives and should be encouraged to engage in physical activities and sports. Only a minority will require some restriction on their physical activity, usually in the form of avoidance of competitive sports.

It is important to emphasize the need for adequate prophylaxis for subacute bacterial endocarditis (SBE) at times of potential bacteraemia. Parents should be informed about the need for antibiotics prior to procedures such as dental extraction (and other minor surgery), and should be instructed to inform the dentist about the presence of the heart disease. Attention to dental hygiene is important.

BEYOND CORE

THE PAEDIATRIC ECG

In general, a paediatric ECG is read according to the same rules as in adults. There are certain characteristics, however, that should be kept in mind:

- There is a prominent sinus arrhythmia.
- The heart rate should always be judged against the age of the patient (Table 7.1).
- The heart axis lies more to the right than in adults. This reflects the thicker right ventricular mass which persists throughout infancy.

- Voltage criteria alone are not enough to diagnose hypertrophy (the chest wall is thin and the different positioning of the heart in the chest cavity may affect the validity of these criteria).
- The T wave is negative in the right ventricular leads, and the presence of a positive T wave in these leads is an important sign of pulmonary hypertension and right ventricular hypertrophy.

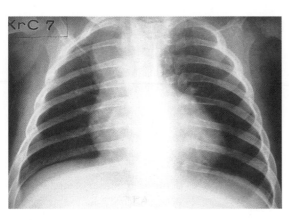

Figure 7.4 The typical appearance on chest radiography in tetralogy of Fallot. A boot-shaped heart and oligaemic lung fields can be seen. (Reproduced by courtesy of TALC)

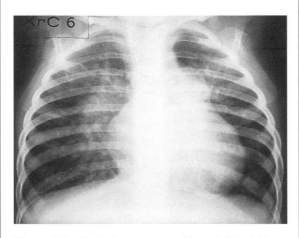

Figure 7.5 Typical appearance of large left to right shunts (in this case a PDA): marked enlargement of the main pulmonary arteries with widening of the main branches on both sides and plethoric lung fields. (Reproduced by courtesy of TALC)

The pharmacological treatment of children with heart disease should be closely supervised. Drugs such as digoxin should be carefully labelled, the dose should be precisely calculated (and double checked) and the amount of syrup to be given should be clearly indicated to the parents with an explanation about the possible side-effects and risks of overdose. It is important to remember that in growing children, drug dosages may be outgrown, and these should be periodically reviewed.

CORE PROBLEMS

Despite the complexity and diversity of the pathology that may affect the cardiovascular system in children, in practice the majority of children with cardiovascular disease present with one or more of the following three clinical problems:

- Murmur
- Cyanosis
- Dyspnoea.

MURMUR

The overwhelming majority of children evaluated because of a heart murmur will turn out to have either an innocent murmur or a small VSD. In either situation these children will remain asymptomatic. Nevertheless, the possibility of a significant underlying heart lesion should be considered and careful attention to history and physical examination is important. Frequently an ECG and chest radiograph are obtained.

History of recurrent chest infections, decreased exercise tolerance and breathlessness may point to the presence of significant left-to-right shunt such as produced by a large VSD. Similar symptoms may be produced by bronchial asthma. Because both asthma and heart murmurs are common in childhood, they can coexist in a particular child, and these symptoms should not automatically be ascribed to the presence of heart disease.

A history of chest pain or fainting on exertion suggests the presence of a significant obstructive lesion such as obstructive cardiomyopathy or aortic stenosis. Though these conditions are relatively rare, it is important not to miss such a diagnosis as it requires close follow-up by a paediatric cardiologist, and some limitation of exercise may be necessary in severe cases. Looking for signs of other specific cardiac lesions is also important (see previous section).

In practice, the commonest situation is an asymptomatic child with a systolic murmur heard at the lower left sternal edge with minimal radiation who otherwise has no signs of cardiovascular disease. The question relevant to further management is whether this is an innocent (functional) murmur or that of a small VSD.

Innocent murmurs

These are by far the commonest variety of murmurs that one is likely to hear in children. They are produced by rapid blood flow and turbulence in the great vessels and across normal valves. As the term implies, these murmurs do not result from cardiac structural abnormalities or from the presence of any other pathology. There are different types of innocent murmurs, heard at different sites (Fig. 7.3) of the precordium.

> **Types of innocent murmur**
> - A venous hum is generated by the blood flow in the great veins, heard at the upper chest; it may simulate a machinery murmur of PDA
> - A flow murmur results from rapid blood flow through a normal pulmonary valve, heard at the upper part of the left sternal edge; it may simulate the short systolic murmur of pulmonary stenosis
> - A musical murmur the commonest variety, best heard at the lower part of the left sternal edge, and is systolic; it may simulate the systolic murmur of a VSD

The only significance of an innocent murmur is that, occasionally, it may not be possible to distinguish reliably from that of organic origin.

> **Characteristics of innocent murmurs**
> - Systolic in timing, short and of low intensity. They are never accompanied by thrills or have significant radiation
> - Tendency to intensify at times of increased cardiac output such as after exercise or during a febrile illness
> - Tendency to change in intensity with change of posture (usually attenuated when sitting), and in the case of venous hum, on changing head position

In many ways it does not matter much to the management or prognosis whether the child has an innocent murmur or that of a small VSD, except for one point. Children with VSDs (regardless of the size of the defect) qualify for SBE prophylaxis as long as they have the defect. This is why a referral for echocardiography is necessary if doubt remains as whether the child has an innocent murmur or that of a VSD. The family should be reassured about the benign nature of both possibilities.

✳ KEY DIAGNOSIS

Ventricular septal defect

As mentioned earlier, this is the commonest congenital cardiac abnormality. It accounts for about 25% of all congenital cardiac disorders. The haemodynamics depend on the size of the defect.

Haemodynamics

A *small VSD* with left-to-right shunt of small magnitude causes no significant haemodynamic disturbance and the child is asymptomatic. However, the jet of blood forced through a small opening causes turbulence and results in a loud and harsh murmur which may be accompanied by a thrill. The murmur may be absent at birth but appears a few days afterwards when the normal fall in the pulmonary artery pressure has occurred.

A *large VSD* results in significant haemodynamic disturbance and the child is likely to be symptomatic. In this situation the fall in the pulmonary vascular resistance normally seen in the first few days after birth takes longer, and it may not take 3–4 weeks for the full pressure gradient to develop. In this period, the baby is usually asymptomatic and the murmur may be faint or absent since the lack of a pressure gradient limits the volume of the shunt.

As the shunt reaches its maximum volume, a considerable proportion of the left ventricular output is diverted to the right ventricle. Consequently, right ventricular output and pulmonary blood flow increase. As a result, pulmonary venous return to the left atrium increases and left ventricular overload occurs. Thus, both ventricles are burdened with increased preloads and, to cope, both undergo hypertrophy.

Clinical picture

In children with small VSDs, the clinical signs are limited to a pansystolic murmur sometimes associated with a thrill (see above). However, some infants with large VSDs develop frank heart failure; they become tachypnoeic, fail to thrive and suffer repeated chest infections. Medical intervention at this stage is necessary (see Cardiac failure, p. 139). Other infants may continue in the compensated state. They may become dyspnoeic on physical exertion (feeding is the major physical activity at this age) and may be prone to recurrent chest infections, which may tip them into heart failure from time to time.

Signs of a large VSD include a bulging precordium with forceful apical beat and a systolic thrill. Characteristically there is a pansystolic murmur heard in the fourth intercostal space at the left sternal edge (Fig. 7.3) and radiating all over the precordium.

Investigation

In the case of a small VSD, the ECG and chest radiograph are normal, whereas in a child with a large VSD, the ECG shows biventricular hypertrophy and the chest radiograph shows cardiomegaly and increased pulmonary vascularity. The diagnosis of VSD, the determination of its size, and the volume of the shunt depends on echocardiography; catheterization is rarely required.

The natural course

A large number of children remain asymptomatic. Another group, children with large defects, manifest the clinical picture of large VSD described earlier. A significant number of all VSDs, however, decrease in size spontaneously and may close completely. Smaller defects are more likely to close, but even large defects may close spontaneously.

In a small number of patients with large VSDs, the exposure of the pulmonary vessels to a chronically increased blood flow leads to Eisenimenger's syndrome. The risk of developing SBE is not dependent on the VSD size. This complication is more likely to occur in older children.

Treatment

Parents should be reassured about the benign nature of small VSDs, and children should be encouraged to lead normal lives. Attention to dental hygiene is important, and antibacterial prophylaxis at times of potential bacteraemia, such as dental extraction, should be provided.

The treatment of infants with large VSDs is directed at the control of congestive heart failure.

Some may respond well to treatment and return to the compensated state. As the natural course of the defect is to become smaller or spontaneously close, conservative management is appropriate. However, in those in whom heart failure is difficult to control, early surgical closure, which carries little risk, is the treatment of choice. For those with large VSDs who do not undergo surgery, close monitoring for early signs of pulmonary hypertension is necessary.

Subacute bacterial endocarditis

All children with structural cardiac defects are at risk of developing this serious complication and qualify for prophylaxis. In some cases the risk may remain even after corrective surgery, and such children should continue to receive prophylaxis.

The prophylaxis regimen consists of administering an appropriate antibiotic at times of potential bacteraemia, such as dental extraction or other surgical procedures such as instrumentation of the bowel or lower urinary tract. The timing, route, dose and choice of the antibiotic varies according to the nature of the procedure. For dental extraction the usual practice is to give a large dose of amoxycillin 1 h prior to the procedure as the involved organism is usually *Streptococcus viridans*.

SBE may present as a fever of unknown origin, with chronic non-specific symptoms, or with a change in the character of the murmur. Confirmation of the diagnosis rests on positive blood cultures. Frequently it is possible to demonstrate bacterial vegetations on the echocardiogram. Treatment involves administering prolonged (4–8 week) intravenous courses of bactericidal antibiotics, and should be supervised by a paediatric cardiologist.

Murmur in a premature baby

This most commonly represents delayed closure of the ductus arteriosus. The murmur is usually systolic or machinery (spilling over into diastole), and is frequently associated with full pulses and other signs of a hyperdynamic circulation. The condition may contribute to the difficulties of ventilating these babies; in

BEYOND CORE

SCANNING MORE DEFECTS (1) OTHER ACYANOTIC DEFECTS

Atrial septal defect

Two types of ASDs are seen. The more common is the isolated ASD with normal atrioventricular valves: the ostium secundum defect. The second type is associated with abnormal atrioventricular valves and an extension of the defect to the ventricular septum: the ostium primum defect or endocardial cushion defect. The latter is a rare condition but is relatively common among children with Down's syndrome. We will briefly discuss the ostium secundum defect.

Haemodynamics

These are generally similar to other conditions with left-to-right shunts. However in ASDs the shunt occurs at the atrial level and most of the burden is on the right ventricle and the left ventricle is spared.

Clinical manifestations

Even children with large ASDs are generally asymptomatic. However, the physical findings are characteristic. There is a systolic murmur which is produced by the increased flow across the normal pulmonary valve and not by the shunted blood across the atrial septum. Hence the murmur is heard over the pulmonary area and is transmitted to the back. The characteristic finding is fixed splitting of the second heart sound. This is explained on the basis of increased flow to the right atrium, which, because of the shunt, persists throughout inspiration and expiration.

Investigations

Cardiomegaly and pulmonary plethora are seen on radiography in large ASDs. The ECG reflects right ventricular hypertrophy and characteristically there is a right ventricular conduction delay. The echocardiogram will demonstrate the defects and allow measurement of the magnitude of the flow.

Treatment and complications

Surgical closure or closure with a device inserted by catheter may be advised even for asymptomatic children if the defect is large. SBE is extremely rare in this condition but untreated, there is a risk of atrial fibrillation and possibly pulmonary hypertension in later life.

Patent ductus arteriosus

The haemodynamics and symptomatology are generally similar to those of VSD. In a large PDA, the clinical features range from no symptoms at one end of the spectrum to frank heart failure at the other (Fig. 7.5). The physical signs of a hyperdynamic circulation are characteristic, and include an active precordium, bounding pulses and wide pulse pressure. The murmur is machinery in type. Treatment is aimed at the control of heart failure when present; the definitive treatment is surgical, though a new device has recently been developed which can be introduced during cardiac catheterization. As pointed out earlier, a PDA in a premature baby reflects delayed closure of a normal ductus. Closure can be expected to happen spontaneously as the baby progresses towards term or it can be accelerated with the help of drugs. In a term baby, a PDA reflects a structurally abnormal duct that is unlikely to close on its own.

Aortic stenosis

In aortic stenosis, the afterload on the left ventricle is increased. This leads to hypertrophy of the left ventricle and sometimes to heart failure. The restricted left ventricular output in severe cases may compromise the blood supply to vital organs, in particular during periods of increased demand such as physical activity. Chest pain and fainting on exercise are recognized features related to poor blood supply to coronary and cerebral arteries. There is a risk of sudden death but it is rare.

The classic sign is a short systolic murmur heard at the base of the heart, usually on the right upper sternal edge, characteristically transmitted to the neck. The pulses in severe cases may be of small volume. Mild degrees of aortic stenosis are asymptomatic. The severity of a lesion may, however, increase with age.

The follow-up of these patients should be supervised by a paediatric cardiologist. Generally speaking, children with aortic stenosis should be allowed to regulate the amount of exercise they undertake, restriction of activity may be required in severe cases.

Coarctation of the aorta

This involves constriction of a length of the aorta, usually just below the origin of the left subclavian artery, leading to hypertension in the upper half of the body while the blood supply to the lower half is compromised. Renal mechanisms involving the renin–angiotensin system contribute to generalized hypertension.

Coarctation of the aorta is an important cause of heart failure in infancy. Beyond this period it is rarely symptomatic. Weakness or pain in the legs after exercise may be present. Coarctation of the aorta is a feature of Turner's syndrome.

The cardinal signs of coarctation of the aorta are either absent or weak femoral pulses, the presence of radiofemoral delay and disparity in the blood pressure between the upper and lower body, being higher in the arms and lower in the legs (the reverse of what is found in normal people when the blood pressure is obtained by the cuff method). A short systolic murmur is often heard at the left sternal edge, and is well transmitted to the back and occasionally to the neck.

The chest radiograph in infancy may show cardiomegaly when heart failure is present. In older children, the left ventricle is prominent. Notching of the inferior border of the ribs from erosion by pressure from enlarged collateral vessels is a late sign on radiography. The ECG reflects left ventricular hypertrophy. The treatment is surgical.

Other obstructive lesions

There are other variants of obstruction to the left side of the heart. Obstructive cardiomyopathy involves subvalvular stenosis. William's syndrome is associated with supravalvular aortic obstruction. Constriction of a significant length of the aortic arch, so-called interruption of aortic arch syndromes, may be viewed as an extreme case of coarctation.

which case it may be appropriate to accelerate the closure of the duct by restricting fluids and administering indomethacin, a prostaglandin inhibitor.

CYANOSIS

Two modes of presentation merit specific attention:

- Cyanosis recognized at birth
- Cyanosis in older infants and children.

Cyanosis at birth

Clinical features and diagnosis
By far the commonest cause of cyanosis in newborn babies is a cold environment. This is particularly true of the fingers and toes, but also applies to the ears and lips. Examination of the tongue may be helpful in making a distinction between central and peripheral cyanosis. However, in neonates the issue may be difficult to resolve. Warming the baby and evaluation with the help of a saturation monitor or arterial blood gases may be necessary.

Cyanosis due to a decrease in oxygen saturation of haemoglobin can be either cardiac or pulmonary in origin or, less commonly, due to neurological causes. Clinical data together with the ECG and chest radiograph should point to the correct diagnosis. Prematurity, respiratory distress and poor expansion of the lungs, may indicate the respiratory distress syndrome or congenital pneumonia as the cause of cyanosis. The presence of heart murmur, oligaemia of the lung fields, abnormal shape of the heart on radiography, or an abnormal ECG points to a cardiac problem. A history of asphyxia or of administration of medication causing central nervous system depression, such as diamorphine, and absence of signs of respiratory distress may indicate respiratory depression as the cause of cyanosis.

The question whether cyanosis is due to respiratory or cardiac causes can be answered by the hyperoxia test. This involves administering 100% oxygen to the cyanotic baby, while monitoring the P_{O_2}; if no significant rise is seen, the presence of a right-to-left shunt is confirmed (see p. 127).

Having established the fact that a baby has cyanotic heart disease, it is important that a more definitive diagnosis is reached quickly. Certain structural abnormalities of the heart with right-to-left shunting may result in a pulmonary flow which is so compromised that the blood flow to the lungs is only maintained by the presence of another shunt in the left-to-right direction through a PDA. However, the duct may follow the normal pattern of closure in the first few days after birth and the blood supply to the lungs may cease, with disastrous consequences. This state of affairs is referred to as duct dependency (see Beyond core: a state of dependency).

Initial management

It may be possible, on the basis of the clinical picture and initial investigations, to determine whether the lesion in a particular baby with a heart defect is likely to be duct-dependent. If it is, patency of the duct must be maintained by prostaglandin infusion until it is possible to perform corrective or palliative surgery. In cyanotic defects, palliative surgery frequently involves the creation of another communication between the right and left side to improve the pulmonary blood supply. This means emergency transfer to a paediatric cardiac centre. Since an increase in P_{O_2} is a stimulant for closure of the duct, care should be taken with oxygen therapy in these babies in the interim. Apart from this, the management of babies with cyanotic heart disease is supportive (see below).

Cyanosis in older babies and children

The differential diagnoses of cardiac, respiratory and neurological disease causing cyanosis still applies. In this group of children, however, enough clinical data is usually available to allow the distinction to be made. Tetralogy of Fallot is the commonest form of cyanotic heart disease.

✳ KEY DIAGNOSIS

Tetralogy of Fallot

Four structural features characterize this condition:

1. Narrowing of right ventricular out flow tract
2. Overriding of the aorta
3. VSD
4. Right ventricular hypertrophy.

Figure 7.6 shows the embryological development of Fallot's tetralogy, the most important feature of which is deviation to the right of the septum, which divides the arterial trunk.

Haemodynamics

The presence of pulmonary stenosis restricts the amount of blood pumped into the pulmonary artery thus increasing the proportion shunted into the overriding aorta. The degree of right ventricular hypertrophy and the volume of the shunt are proportional to the degree of narrowing at and below the pulmonary valve.

Clinical features

Babies with tetralogy of Fallot are usually pink at birth. Cyanosis develops gradually over the following weeks and months. These infants are, however, prone to episodes when cyanosis suddenly increases and they become dyspnoeic, irritable and, on occasion, unconscious. Such episodes, called hypercyanotic or blue spells, are thought to be triggered by a reduction in the systemic vascular resistance resulting in an increase in the right to left shunt. Children with tetralogy of Fallot also have reduced exercise

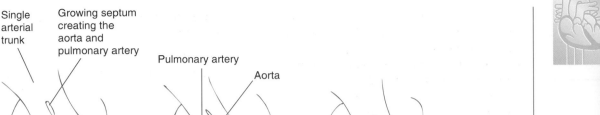

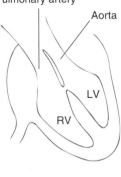

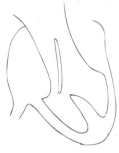

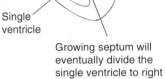

Single arterial trunk

Growing septum creating the aorta and pulmonary artery

Single ventricle

Growing septum will eventually divide the single ventricle to right and left ventricles

Pulmonary artery

Aorta

LV

RV

The two correctly aligned septa result in normal anatomy

Deviation of the vascular septum to the right results in all the features of ToF
- overriding aorta
- VSD
- right ventricular outflow obstruction
- subsequent right ventricular hypertrophy

Figure 7.6 Embryology of Fallot's tetralogy. In the embryo the two ventricles originate from a single ventricle which is divided by the ventricular septum into right and left ventricles. The pulmonary artery and aorta originate from a single arterial trunk that is also divided by a septum. Normally the two septa meet. In tetralogy of Fallot, all the features can be explained on the basis of a deviation to the right of the septum that divides the arterial trunk. LV, left ventricle; RV, right ventricle

tolerance. In toddlers and young children with significant right-to-left shunt, hypoxia may be exaggerated during physical activity. Feeling more breathless, these children learn the habit of squatting: flexing the thighs and knees raises the systemic vascular resistance, thus reducing the right-to-left shunt and improving oxygenation.

On examination, there is clubbing of fingers and toes. Growth is usually poor. Right ventricular heave, often associated with a systolic thrill, is found on palpation. Auscultation reveals a single second heart sound and a systolic murmur over the pulmonary area (see Fig. 7.3).

Complications
Chronic hypoxia stimulates haemopoietic activity of the bone marrow, and polycythaemia results. This leads to increased blood viscosity and a hypercoagulable state. Children with tetralogy

of Fallot are also at risk of developing bacterial endocarditis and cerebral abscess. Heart failure is rare.

Investigation
The chest radiograph shows the characteristic boot-shaped heart and oligaemia of the lung fields (see Fig. 7.4). The ECG reflects right ventricular hypertrophy, and echocardiography confirms the diagnosis.

Management
The definitive treatment for tetralogy of Fallot is corrective surgery. The optimal timing for such major surgery is later in infancy when the affected babies are bigger and stronger. However, with modern surgical techniques, early corrective surgery is becoming a realistic option in many centres.

In certain cases the severity of the structural lesions is such that it is difficult to maintain the general health of these infants for any length of time. The decision is then whether to perform the corrective surgery at an early age, if the risks are considered favourable, or to undertake a palliative procedure. The latter usually involves creating an artificial shunt to improve pulmonary flow (the traditional procedure is the Blalock–Taussig shunt between the pulmonary artery and the subclavian artery). In extreme cases, a shunting procedure such as this may be required as an emergency (see Beyond core: a state of dependency).

Medical management of stable infants awaiting corrective surgery involves careful observation and avoidance of complications. These infants are at risk of cerebral thrombosis, a complication which is more common in the presence of marked polycythaemia. Dehydration should be promptly corrected.

Hypercyanotic (blue) spells are managed in the following manner:

- Calm and reassuring behaviour
- Knee–chest position
- Oxygen
- Pharmacological treatment (diamorphine, sodium bicarbonate, β blockers).

In spite of the dramatic nature of these spells, a fatal outcome is rare.

Iron deficiency seems to increase the risk of thrombosis in children with untreated cyanotic heart disease. It may also increase the frequency and severity of the blue spells. Because of the accompanying polycythaemia, iron deficiency may exist at haemoglobin values in the normal range. Attention to diet, iron supplements and maintenance of the red blood cell indices in the normal range are important steps in the management of these children.

Children with cyanotic heart disease, as with other children with structural heart defects, are at risk of developing SBE and measures to prevent this complication should be observed (see Ventricular septal defect, p. 133).

DYSPNOEA

Overt heart failure is a well-recognized cause of respiratory distress in children. When the presence of a pre-existing cardiac pathology is known, or when the full blown picture is present,

BEYOND CORE

SCANNING MORE DEFECTS 2 – TRANSPOSITION OF THE GREAT ARTERIES

This is the second most common form of cyanotic congenital heart disease. In this condition the aorta arises from the right ventricle and the pulmonary artery from the left ventricle. The venous return to the atria remains in the normal relationship. Desaturated blood is ejected from the right ventricle into the aorta, whereas the oxygenated blood delivered to the left atrium and ventricle simply returns to the lungs. Thus the systemic and pulmonary circulations operate as two parallel and separate circuits. In this situation, survival is only possible because of the presence of a patent foramen ovale, usually together with some other communication such as a VSD or a PDA.

Transposition of the great vessels presents with cyanosis and tachypnoea at birth. Untreated, the majority of babies would not survive beyond the neonatal period. The condition is a medical emergency, and early appropriate intervention may be life-saving. Treatment involves maintaining the patency of the duct by means of a prostaglandin infusion until a palliative operation is possible, which usually involves creation of a bigger communication between the two sides through a septostomy (creating a defect in the atrial septum). The definitive treatment is correction of the anatomical relationships at open heart surgery.

A STATE OF DEPENDENCY

Duct dependency is generally seen when either the systemic or pulmonary circulation is dependent on the blood flow through a patent ductus arteriosus. It is also seen in those situations where the systemic and pulmonary circulations operate in isolation from each other and mixing mainly happens through a patent duct, as seen in certain cases of transposition of great vessels (see Beyond core: scanning more defects 2 – transposition of the great vessels).

In conditions with a pulmonary flow dependent on a patent duct, babies usually present with cyanosis at or soon after birth, and their chest radiographs show marked oligaemia. Examples are pulmonary atresia (with obligatory ASD or VSD) and severe tetralogy of Fallot. In both situations an intracardiac right-to-left shunt results in cyanosis, and the pulmonary blood flow is dependent on a left-to-right shunt through a patent duct.

The systemic circulation becomes dependent on blood flow through a patent duct in those situations where there is a severe degree of obstruction on the left side of the heart. Two such conditions are hypoplastic left ventricle and severe coarctation of the aorta. In the former, all of the blood is diverted from the left atrium to the right atrium (via an obligatory ASD), and all the systemic flow is dependent on a right-to-left shunt through a patent duct. Clinically, these babies have weak or absent pulses, and their colour is 'earth grey' as a result of the combined effects of hypoperfusion and cyanosis.

In severe coarctation, the blood supply to the lower half of the body is derived from a right-to-left shunt via a patent duct, while pure oxygenated blood is supplied to the upper half, normally, from the aorta (above the level of the coarctation). This results in a peculiar state of differential cyanosis, with the upper half of the body pink and the lower half blue.

The possibility of a duct-dependent heart lesion should be suspected when there is a rapid deterioration in the condition of a baby in the first few days of life (as the duct closes). In a baby that collapses it may then be necessary to consider this scenario as part of a differential diagnosis that includes sepsis and metabolic disorders.

Even if duct dependency has been diagnosed retrospectively (i.e. after the duct has started to close and clinical deterioration began) there is still a case for starting a prostaglandin infusion since this may slow the closure process or even reopen a closed duct, thus buying time until a palliative or definitive surgical procedure can be performed.

the diagnosis should be straightforward. However, occasionally the diagnosis may not be clear, and careful evaluation is necessary (see Ch. 6 for the differential diagnosis of dyspnoea in children).

Cardiac failure

Aetiology and pathogenesis

Heart failure in children is usually related to the presence of an underlying significant left-to-right shunt such as that produced by a large VSD. Sometimes an infant with a VSD in the compensated state may be tipped into heart failure by an intercurrent chest infection.

Less commonly, the underlying pathology is an obstructive lesion. Coarctation of the aorta is the most important of these (it is the commonest cause of heart failure in the neonatal period). Four-limb blood pressure is mandatory in all infants presenting in heart failure.

Acquired cardiac disease is usually the result of cardiac involvement in other systemic illnesses, such as viral and bacterial infections and connective tissue disorders. These may progress to, or even present in, heart failure. Hypertension and fluid retention accompanying renal disease can also lead to heart failure.

Rarely, rhythm disturbances, most notably supraventricular tachycardia, in a structurally normal heart may result in cardiac failure. This diagnosis should be considered in infants and children with particularly fast heart rates, i.e. above 250 beats/min.

One further situation worth mentioning is overloading the circulation with intravenous fluids, which can result in congestive heart failure. This possibility should always be considered in children with previously normal hearts who develop heart failure while on intravenous fluid therapy. It highlights the need to take extra care and precision in calculating and prescribing intravenous fluid therapy for children.

Clinical picture

The cardinal manifestations of heart failure in children are:

- Tachypnoea (frequently with other signs of respiratory distress)
- Cardiomegaly
- Hepatomegaly.

Cyanosis, basal crepitations and increased sweating are other important signs.

Frequently, frank heart failure is preceded by a period of decreased tolerance of physical activity. This may be difficult to elicit in children and particularly in infants. However, certain behavioural patterns may be suggestive.

In infants, a characteristic feeding cycle may be seen. Because the physical effort involved in feeding cannot be maintained, these infants take less volume per feed. Because of the extra work of breathing while sucking, they characteristically sweat profusely. Exhausted, these infants fall asleep inadequately fed, only to be awakened by hunger. After a short while the cycle is repeated. Such a pattern may be misinterpreted as colic, other feeding problems or even overfeeding.

The combination of poor feeding and increased demands imposed by the extra work required from the heart, functioning in an abnormal haemodynamic situation, results in a poor nutritional state with failure to thrive and, in extreme cases, emaciation. In toddlers, a decreased level of activity may reflect reduced exercise tolerance. In older children, similar information is obtained from a knowledge of their behaviour in play, sport, etc.

Management

Diuretics are the most commonly used drugs in the treatment of cardiac failure in children. Digoxin is indicated in cases with poor ventricular function. The small doses involved and the narrow margin of safety of digoxin warrants extra care when calculating the dose of and administering this drug to children. Angiotensin-converting enzyme (ACE) inhibitors are used to decrease the pre- and after-loads, as are other vasodilators.

HIGHLIGHTS AND HYPOTHESES

BARKER'S HYPOTHESIS

Adult heart disease – a matter of indulgence or a sealed fate?

Having made the observation that areas in England and Wales which at present have a higher incidence of ischaemic heart disease used to have a high infant mortality in the past, Professor D.J.P Barker, of the University of Southampton, and his team undertook a series of retrospective longitudinal studies.

Their aim was to define and explain the possible link between events early in life and the later development of adult disease. They utilized data that spanned 50 years or more.

The team was able to access the health records of a large group of people born in certain areas of England in the late 1920s. It was possible to obtain from those records details of the pregnancy, maternal health, delivery, weight at birth and feeding in early infancy,

all meticulously recorded and carefully kept. The team then succeeded in tracing a significant number of these people. They were contacted and their present state of health assessed.

The association between birth weight (hence fetal nutrition) and weight at 1 year of age with later development of ischaemic heart disease and hypertension was strong and independent of any other variable, including smoking and other environmental effects.

HIGHLIGHTS AND HYPOTHESES *cont'd*

In an attempt to explain these associations, an intriguing hypothesis was put forward. In essence, it claims that during fetal life and early infancy, certain programming of various body structures and organs takes place. Nutritional shortages at this crucial time may alter such programming for ever. Thus, poor nutrition in late pregnancy may set off the programming of the liver in such a way that its handling of lipids later in life may be the cause of hypercholesterolaemia, etc.

As might be expected, Professor Barker's views are disputed, and alternative arguments in favour of the environmental effects on the development of these diseases are cited. The controversy is likely to go on.

The additional value of Professor Barker's work lies in the ingenuity of the research and the skilful design of the studies. Such work, however, would not have been possible without the meticulousness and dedication of the health workers in the early years. Those men and women who painstakingly recorded all the possible details about their patients. It is difficult now to imagine what purpose they thought they were serving in recording the weights of the placentas, the circumferences of the abdomen, etc. Could it be faith that science and scientific methods will always benefit from adequately collected data?

FURTHER READING

Behrman R E, Kliegman R M, Arvin A M 1996 Nelson textbook of paediatrics, 15th edn. Saunders, London

Roberton N R C 1994 Roberton's manual of neonatal intensive care. Edward Arnold, Edinburgh

CHAPTER 8

The renal system

D. D. Ratnasinghe   D. F. Haddad

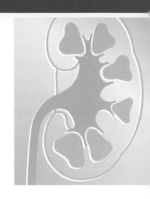

CORE PROBLEMS OF THE RENAL SYSTEM

KEY PROBLEM	KEY DIAGNOSIS	RELATED TOPICS
• Urinary tract infection	Vesicoureteric reflux	Obstructive lesions of the renal tract
• Generalized oedema	Minimal-change nephrotic syndrome	Acute glomerulonephritis Other glomerular disorders (Heart failure)
• Haematuria	Acute glomerulonephritis	Urinary tract infection Henoch–Schönlein purpura IgA nephropathy (Wilms's tumour)
• Acute renal failure	Haemolytic (uraemic syndrome)	Acute glomerulonephritis Tubular damage

ESSENTIAL BACKGROUND

INTRODUCTION

The renal system can be involved in a number of different types of pathology which together make a major contribution to morbidity in the paediatric age group.

Congenital abnormalities of the renal system are among the most common congenital defects diagnosed in children. Many of these can be picked up on prenatal ultrasonography, which is nowadays a routine part of antenatal care. The significance of congenital abnormalities of the renal tract relates to their potential to damage renal function (e.g. by obstruction or predisposition to infection) and also to the fact that they may be associated with other congenital abnormalities and may point to a particular diagnosis or syndrome.

Infections of the urinary tract are common and pose special problems in children both in terms of diagnosis and of management. Inadequate treatment may lead to serious long-term consequences for renal function, and thus awareness of these considerations is mandatory for all those working in the field of paediatrics.

The unique arrangement of the microcirculation in the glomerulae, with very high blood flow rates and highly permeable capillary walls, facilitates filtration by bringing large volumes of plasma into close proximity to the glomerular basement membrane. This allows the kidneys to execute their excretory function efficiently but renders the glomerulae particularly susceptible to immune injury and immune complex disease. The mesangium, which comprises the mesangial cells closely applied to the glomerular capillary walls, plays an important role in removing macromolecules such as immune complexes and becomes damaged in certain forms of glomerular disease.

The clinical presentation of glomerular disease is variable, ranging from the nephritic and nephrotic syndromes at one extreme (see below) to microscopic haematuria and/or proteinuria at the other (Table 8.1).

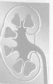

Finally, the renal system is frequently involved in the late stages of severe illness arising elsewhere in the body. Septicaemia, hypotension, inappropriate secretion of adrenocorticotrophic hormone (ADH) are examples of pathophysiological pathways that lead to disturbances in renal function. Attention to such disturbances is an important part of the care of the acutely ill child.

ANATOMY AND PHYSIOLOGY

Development of the renal tract

Embryologically, the kidneys develop from the union of the nephrogenic mesenchyme with the ureteric bud. Nephrons (glomerulae and tubules) originate from the nephrogenic mesenchyme, while the ureteric bud gives rise to the collecting ducts, calyces, pelvis and ureter (Fig. 8.1). Subsequent caudal migration of the kidneys results in their final position in the fetus. After 36 weeks, when the total complement of nephrons is complete, nephron mass increases as a result of glomerular and tubular growth.

Although the formation of nephrons is complete at birth, the glomerular filtration rate (GFR) is only about a third of that expected for an adult. By the second year of life the GFR reaches 120 ml/min/1.73 m^2, similar to that of the adult (normalized for size).

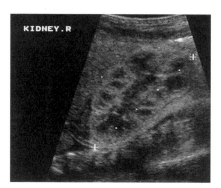

Figure 8.1   An ultrasound examination of a normal neonatal kidney. At this age there is increased echogenicity of the cortex relative to the medulla, demonstrating the normal calyceal system. The echnogenicity pattern reverses around the age of 2 years

The kidneys lie in a retroperitoneal position and have two layers: an outer *cortex* and an inner *medulla*. The cortex contains the glomerulae, proximal and distal convoluted tubules and collecting ducts. The medulla contains the loops of Henle, the vasa recta and terminal collecting ducts, which open into the calyces and conduct urine into the renal pelvis on either side. The ureters then take a course caudally and insert into the bladder at the trigone. The urethra opens to the outside and negotiates a considerably shorter distance in the female than the male.

Abnormalities in the development of the kidneys vary in severity and functional significance (see Beyond Core: congenital malformations of the renal tract). At one extreme, complete failure of renal development 'bilateral renal agenesis', is not compatible with life; at the other, there is a large number of minor aberrations, such as discrepancies in the size of the kidneys or mild degrees of dilatation of the renal tract, which may only come to light when the patient undergoes investigations for some other reason.

The point at which the renal pelvis connects to the ureter at the pelviureteric junction (PUJ) is an important area of potential obstruction. Another point of potential malfunction is where the ureters insert into the bladder. Normally insertion is at an angle, and the ureters take a long intramural course, thus creating an effective valve mechanism. A structural anomaly where the ureters are laterally displaced and take a direct, shorter course through the bladder wall can lead to reflux of urine (vesicoureteric reflux (VUR), see p. 151). However, mild degrees of VUR are common in young children, of doubtful pathological significance, and can be thought of as a developmental stage.

HISTORY AND EXAMINATION

A salient feature of renal tract disorders in young children is the non-specific nature of the symptoms. This is particularly true of urinary tract infections, and emphasizes the need for a high index of suspicion.

Prolonged jaundice in a neonate, slow weight gain, or a septicaemic illness may be caused by urinary tract infection (UTI). Symptoms of fever,

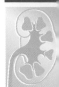

irritability, failure to thrive, vomiting and diarrhoea may also be presenting complaints of UTI.

Febrile illness without an obvious cause is an important presentation of UTIs in infants and young children (see Ch. 14). Other accompanying features may include vomiting with or without diarrhoea, poor appetite, with the child being generally 'off food' and 'off colour'. Such an episode may erroneously be attributed to a viral illness. In some children with UTI, the illness may pass unnoticed.

More specific symptoms should be inquired about by direct questioning. A change in the appearance or smell of the urine, pain on passing urine or an increase in frequency of urination can all be relevant and indicative of an underlying UTI. However, similar symptoms may result from local skin irritation in the genital area (e.g. phimosis and balanitis in boys and vulval irritation in girls), and it is unwise to diagnose a UTI without urine microscopy and/or culture. Inspection of the perineum in these cases may establish the diagnosis and spare the child the unnecessary treatment and investigations for a presumed UTI.

The onset of bedwetting in a child who has already achieved bladder control and come out of nappies (secondary enuresis, see Ch. 18), particularly if associated with daytime incontinence, may occasionally be secondary to a UTI.

Renal disease is an important cause of generalized oedema in children. The fluid retention can be due to a decrease in the excretory function of the kidneys or it may be secondary to hypoproteinaemia and reduction of plasma oncotic pressure (see p. 153). Mild degrees of generalized oedema can be difficult to identify. A puffy face in the morning is one of the early clues to developing generalized oedema in children.

Palpation of the kidneys, including balloting, and assessment of renal angle tenderness should not be forgotten. Checking for pitting oedema or signs of ascites, such as a fluid thrill or shifting dullness, may also give valuable clues. Scrotal oedema in boys is a feature of severe generalized oedema and ascites.

Blood pressure measurement (see Ch. 7) is an important part of the physical examination since hypertension may be the only indication of unilateral renal disease; plotting the child's growth on an appropriate chart (see Ch. 2) may reveal any deviations due to chronic disorders of the renal tract such as unrecognized chronic urine infection.

INVESTIGATION

Urinalysis

Testing a sample of urine by dipping a multiple reagent strip has become an almost universal routine in the medical evaluation of children irrespective of whether there are features suggestive of renal disease. Nevertheless, urine dipstick testing should not be undertaken casually and requires a degree of care in following the manufacturer's instructions. In infants and young children, there is the added concern of ensuring that the urine sample is collected adequately and is not contaminated with other materials (e.g. stool, nappy creams, etc.), although for dipstick testing this is not quite so important as for culture.

Urine testing by multiple reagent strips can yield useful information regarding:

- *Glycosuria.* This may be due to hyperglycaemia or absorption defects in the renal tubules.
- *Proteinuria* (Table 8.1). Small amounts (trace, +1) are acceptable, particularly if the sample is concentrated, collected later in the day or during febrile illnesses.
- *Haematuria.* Small amounts of blood (trace, +1) are acceptable if transient, particularly during a febrile illness or following exercise. The commonest cause of significant haematuria is UTI but further tests to rule out other causes need to be considered (Table 8.1). The presence of red cells should be confirmed by microscopy.
- *pH and osmolality.* The urinary pH varies between 5 and 7. Formal investigation for renal tubular disorders that result in acidosis requires an acidification test. A urine sample first thing in the morning after overnight fasting is useful in screening for concentrating defects; a value above 800 mOsm/kg (specific gravity >1020) is a normal result.

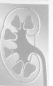

Table 8.1 Causes of haematuria, proteinuria and oedema[a]			
Aetiology	Haematuria	Proteinuria	Oedema
Infection, idiopathic,[b] IgA nephropathy, sickle cell anaemia, tumour, trauma	–	–	–
Henoch–Schönlein purpura, haemolytic uraemic syndrome, systemic lupus erythematosus	+	+	±
Acute glomerulonephritis Membranoproliferative glomerulonephritis	+	+	+
Minimal-change nephrotic syndrome Focal segmental glomerulosclerosis	–	+	+
Orthostatic, exercise, fever	–	+	–

[a] Typical forms of presentation are listed but other presentations are possible. For example, the urinary findings in infection and IgA nephropathy may include proteinuria, and in exercise may include haematuria (or haemoglobinuria); systemic lupus erythematosus may present without haematuria and glomerulonephritis (acute and membranoproliferative) without oedema

[b] Idiopathic haematuria may be familial or non-familial. The former includes benign familial haematuria (non-progressive, autosomal dominant) and Alport's syndrome (progressive renal failure and high-tone deafness). The prognosis for the non-familial and non-Alport's disorders is excellent

- *Pyuria*. 2+ on the test strip is roughly equivalent to 75 leucocytes/µl, and is an indication for proper sample collection and culture (see below). Absence of leucocytes in a urine sample is strong evidence against the presence of a UTI.
- *Nitrite*. In UTI, urinary nitrate is reduced by the infecting bacteria to nitrite, which can be detected by the reagent strip. Although of poor sensitivity (approximately 30%), the nitrite test is highly specific, particularly in girls, in whom a positive test obtained from freshly voided urine is almost diagnostic. In boys, nitrite produced by the action of skin bacteria may accumulate under the prepuce, reducing the specificity of the test. Also, contaminating bacteria will produce nitrite if the urine sample is allowed to stand longer than 4 h before testing.

Urine microscopy and culture

The diagnosis of UTI, by far the most common pathology of the renal tract in children, hinges on a positive urine culture. As a laboratory technique, urine culturing is generally an inexpensive and straightforward test. However, the method by which the urine is collected greatly influences the reliability of the results obtained, particularly if positive. A midstream, clean-catch urine specimen is good enough in most patients and has only a small chance of being contaminated. This technique, however, requires some degree of cooperation from the child, and is therefore not practicable in the very young in whom the alternative is to use a bag stuck to the cleaned and dried perineum. The results from bag urine samples need to be interpreted with caution as the potential for contamination is high, often yielding a mixed growth. The ideal method for a sterile sample collection is to perform a suprapubic aspiration.

Microscopy of the urine may be very helpful diagnostically. The presence of pus cells and/or microorganisms on a Gram stain are indicative of infection. Granular (white cell) and red cell casts are found in acute glomerulonephritis, while hyaline (proteinaceous) casts are typical of the nephrotic syndrome.

Culture of the urine will yield useful information regarding the presence of infection, the microorganism and its antibiotic susceptibility.

Blood biochemistry

Urea is filtered in the glomerulus but absorbed and secreted by the renal tubules, and thus is not a reliable indicator of the GFR. A rising serum urea level from the normal value of less than 5 mmol/l can be seen in cases of dehydration and gastrointestinal bleeding. In infants, on the other hand, blood urea levels may remain initially low despite significant reduction in glomerular filtration because the balance between the anabolic and catabolic metabolism is shifted in favour of the former and thus the production of urea at the cellular level is reduced. A rise in the serum creatinine level, however, is significant and points to a considerable reduction (>30%) in the GFR. It is also important to note that normal serum creatinine levels in children are lower than those in adults (reflecting the proportionately lower muscle mass) and, while an upper limit of 120 µmol/l is acceptable in an adult male, the normal range varies in children according to age. In infants (beyond the neonatal period) the upper limit of the range may be as low as 35 µmol/l, depending on the method of estimation.

Hyponatraemia (plasma Na^+ level < 135 mmol/l) is a relatively common pathological finding in sick children. As is the case in adults, hyponatraemia can be spurious, reflecting poor sampling (sampling site proximal to an intravenous fluid line, sample haemolysis) or gross hyperlipidaemia. The latter is not uncommon in infants receiving total parenteral nutrition (TPN) where part of the sample volume is taken up by the lipids so that, despite a normal level of sodium in the plasma, a low result is obtained because the calculation is made on the basis of the total volume of the sample. Genuine hyponatraemia may reflect greater loss of sodium relative to water as in certain cases of dehydration and diuretic therapy, or a relative excess of water

as seen in the various conditions with water retention (e.g. renal failure, fluid overload). A special case of dilutional hyponatraemia is that arising from inappropriate anti-diuretic hormone secretion (syndrome of inappropriate ADH secretion (SIADH), see Ch. 10).

Hyperkalaemia arising from renal failure can be rapidly lethal.

Imaging

Ultrasound scanning

Ultrasound, because of its non-invasive nature and ease of use, is the investigation of first choice when an anatomical image of the renal tract is desired. However, it requires a skilled operator and gives little information on function.

Radioisotope scanning

The use of radionuclides, usually technetium-99-tagged molecules, can provide information of both structure and function as long as the child is more than a few weeks old. It also exposes the patient to less radiation than X rays.

DMSA, because of its property of binding to functional renal tissue, will allow the investigator to obtain static images which define the presence and extent of renal scars.

MAG-3 and DTPA are isotopically labelled substances that are excreted in the glomerular filtrate and give information regarding renal blood flow, renal function (GFR) and urine flow from the level of the calyces. A late image, when the excreted isotope has collected in the bladder, can also provide an indirect method of assessing vesicoureteric reflux if the child is old enough to cooperate by voiding the bladder when asked to do so. Neither isotope can provide the necessary definition to delineate renal scars, and DMSA remains the radioisotope of choice in this respect.

Micturating cystourethrography (MCUG)

In MCUG the bladder is catheterized and contrast medium instilled to outline the bladder and detect any vesicoureteric reflux. Cooperation of the patient is not necessary, but it is important to obtain further images when the bladder is being voided, after the catheter is removed, in order to identify any obstruction of the urethra such as posterior urethral valves.

Intravenous urography (IVU)

IVU is not commonly undertaken in childhood except in situations where detailed images of the calyces and ureter are required.

Tests of renal function

Apart from functional renal scanning (DPTA), a simple biochemical measurement of the plasma creatinine concentration can give useful information. This rises when renal function has fallen to less than 70% of normal. The upper limit of the normal range increases in childhood with increasing height and muscle bulk.

An estimate of the GFR can be obtained using

$$\frac{height\ (cm) \times 40}{plasma\ creatinine\ level\ (\mu mol/l)}$$

Creatinine clearance is rarely measured in children as it is often very difficult to obtain an accurate, timed sample of urine.

CORE PROBLEMS

URINARY TRACT INFECTION

The significance of UTI in children stems from the following:

- UTI is a relatively common cause of morbidity in children. However, since specific symptoms

BEYOND CORE

CONGENITAL MALFORMATIONS OF THE RENAL TRACT

In recent years, abnormalities of the renal tract are being detected quite commonly during the antenatal period (approximately 1 in 400 fetuses). This is due to advances in the use of ultrasonography. Many of the abnormalities are not functionally significant, but some are important as they may be associated with, or result in, loss of function.

Renal agenesis and dysgenesis

Renal agenesis. Bilateral failure of the union of the ureteric bud with the nephrogenic mesenchyme produces two cystic masses that have no recognizable excretory function and no connections with the bladder. As two-thirds of the amniotic fluid is formed by fetal urine, this leads to oligohydramnios and compression of the fetus. The resulting Potter's syndrome is characterized by epicanthic folds, broad flattened nose, large low-set ears, severe talipes and lung hypoplasia (see Ch. 6). The neonate may be stillborn or die soon after birth from respiratory failure.

Renal hypoplasia and dysplasia. A unilateral cystic mass, which can vary from a large single cyst to multiple small cysts, results in a condition called multicystic disease due to an aberration in the union and subsequent development of the renal mesenchyme and ureteric bud. A particular extreme of this aberration may result in a small, poorly functioning dysplastic kidney that contains tissue such as hair and cartilage. Severe hydronephrosis has to be excluded, and the contralateral kidney should be investigated to ensure that it is normal.

Polycystic disease of the kidneys can be due to an autosomal recessive infantile disease or autosomal dominant adult-type polycystic disease. Associated cystic changes in the liver and other viscera may also be found. These conditions appear quite distinct from multicystic disease on imaging, and there is always at least some renal function.

Congenital abnormalities that can result in obstruction

Pelviureteric junction obstruction, which is the most common cause of hydronephrosis, and *Posterior urethral valves,* which are important because of the

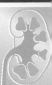

high risk of severe renal damage if not diagnosed and treated early, are discussed on p. 153. Other congenital anomalies associated with renal tract obstruction include horseshoe kidneys, duplication of the ureter and ureterocoele.

Horseshoe kidneys occur when the two kidneys are joined at the lower poles, and are usually not of any great consequence unless PUJ obstruction, with which it is sometimes associated, is present. Associated dysmorphic syndromes such as Turner's (see Ch. 9) are worth remembering.

Duplication of the ureters can occur but the ureter is more often bifid rather than completely duplicated. The ureter draining the upper portion of the kidney inserts lower in the bladder than the ureter that drains the lower moiety. Since the intravesical course of the lower ureter is longer, this can result in obstruction, and therefore hydronephrosis of the upper renal moiety. Conversely the upper ureter may reflux due to its shorter course and thereby pose a risk from infection to the kidneys.

Ureterocoele results when an expanded end of a normal ureter or an ectopic ureter prolapses into the bladder. It can predispose to urinary tract infection or symptoms due to inability to completely empty the bladder.

Abnormalities from the failure of complete fusion of the midline structures below the umbilicus result in an exposed bladder: *mucosa–bladder exstrophy*. Associated epispadias, where the urethra opens on to the ventral part of the penis as well as unfused pubic bones can make definitive treatment of this problem all the more difficult. In the *prune belly syndrome*, absent abdominal musculature is associated with a large bladder, dilated ureters and undescended testis.

Due to the fact that key events in development of the renal tract and auditory system in embryonic life occur at the same time, it is wise to look out for defects in hearing when a renal abnormality is found.

A baby born following antenatal detection of renal pelvis dilatation should be placed on prophylactic antibiotics from birth while undergoing a full diagnostic work-up.

are frequently lacking, the diagnosis requires a high index of suspicion.

- Untreated UTI may cause permanent damage to the kidneys and renal failure. In early infancy, a UTI may be associated with septicaemia.

Furthermore, a significant proportion of children with UTI have an underlying structural or functional abnormality of the renal tract which predisposes to recurrent UTIs or may, on its own, result in renal scarring and damage.

Up to 3% of girls and 1% of boys have had a UTI by the age of 11 years. In early infancy, the bacteria reach the renal tract by haematogenous spread and the incidence of UTI, as with many other infections, is higher in boys than in girls, and both Gram-negative and -positive bacteria (including *Staphylococcus aureus*) are implicated. From late infancy onwards, a UTI usually represents an ascending infection, and Gram-negative bacteria are the predominant pathogens involved. Reflecting the anatomical differences between the two sexes, the incidence of UTIs is higher in girls.

Clinical features

Manifestations of UTI can be specific or non-specific; the latter are usually the only feature of UTI in infancy.

Non-specific features of UTI
- In neonates – jaundice, poor feeding, vomiting and slow weight gain
- Septicaemia
- Fever with no obvious cause, some times in association with vomiting and lethargy simulating central nervous system infection
- Irritability, poor appetite and generally being unwell with or without vomiting and diarrhoea; a presentation which can be mistaken for gastroenteritis

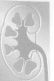

> **Specific features of UTI**
> - Irritability, discomfort or pain on passing urine which may be followed by refusal to urinate and urinary retention, frequency and urgency with or without loss of bladder control, colic and abdominal pain.
> - Change in the colour or smell of the urine/wet nappy
> - Loin pain and tenderness with rigors; features which point to renal involvement (pyelonephritis) as opposed to cystitis

Rarely, chronic (recurrent) UTI may not be suspected until the child presents with failure to thrive or hypertension. An extreme example, and a constant reminder of the importance of having a high index of suspicion for the diagnosis of UTI, is the child with previously unrecognized UTI who presents with end-stage renal failure.

Diagnosis

If a UTI is suspected, it is important to obtain a clean-catch urine specimen or a suprapubic aspirate for microscopy and culture. The sample should be plated out with the minimum of delay in order to prevent the overgrowth of any contaminating bacteria. The presence of pus cells alone in the urine is not reliable as this can be caused by pyrexia without UTI.

Dipstick testing for nitrite and white cell enzymes may be carried out, but false-negative results are common.

Culture resulting in more than 10^5 colony forming units of a single species of bacteria per millilitre indicates a very high probability of infection. This is also known as 'significant bacteriuria'. If any doubt exists, a further urine culture is advised.

Bacteria derived from the gastrointestinal system are responsible for most urinary tract infections. *Escherichia coli*, *Proteus species* and *Pseudomonas species* are the three that are mostly cultured in descending order of frequency. *Proteus* species are commoner in boys, probably because these organisms tend to reside under the prepuce. *Pseudomonas* infection raises the possibility of there being an underlying structural abnormality.

Management

Treatment of a UTI depends on the age and severity of presentation. Thus in infancy, and in the older child with associated pyelonephritis, admission to hospital may be required for intravenous antibacterial treatment, at least initially. However, oral antibiotics at home are adequate in most other situations. Monitoring of hydration and encouraging fluid intake are also important and, at least at presentation, blood pressure should be measured. The duration of treatment varies according to the child's response but usually 7–10 days will be sufficient. Co-amoxiclav, a cephalosporin or trimethoprim is a reasonable choice for initial antibacterial therapy, but this should be modified according to the sensitivity profile of the cultured microorganism. A further culture after the conclusion of treatment should be undertaken to check that complete clearing of infection has occurred.

An important aspect of the management of UTIs is to assess the risk of an underlying structural abnormality of the renal tract and hence of complications and recurrence of the infection; the greater the risk, the more extensive is the series of investigations. The following factors are helpful in the assessment:

- *The child*. The younger the child the more likely is the presence of underlying abnormality and the greater the potential of UTIs to result in renal scarring. It is also important to consider any family history of renal disease or past medical history of possible UTI episodes.
- *The infection*. A severe course, particularly if features of pyelonephritis are present, is more likely to be associated with both structural abnormalities and renal scarring. This association is also true of infections that are difficult to treat and where there are recurrences.
- *The bacteria*. Certain bacteria are unusual pathogens of the normal renal tract, and their presence suggests the possibility of an underlying structural abnormality. This is particularly true of *Pseudomonas* infections.

If there is a significant risk of an underlying abnormality, the child should be given daily prophylactic treatment (usually trimethoprim 2 mg/kg at night) in order to prevent further infection and possible renal damage during the time it takes to complete the diagnostic work-up.

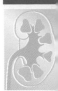

Antibiotic prophylaxis may be continued if an underlying abnormality is detected (e.g. VUR, see below) or if recurrences are frequent even in the absence of an underlying abnormality. Other important aspects of management include avoidance of constipation, good hygiene and complete voiding before going to bed at night.

The range of investigations which are usually considered in evaluating children with a history of UTI include:

- Ultrasound to give an assessment of size, presence of scarring and to identify any hydronephrosis
- MCUG to identify reflux or posterior urethral valves in infancy and in preschool children unable to cooperate for indirect cystography (see below)
- DMSA (static) scanning to look for renal scars
- DTPA or MAG-3 (dynamic) scanning to detect ureteric obstruction or for indirect cystography to check for reflux in school-age children
- DTPA scanning for measurement of the GFR where renal abnormality has been demonstrated.

The choice and extent of investigations, undertaken in a particular case, are based on the age of the child and the risk assessment as discussed previously. Initial investigations are as follows:

Age	Investigation
Infants (under 1 year of age)	Renal ultrasound scan, DMSA scan, MCUG scan
Preschool age	Renal ultrasound scan, DMSA scan
School age	Renal ultrasound scan

The rationale for the diminishing scope of the initial investigation of UTIs with age is that the risk of an underlying abnormality and of scarring declines with age and that, in the older child, a normal ultrasound scan (obtained by an experienced radiologist) virtually excludes a clinically significant anatomical or functional abnormality. An abnormal scan is usually an indication for further investigation, continued antibiotic prophylaxis and, on occasion, surgical intervention. Recurrent UTIs, even in the absence of underlying abnormality, are an indication for a prolonged course of antibiotic prophylaxis (6 months to 1 year), following which there is usually a 'carry-over' of the protective effect.

Two categories of renal tract abnormalities are associated with UTI and further complications: VUR, (see below) and obstructive lesions (see p. 153 and Beyond core: congenital abnormalities of the renal tract).

(see p. 153 and Beyond core: congenital abnormalities of the renal tract).

✱ KEY DIAGNOSIS

Vesicoureteric reflux

VUR occurs when the ureter takes a shorter than normal intramural course through the bladder. It is a developmental anomaly, and may be unilateral or bilateral (see Fig. 8.2). Transmission of bladder hydrostatic pressure to the kidneys may give rise to varying degrees of hydronephrosis.

Classification of severity of VUR	
Mild reflux:	affecting the ureter only
Moderate reflux:	dilatation of ureter and pelvis
Severe reflux:	gross dilatation of ureter, renal pelvis and calyces

Because reflux can be a familial problem it is appropriate to screen other family members by ultrasound when a case of severe VUR is identified. As the child grows, VUR tends to reduce in severity. Thus the more severe categories become less severe, and in 10% of affected children it resolves completely each year.

VUR is important because it encourages infection by incomplete bladder emptying. Furthermore, it facilitates ascending infection with the risk of pyelonephritis, and the transmission of bladder pressure to the renal papillae adds to renal damage, particularly in infancy. Renal tissue that has been destroyed usually manifests as a scar in the cortical region. This may produce excessive amounts of renin, resulting in hypertension. If the scarring process continues unchecked, the affected kidney becomes shrunken and poorly functioning; if bilateral and severe, end-stage renal failure may develop.

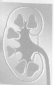

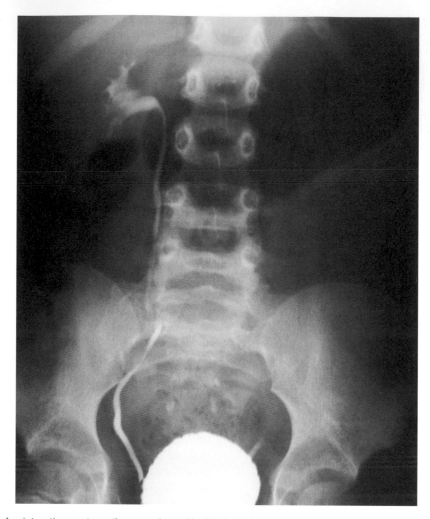

Figure 8.2   A micturating cystourethrogram in a girl with right-sided grade 3 reflux

Management

In children in whom reflux is identified, investigations should be repeated every 2 years or so in order to monitor resolution of the reflux, new scar formation, renal growth and function. The formation of new scars can be prevented by prophylactic antibiotic treatment, which should be continued until resolution of the reflux or 10–12 years of age when renal growth has stopped. There should be regular follow-up with urine culture and measurement of blood pressure.

In the minority of cases with severe reflux associated with recurrent breakthrough UTIs and appearances of new renal scars, surgical reimplantation of the ureters may be indicated.

Obstructive lesions of the renal tract

Obstruction of the flow of urine will result in dilatation of the urinary tract proximally. When this involves the kidneys it is known as hydronephrosis (Fig. 8.3). A dilated, lax tortuous ureter is called a hydroureter.

PUJ obstruction is the commonest obstructive cause of hydronephrosis, and may be due to a functional defect in the area, a stenosis of the wall or an abnormal course of an artery or fibrous

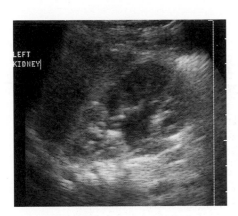

Figure 8.3   A renal ultrasound scan showing hydronephrosis in a 1 year old child with a dilated renal pelvis and calyses

band. Surgical release of the obstruction by pyeloplasty is the treatment of choice.

Posterior urethral valves occur in male infants as a result of mucosal folds or a membrane in the proximal part of the urethra. This results in poor renal growth bilaterally, hydronephrosis and a decreased volume of amniotic fluid. The diagnosis is usually suggested by abnormal antenatal or postnatal ultrasound scans. Previously undiagnosed cases may be suspected after birth on the basis of a palpable bladder or a poor urine stream. Subsequent confirmation by an MCUG scan (see above) carried out promptly allows the obstruction to be relieved as an urgent procedure

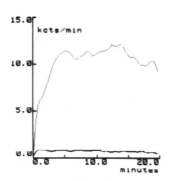

Figure 8.4   A renal isotopic examination (DTPA) of a boy diagnosed with posterior urethral valves at the age of 2 months. At the age of 2 years he required a left nephrectomy (demonstrated by no isotope in the left kidney). The right kidney shows a marked delay in excretion, confirming chronic renal failure

by ablation of the valve(s). Associated VUR is common, and it is advisable to commence the child on prophylactic antibiotics soon after birth. Progression to chronic renal failure is still a possibility and depends on the amount of residual renal tissue and the presence of dysplastic change (Fig. 8.4).

GENERALIZED OEDEMA

Oedema is the clinical manifestation of excessive accumulation of interstitial fluid. It can be differentiated from other causes of tissue swelling by 'pitting': a depression created in the skin by applying sustained pressure with the finger and thus displacing the interstitial fluid. The depression disappears after the pressure has been removed.

Oedema can be localized or generalized; localized oedema is usually due to local exudation arising as a result of infective, traumatic or allergic factors. Localized oedema may also be an early manifestation of generalized oedema: local tissue tension and gravitational forces influence the distribution of the excessive interstitial fluid. In children, periorbital oedema in the morning is frequently the earliest manifestation of generalized oedema.

The pathophysiological mechanisms leading to generalized oedema involve a disturbance to mechanisms regulating transcapillary fluid transfer such that filtration into the interstitial space is increased due to:

- Decreased plasma oncotic pressure (e.g. protein loss due to nephrotic syndrome, see below)
- Increased capillary hydrostatic pressure (e.g. increased total body water due to the fluid retention, heart failure)
- Increased capillary permeability.

Disease states giving rise to generalized oedema include renal, cardiac, hepatic and nutritional disorders. More than one of the above-listed mechanisms may be involved in the development of generalized oedema. By far the commonest cause of generalized oedema in childhood is the nephrotic syndrome, which is characterized by heavy proteinuria and hypoalbuminaemia. Generalized oedema,

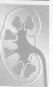

although not usually so severe, is also a common feature of the acute nephritic syndrome in which there may be variable proteinuria, haematuria, oliguria and hypertension (see below). Both the nephrotic syndrome and the acute nephritic syndrome are manifestations of glomerular damage, and it is not surprising that there may be overlap in clinical presentation. Thus, the nephrotic syndrome may sometimes present with nephritic features.

The idiopathic nephrotic syndrome refers to cases of where there is no association with systemic illness and there is usually no other major manifestation of glomerular disease (i.e. no gross haematuria or nephritic features). In the 90% of all cases fulfilling these criteria, the underlying pathological picture is consistent with minimal-change disease (MCD) in about 85%, focal segmental glomerulosclerosis in 10% and membranoproliferative glomerulonephritis in 5% (see Other glomerular disorders presenting as the nephrotic syndrome, below).

More important than the pathological categorization of the glomerular lesion is the response to steroid therapy. The steroid-sensitive nephrotic syndrome generally carries a good prognosis whether due to MCD or not. A significant number of children with the steroid-resistant nephrotic syndrome will have a progressive course leading to end-stage renal failure, and their management should be supervised by a paediatric nephrologist. A renal biopsy to determine the nature of the underlying pathology is usually indicated.

In addition to steroid responsiveness, indicators of the presence of an underlying pathology other than MCD include:

- Age of onset < 2 years or > 10 years.
- Presence of features of the acute nephritic syndrome.
- Low complement (C_3) levels at any stage of the illness.

✱ KEY DIAGNOSIS

Minimal change nephrotic syndrome

This condition is a triad of gross urinary protein loss, low plasma albumin levels and oedema. Although relatively uncommon, with an incidence of 2–4 per 100 000 children per year, it is about four time more frequent in the Asian population. Males are more commonly affected than females, and the peak age is between 1 and 5 years. MCD accounts for approximately 80% of all cases of the nephrotic syndrome presenting in childhood.

Aetiology and pathogenesis

The cause of MCD is unknown; the renal biopsy findings are a grossly normal glomerular appearance on light microscopy with only 'minimal-change'. Fluorescent microscopy in these children is also negative, but electron microscopy reveals the nonspecific finding, common to other conditions with heavy proteinuria, of fusion of the glomerular epithelial cell foot processes. This histopathological picture is associated with 95% steroid responsiveness.

The pathogenesis of this condition relates primarily to the glomerulae, which become permeable to albumin to such a degree that neither tubular absorption of the filtered albumin nor a compensatory increase in hepatic synthesis of albumin can keep up with the urinary loss, and consequently the plasma albumin level drops. This leads to a reduction in plasma oncotic pressure, disturbing the balance of oncotic and hydrostatic pressures across capillary walls (the Starling forces) and a progressive loss of fluid from the intravascular space into the interstitium. Hence, even though the child may look fluid overloaded, the circulation can be critically volume depleted. Oedema becomes apparent when the plasma albumin level drops below 20–25 g/l.

Clinical features

The characteristic feature is generalized oedema (periorbital and dependent, with ascites), and in boys, scrotal oedema. There is often a preceding history of a respiratory illness. Abdominal pain (probably secondary to impairment of intestinal circulation and thus a warning sign of hypovolaemia), vomiting, diarrhoea and breathlessness (due to pleural effusions) may also be present. Frothing of the urine may be noticed.

Blood pressure measurement, urine dipstick testing for protein and blood, and assessment of the degree of oedema (including weighing) should be part of the initial assessment.

There is a risk of acute circulatory collapse due to hypovolaemia, and this may be exacerbated by vomiting and diarrhoea. Children with the nephrotic syndrome have an increased vulnerability to infection, particularly primary pneumococcal peritonitis. This may be related to loss of antibody, complement components and other immune proteins, as well as treatment with steroids and the presence of ascites. Because of the modifying effects of steroids, children on treatment for the nephrotic syndrome (see below) who develop peritonitis may have surprisingly few signs and symptoms.

Investigation

Urinalysis and regular investigation of serum electrolytes and albumin are essential in the acute phase of the disease. A 24 h urine collection will show proteinuria in excess of $1 \ g/m^2$ and a spot urine more than 200 mg per 1 mmol of creatinine. Serial haematocrit measurement is a useful method of monitoring the circulatory volume and getting advance warning of any adverse trend (rising haematocrit).

Plasma cholesterol and triglyceride levels are elevated. Unlike many other forms of glomerular disease, the complement levels (C_3, C_4) are not low in MCD at any stage of the illness.

Renal biopsy is not routine, but patients who have atypical 'nephritic' features (e.g. haematuria, hypertension, low C_3 levels) aged under 6 months or who fail to respond to a 4 week course of steroids require a renal biopsy to look for an alternative diagnosis.

Management

Children with the typical picture of the nephrotic syndrome who manifest no features to suggest that the condition has arisen secondarily to more serious renal or generalized pathology (i.e. who manifest no nephritic features, intrinsic renal failure, or features of systemic disease such as systemic lupus erythematosus) are assumed to have MCD and hence are assumed to be steroid-responsive. Oral steroids are the mainstay of treatment in these circumstances.

There are several regimens of steroid therapy in this condition, reflecting the difficulty in reconciling the aim to achieve high levels of efficacy (including minimizing the chance of relapse) with the need to avoid side-effects. The usual practice is to start prednisolone at 2 mg/kg/day as a single daily dose. The first sign of response is a diuresis as the plasma albumin level rises and fluid moves back into the vascular compartment. The urine usually becomes protein-free (remission) within 2 weeks of starting this treatment. After being in remission for 3 days the steroid dose is gradually reduced and stopped over a 6 week period. The condition is considered to be steroid-resistant if there is no response within 4 weeks.

Accurate intake and output charting as well as serial measurements of body weight are essential. A diet with no added salt helps control the oedema. In the patient with impending circulatory collapse the cautious use of albumin infusions together with diuretics may be considered.

As a prophylaxis against pneumococcal infections, it is recommended that oral penicillin be given during the hypoalbuminaemic phase. Some authorities also advocate the use of the polyvalent pneumococcal vaccine during remission as an added protection during any future relapses. Measles and chickenpox are two other types of infection that may have devastating consequences in children on steroid/immunosuppressive therapy. The immune status for these two infections should be checked in children with the nephrotic syndrome at presentation; exposure in a non-immune subject warrants the administration of prophylactic immunoglobulins (zoster immunoglobulin (ZIG) in the case of chickenpox)

Prognosis

The ultimate prognosis for renal function in MCD is excellent. However, three-quarters of steroid-responsive children will have at least one relapse. Frequent relapses (>2 per 6 months) may be controlled by alternate-day steroids, or a brief

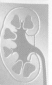

course of cyclophosphamide if steroid toxicity occurs. Cyclophosphamide may also be indicated in those children who cannot be weaned off steroids (steroid dependency). However, there is a danger of diminished fertility in boys so treated.

Other glomerular disorders presenting as the nephrotic syndrome

Of all children exhibiting the clinical features of the nephrotic syndrome (the 90% of cases meeting the criteria of the idiopathic nephrotic syndrome *and* the 10% who do not), 20–25% may have an underlying renal pathology different to that of MCD. The histopathological picture is usually consistant with one of the following:

- Focal segmental sclerosis (FSGS) accounts for about 10% of cases of the nephrotic syndrome and may be part of a continuum with MCD. However, although the electron microscopy findings are similar, light microscopy shows a focal pattern of obliteration of Bowman's space with proteinaceous deposits (hyalinosis). The prognosis is considerably worse than MCD, and 80% are steroid-resistant.
- Membranoproliferative glomerulonephritis (MPGN) may occur in isolation or as part of a systemic disorder such as systemic lupus erythematosus, Henoch–Shönlein purpura (see Ch. 11) or chronic infection (e.g. subacute bacterial endocarditis, hepatitis B, malaria). The most consistant histological pattern is a generalized proliferation of the mesangial cells (see p. 143). It has a poor prognosis, with 50% of patients in end-stage renal failure within 10 years.
- Membranous glomerulonephritis is the most common cause of the nephrotic syndrome in adults, but is rare in children, in whom it accounts for less than 1% of cases, mostly in the second decade of life. It may sometimes be the result of drug therapy or, as in MPGN, part of a systemic disease.
- The congenital nephrotic syndrome is a rare autosomal recessive condition but may be sporadic. It presents at birth or develops in the first year of life, and is associated with early end-stage renal failure.

HAEMATURIA

Red or brown discoloration of the urine of a child is an alarming observation for the parents, and medical advice is usually sought without delay. In addition to macroscopic haematuria, possible causes of red/brown discoloration of the urine include ingestion of certain foods (beetroot, berries, food colourings), drugs (rifampicin, phenothiazines), bilirubinuria and myoglobinuria. In infants, nucleic acid metabolism is highly active because of the high rate of cell turnover, and thus the production (and hence urinary excretion) of urate is increased. Oxidized urate crystals may give a pink tinge to a wet nappy that has been exposed to the air for some time. Use of the term 'microscopic haematuria' implies that there is no suggestion of haematuria on naked-eye examination.

The presence of blood in the urine can be confirmed by both dipstick testing and visualization of red blood cells under the microscope. However, care should be exercised in interpreting positive results on urine dipstick testing; the method is sometimes too sensitive, and false-positive results can occur. The strip reagent also reacts with myoglobin, haemoglobin (in addition to intact red blood cells) and other oxidizing agents. Readings of 'small' or 1+ are generally insignificant unless they persist on repeated testing. On microscopy, the presence of more than five red cells per 1 mm^3 of the unspun urine sample is a positive finding for haematuria, and may warrant further evaluation if it persists on repeated testing.

Whether macro- or microscopic, the source of haematuria can be the upper or lower renal tract. Haematuria at the glomerular level (e.g. glomerulonephritis, IgA nephropathy, see below) is suggested by a brown colour to the urine and the presence of red cell casts. The red cells are deformed, and there is often accompanying proteinuria. In lower renal tract haematuria (e.g. cystitis) the urine is usually red and not associated with proteinuria. Red cells more or less retain their usual shape with little deformity, and red cell casts are absent.

The commonest cause of microscopic haematuria in children is infection, and is suggested by additional pyuria and bacteriuria. However, IgA nephropathy (Berger's disease) is the most common cause of recurrent macroscopic haematuria and persistent microscopic haematuria in children. Other causes of haematuria are listed in Table 8.1.

Haematuria due to glomerular disease is frequently associated with oedema, hypertension and a degree of renal insufficiency. Together, these findings constitute the 'acute nephritic syndrome'. In children, the commonest form of this syndrome is acute glomerulonephritis.

✳ KEY DIAGNOSIS

Acute glomerulonephritis

Acute postinfective glomerulonephritis affects predominantly school-aged children, and there is usually a history of an upper respiratory tract infection 1–2 weeks previously. Although most commonly caused by group A β-haemolytic streptococci, infection by viruses, and bacteria other than streptococci are increasingly implicated.

Soluble immune complex-mediated injury to the glomerulae leads to proliferative changes within the glomerulus capillaries and impairment of the blood flow and filtration. This in turn can cause a reduction in urine output, volume overload, hypertension, oedema and haematuria.

Clinical features

Common complaints include malaise, headache and vague loin discomfort, but many affected children are asymptomatic. Frequently it is the smoky brown colour of the urine that causes concern. Examination may reveal oedema of the dorsum of the hands and feet. The reduction in urine output (oliguria) is usually mild, but severe fluid retention can give rise to acute severe hypertension with encephalopathy, seizures and heart failure.

Investigations include urine microscopy to confirm haematuria and to look for red cell casts. Urinalysis shows haematuria and moderate proteinuria ($0.5–1$ g/m²/day). Blood should be obtained to measure the anti-streptolysin O titre and complement levels. The former is usually high (above the normal level for a particular age group; it tends to be higher in older children) and the latter (C_3, C_4) are transiently low. A throat swab may confirm persistence of streptococcal carriage.

Management

Post-streptococcal glomerulonephritis has an excellent prognosis. However, close attention to fluid and electrolyte balance and the monitoring of blood pressure and renal function will require hospital admission for all but the mildest cases. Serial measurements of the plasma creatinine level as well as daily weights and accurate fluid balance charts are essential aspects of management.

Oliguria, provided that there is no prerenal cause (i.e. fluid deficit), is managed by restriction of fluid intake to the urine output assessed every 4 h and insensible losses (400 ml/m²/day). Salt intake also needs to be minimized. Hypertension occasionally requires the use of diuretics and antihypertensives. Rarely, peritoneal dialysis may be necessary in the acute stage.

It is usual to give a 10 day course of penicillin in order to eradicate any persisting streptococci in the nasopharynx.

In most cases (approximately 95%) glomerular function returns to normal in about 2 weeks, with improvement in the urine output, blood pressure and symptoms. A renal biopsy is indicated only if the oliguria persists or, progresses to anuria, in order to identify the precise nature of the glomerular lesion. Fortunately, this scenario is rare in childhood.

IgA nephropathy

IgA nephropathy is generally a benign disease in children and there are few symptoms apart from recurrent haematuria. Although the pathogenesis of this disorder is not clear, affected individuals have an abnormality of immune system regulation leading to excessive synthesis of IgA in response to infections and other triggers. IgA and IgA immune complexes are then trapped by the glomerular mesangium, where they activate the alternative complement pathway and initiate the reactions leading to glomerular injury. The pathological picture in IgA nephropathy is characterized by mesangial proliferation, and bears resemblance to the glomerular involvement in Henoch–Schönlein purpura.

The clinical picture is characterized by recurrent episodes of gross haematuria, usually 1–4 days following an upper respiratory tract infection. The shorter time interval between the upper respiratory tract infection and the haematuria, and lack of other nephritic features, helps to differentiate IgA nephropathy from postinfective glomerulonephritis. The complement levels are normal, and in some children the serum IgA levels may be elevated. No treatment is required but, although the course in children is usually benign, some children may have progressive disease, and periodic assessment is required.

ACUTE RENAL FAILURE

Acute renal failure may be prerenal (poor perfusion due to hypovolaemia or cardiac failure), postrenal (due to obstruction, e.g. posterior urethral valves or ureteric obstruction) or renal (intrarenal).

Causes of acute renal failure

- Vascular
  - Haemolytic uraemic syndrome
  - Arteritis (e.g. Henoch–Shönlein purpura)
  - Renal vein thrombosis
- Glomerular
  - Acute glomerulonephritis
- Tubular
  - Nephrotoxins (particularly drugs)
  - Myoglobinuria and haemoglobinuria
  - Secondary to prerenal failure (acute tubular necrosis)

✱ KEY DIAGNOSIS:

Haemolytic uraemic syndrome (HUS)

HUS is one of the main causes of acute renal failure in children. The syndrome is characterized by the triad of acute renal failure, microangiopathic haemolytic anaemia and thrombocytopenia. These manifestations usually follow an episode of bloody diarrhoea caused by *E. coli* O157.

Aetiology and pathophysiology

HUS is not a single disease but comprises a number of disorders which, probably through different mechanisms, lead to endothelial cell injury which is central to the pathophysiology of the syndrome and gives rise to the major manifestations. In those cases preceded by bloody diarrhoea, the verocytotoxin produced by *E. coli* O157 causes endothelial damage liberating endothelin, reducing endothelial NO and thus promoting vasoconstriction. There is also activation of neutrophils, platelets, and the coagulation pathway leading to enhanced thrombosis and microangiopathy, which is most prominent in the kidneys. The haemolytic anaemia in these cases results from the passage of the red blood cells through the narrowed and deformed vascular channels.

In cases of HUS which follow prodromal respiratory and gastrointestinal infections caused by other bacteria, such as *Streptococcus pneumoniae*, and viruses, the manifestations of HUS may be mediated by different toxins (e.g. neuraminidase removing sialic acid residues and exposing certain autoantigens on the surfaces of red blood cells, platelets and in the glomerulus). Rarely, familial and recurrent cases occur in which abnormalities in prostacyclin production may be involved.

Clinical features

The prodromal illness, usually bloody diarrhoea, is followed by sudden pallor and oliguria. The child is irritable or drowsy, looks unwell and may have an elevated blood pressure. The blood picture is characteristic of microangiopathic haemolytic anaemia with fragmented red blood cells, an elevated reticulocyte count and negative Coombs's test. There is also thrombocytopenia and neutrophilia. Blood chemistry reveals reduced renal function with high urea and creatinine levels. Electrolyte imbalances, including hyperkalaemia, may occur. Findings on urinanalysis are surprisingly scanty and are frequently limited to moderate haematuria and mild proteinuria.

Extrarenal involvement may occur and present with haemorrhagic colitis, seizures and other central nervous system syndromes, and myocardiopathy. Heart failure may develop because of fluid overload.

Management

The diagnosis should be suspected in any child with bloody diarrhoea and included in the diagnosis of acute renal failure in a previously healthy child. Treatment is mainly supportive, with careful attention to fluid and electrolyte balance. Children requiring dialysis, or with other severe manifestations, are best managed at a paediatric nephrology centre. Epidemic HUS affecting younger children following an episode of infective bloody diarrhoea generally carries a favourable prognosis.

Infection with *E. coli* O157 is most frequently transmitted via undercooked minced meat or cold meats contaminated by fresh meat. Following the recent epidemics in Scotland, a major review of husbandry and meat-handling practices was launched, and its numerous recommendations should improve the standard of hygiene in the meat industry.

FURTHER READING

Kumar V, Cotran R S, Robbins S L 1997 Basic pathology, 6th edn. Saunders, London
Postlethwaite R J 1994 Clinical paediatric nephrology. 2nd edn. Churchill Livingstone, Edinburgh

CHAPTER 9

The endocrine and metabolic system

S. A. Greene

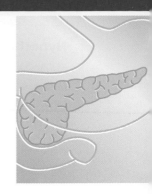

<table>
<tr><td colspan="3">

CORE PROBLEMS OF THE ENDOCRINE AND METABOLIC SYSTEMS

</td></tr>
</table>

CORE PROBLEM	KEY DIAGNOSIS	RELATED TOPICS
• Hormone dysfunction	Type I diabetes	Hypothyroidism Hyperthyroidism
• Growth disorder	Short stature	Growth hormone deficiency
• Metabolic disturbance	Hypoglycaemia	Obesity

Table 9.1 Incidence and prevalence of the common endocrine and metabolic problems in childhood

Diagnosis	Incidence	Prevalence
Type I diabetes	1.4–1.5/1000	25/ 00
Hypothyroidism Congenital	1/4000 live births	1.3/1000
Congenital adrenal hyperplasia		0.1/1000
Growth hormone deficiency		1/5000 to 1/10 000
Addison's disease		0.05/1000
Glycogen storage disease (type I)		0.08/1000

ESSENTIAL BACKGROUND

INTRODUCTION

While the endocrine and metabolic systems are fundamental to the growth and development of the child (see Ch. 2), major pathophysiological abnormalities are relatively rare (Table 9.1). Growth disorders are dominated by extreme but normal variations of the pattern of growth, where the underlying hormone systems are intact. Organic disorders account for less than 10% of children presenting with growth abnormalities, whereas type I diabetes and thyroid disorders alone account for 80% of paediatric endocrine problems. The rarer deficiencies in specific hormones occur with usually serious consequences and often severe and life-threatening illness. The understanding of endocrine and metabolic disorders has advanced rapidly over the last three decades with the developments in biochemical methodology (e.g. steroid biochemistry, radioimmunoassay) and, recently, molecular and genetic technology. A fuller understanding of the complex hormone and metabolic systems has emerged, with the result that specific syndromes can be defined by the linkage of specific hormone deficiency/excess or intermediate metabolites with their specific gene defects.

ANATOMY AND PHYSIOLOGY

Hormone action and function are described in Chapter 2. Central to clinical abnormalities in children and adolescents is the hypothalamic–pituitary–endocrine gland axis and the mechanisms involved in glucose homoeostasis.

Hypothalamic–pituitary gland axis

The main endocrine glands are operating by feedback systems (usually negative) through the hypothalamus and/or pituitary gland. Loss or overproduction of a hormone results in compensatory action from the feedback system, which in itself may induce pathophysiological change. A prime example of this is seen in congenital adrenal hyperplasia (CAH), which will be described in some detail to give a general understanding of the way in which endocrine systems are regulated.

The commonest type of CAH is a genetic disorder, in which abnormalities of chromosome 6 produces loss of an enzyme system – 21-hydoxylase – resulting in abnormal biosynthesis of adrenal gland hormones. This enzyme is responsible for a hydroxylation step in the cascade of converting cholesterol to the adrenal hormones cortisol and aldosterone (Fig. 9.1).

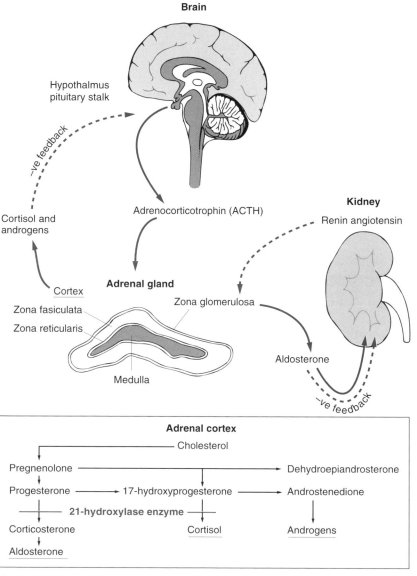

Brain

Hypothalmus pituitary stalk

–ve feedback

Cortisol and androgens

Adrenocorticotrophin (ACTH)

Kidney

Renin angiotensin

Adrenal gland

Cortex

Zona fasiculata

Zona reticularis

Zona glomerulosa

Medulla

Aldosterone

–ve feedback

Adrenal cortex

Cholesterol

Pregnenolone ———————————————→ Dehydroepiandrosterone

Progesterone ——→ 17-hydroxyprogesterone ——→ Androstenedione

21-hydroxylase enzyme

Corticosterone   Cortisol   Androgens

Aldosterone

Figure 9.1   The control through a negative-feedback system of the hypothalamic–pituitary–adrenal axis

Deficiency of the enzyme results in overproduction of an intermediate metabolite: 17-hydroxyprogesterone. Loss of cortisol production activates the negative-feedback system to signal to the hypothalamus to increase secretion of pituitary adrenocorticotrophin (adrenocortrophic hormone, ACTH). Overproduction of ACTH leads to hyperplasia of the adrenal gland and excess production of other adrenal hormones (e.g. oestrogen and testosterone, Fig. 9.1). Excess production of testosterone in the female fetus leads to abnormal virilization in the first trimester of development with the phenotype of 'ambiguous genitalia': i.e. on physical inspection, because of clitoral hypertrophy and labial fusion, it is difficult to identify the baby as male or female.

The complex problem of CAH identifies some key features in abnormalities of paediatric endocrine and metabolic disorders:

- The hypothalamic–anterior pituitary gland axis has a central role in regulating the various endocrine glands (Table 9.2).
- The underlying cause is frequently a single hormone or enzyme deficiency secondary to a gene defect(s).
- The defect may be primary (i.e. abnormality of the endocrine gland), secondary (abnormality of the pituitary gland) or tertiary (abnormality of the hypothalamus).
- Complex and widespread physical changes may result from a specific hormone deficiency (Table 9.3).
- Changes in biochemical and physiological homoeostatic mechanisms, secondary to imbalance in the feedback controlling systems, may be the cause of the major pathophysiological changes, e.g. testosterone overproduction in CAH.

Table 9.2   Regulation of hormone secretion by the hypothalamic–pituitary gland axis

- Thyroxine production from the thyroid by thyroid-stimulating hormone (TSH)
- Cortisol production from the adrenal gland by adrenocorticotrophin (ACTH)
- Sex steroids from the gonads (oestrogen/ovary; testosterone/testis) in response to luteinzing hormone (LH) and follicule-stimulating hormone (FSH)
- Human growth hormone (hGH) produced from the pituitary in response to hypothalamic gonadotrophin-releasing hormone (GnRH)
- Insulin-like growth factor 1 (IGF-1) produced in the liver in response to hGH.
- Vasopressin (antidiuretic hormone, ADH) directly from the postpituitary gland to act on the proximal tubule of the renal nephron

Table 9.3   Clinical effects of hormone deficiency

Hormone	Effect of deficiency
Cortisol	General malaise, decreased resistance to infection, hypotension
Thyroxine	Malaise, poor growth, deterioration in mental functioning (depression, reduced cognition), hair loss, skin changes
Aldosterone	Hypotension, hyponatraemia, hyperkalaemia, polyuria
Growth hormone	Short stature, growth failure, increased fat mass, hypoglycaemia
Gonadotrophin	Delayed puberty, primary gonadal failure
Vasopressin	Polyuria and nocturia, dehydration, shock

Glucose homoeostatic mechanisms

A continual supply to the brain of glucose (6 mmol/l/kg body weight/min) is essential for its normal functioning. Complex homoeostatic mechanisms exist to ensure this supply, taking into account glucose and carbohydrate stores, fed or fasting state and the needs of energy for exercise. The major hormones controlling this balance are insulin, as an anabolic hormone, and the counter-regulatory catabolic hormones adrenaline, noradrenaline, cortisol, growth hormone and glucagon (Fig. 9.2).

Diabetes mellitus is the most common abnormality of glucose homoeostasis. Insulin deficiency (type I diabetes; see below) or insulin resistance (type II diabetes in the older person) produces persistent hyperglycaemia (random blood glucose level >11.0 mmol/l; fasting blood glucose level >7.0 mmol/l). This can be tolerated for a period but ultimately will lead to severe symptoms when the metabolic buffering systems become overwhelmed. Unchecked glycosuria leads to dehydration, and insulin deficiency produces ketonaemia and acidaemia. Finally, diabetic ketoacidosis produces hypovolaemia, shock and coma; death results if left untreated (Fig. 9.3).

Hypoglycaemia (defined as a blood glucose level <3.5 mmol/l) produces adrenergic and neuroglycopenic symptoms. The former is secondary to the secretion of the counter–regulatory hormones (especially catecholamines), which are secreted in high concentration in an attempt to increase the circulating blood glucose concentration by gluconeogenesis and glycogen breakdown (Fig. 9.4). This produces the secondary

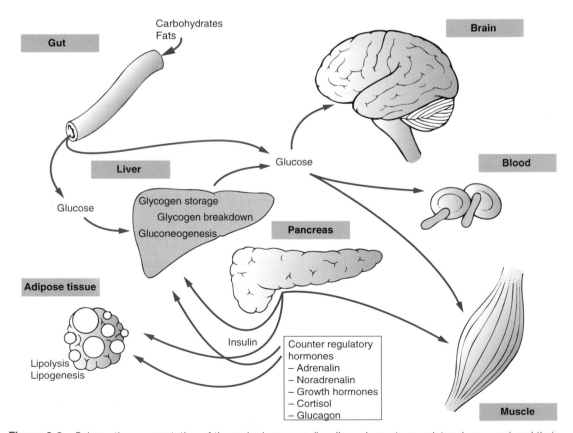

Figure 9.2   Schematic representation of the major hormones (insulin and counter-regulatory hormones) and their role in the homoeostatic control of glucose metabolism

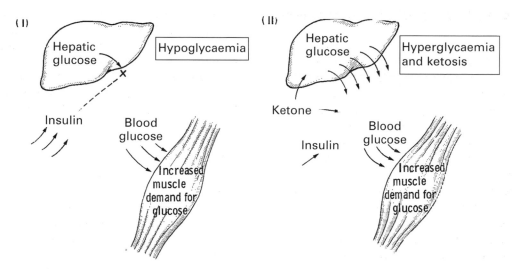

Figure 9.3 Schematic representation of the major role of insulin in the production of hypoglycaemia and hyperglycaemia and ketosis. (I) Insulin excess blocks hepatic glucose production and increases muscle glucose uptake, resulting in hypoglycaemia. (II) Insulin deficiency leads to excessive liver glucose production and decreases muscle uptake. The culmination of hyperglycaemia ketosis and dehydration leads to diabetic ketoacidosis

symptoms of tachycardia, sweating, and agitation. If the hypoglycaemia persists or indeed worsens, then the symptoms of neuroglycopenia develop (headache, light-headedness, abdominal pain), which will then lead to change in consciousness level and ultimately convulsions and coma. If the blood glucose level falls quickly, the symptoms merge rapidly, with coma developing suddenly. In the neonate (see Ch. 4) or young child, physical symptoms maybe difficult to identify before convulsions or coma develop.

HISTORY AND EXAMINATION

As in all childhood illnesses, a detailed and comprehensive history and careful examination are essential. Particular attention should be paid to the following features which may indicate certain syndromes and diseases:

- Family history: autoimmune disease (type I diabetes, thyroid disease, Addison's disease, vitiligo); known endocrine disorders (CAH, glycogen storage disorders, phenylketonuria, hypoglycaemia).
- Pregnancy: exposure to steroids (ambiguous genitalia).
- Neonatal period: hypoglycaemia, optic atrophy (congenital hypopituitarism); abnormal neonatal screening test prolonged jaundice (congenital hypothyroidism); ambiguous genital development (CAH).
- Early childhood: failure to thrive, delayed neurodevelopment (thyroid disorders); polyuria and polydipsia (type I diabetes – at any age).
- Mid-childhood: falling away from growth centiles (human growth hormone (hGH) deficiency isolated or part of hypopituitarism); educational difficulties, behavioural changes (hypothyroidism); abnormal fat distribution (Cushing's syndrome); low blood pressure, skin pigmentation (Addison's disease).
- Adolescence: delayed or early onset of puberty (idiopathic, hypopituitarism).

Specific points in the clinical examination include:

- Growth: screening for growth failure is mandatory (see Ch. 2)
- Genital examination (particularly in the newborn)

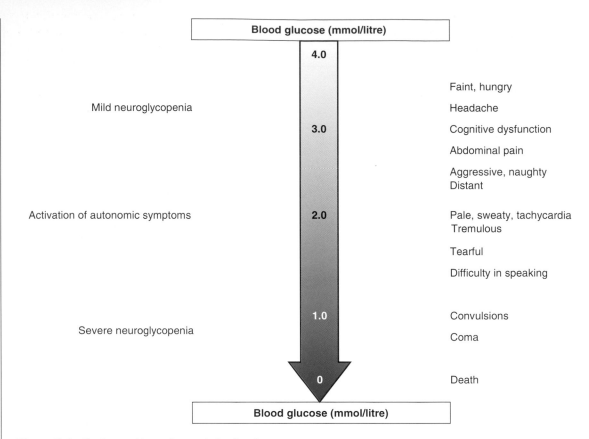

Figure 9.4 Features of hypoglycaemia leading to coma

- Puberty assessment (according to Tanner, see Ch. 2)
- Presence of a goitre
- Collection of dysmorphic features and/or disproportion to indicate specific syndromes (Turner's syndrome, Down's syndrome, Russell–Silver syndrome, Achondroplasia).

PRESENTATION OF ENDOCRINE AND METABOLIC DISORDERS

Endocrine and metabolic disorders can often present acutely and severely (e.g. CAH, hypoglycaemia) or chronically over a few weeks (e.g. type I diabetes, hyperthyroidism) or several months or indeed years (e.g. hypothyroidism). Some problems (e.g. hypopituitarism) can have varied presentation: acute life-threatening hypoglycaemia in the neonatal period or poor growth in childhood with delayed puberty.

Rapid assessment with some basic hormone tests can often lead quickly to the diagnosis, e.g.

- Random or fasting blood glucose level for type I diabetes
- Plasma free-thyroxine and thyroid-stimulating hormone levels for hypothyroidism
- Plasma 17-hydroxyprogesterone level in a suspected neonatal presentation of CAH
- Plasma cortisols levels (assessing diurnal variation) in Cushing's syndrome and Addison's disease.

Most of the rarer endocrine and metabolic disorders will require some form of dynamic testing procedure in which the response to hormone or physiological challenge is measured.

This requires special facilities and experience in performing the tests that are usually available only in special laboratories

NEONATAL SCREENING – THE GUTHRIE TEST

Children born in the UK have a blood sample test (usually a heel prick capillary sample) taken in the newborn period. For most babies this is on day 6 or 7, provided normal breast or formula milk feeding has been established. Approximately 10 µl of blood is placed on to a special blotting paper card, which is posted to a central laboratory serving several clinical centres. Currently in the UK each blood spot is analysed for the level of phenylalanine (to screen for phenylketonuria) and thyroxine and/or (thyroid-stimulating hormone, TSH) (to screen for congenital hypothyroidism). While other diseases have been screened for on occasion (e.g. CAH, cystic fibrosis), they have not fully conformed to the requisites of a successful screening programme (high specificity and sensitivity, with a simple effective remedy started early in life).

CORE PROBLEMS

HORMONE DYSFUNCTION

✳ KEY DIAGNOSIS

Type I diabetes

Aetiology

Type I diabetes insulin-dependent diabetes mellitus, (juvenile diabetes, ketosis prone diabetes) is an 'ancient' disease, with records in Greek and Egyptian writings. The modern era of diabetes started in 1921 with the discovery of insulin by Banting and Best in McCleod's laboratory in Toronto, Canada. It is an autoimmune disease usually occurring under the age of 40 years, with a peak onset in early adolescence.

Recently there has been a well-documented evidence of a rise in incidence throughout the world. In Scotland, for instance, there has been a near tripling of new cases per year since the early 1970s. There is a well-recognized variation in the world in the prevalence and incidence of diabetes, with Scandinavia and North Europe having the highest rates. This 'explosion' of diabetes cannot have occurred by genetic influences alone. Environmental changes have played a part and, while many suggestions have been made (e.g. specific virus infections, dietary ingredients, pesticides), as yet no single agent has been confirmed. The cause of diabetes is almost certainly an example of the classical 'double-hit theory'; in this case genetic predisposition and antigen stimulation. It is probable that the auto-immune reaction, in this case the development of chronic β islet cell inflammation, is initiated in a genetically at-risk person with possibly several different forms of antigen stimulation acting through common molecular immune pathways (see Highlights and Hypotheses: type I diabetes).

Clinical presentation

Insulin deficiency leads to chronic hyperglycaemia (Fig. 9.4). Classically, diabetes presents with the symptoms of persistently raised blood glucose levels: polyuria, polydipsia, weight loss and general malaise. An abnormal blood glucose level (random >11.0 mmol/l) confirms the diagnosis. If these symptoms remain unrecognized or proceed rapidly, diabetic ketoacidosis (DKA) will develop (acidaemia, dehydration, shock and coma). Most children and older teenagers are diagnosed relatively early by recognition of the symptoms and rapid assessment of the blood glucose concentration; newly diagnosed children under the age of 5 years appear to present more commonly with DKA.

Management

The aim of therapy is to 'normalize' the blood glucose concentration. However, replacement of the complex homoeostatic mechanisms controlling blood glucose levels is extremely difficult with the tools available to the clinician and the patient. Insulin can be replaced but it is delivered in to the peripheral, not the hepatic circulation, and is not connected to a negative-feedback system, i.e. insulin secretion from the β cells of the pancreas is not titrated against the

TYPE I DIABETES

What is its cause?

The exact cause of type I diabetes at present remains elusive, although a considerable volume of research in the last 20 years has uncovered many of the mechanisms that lead to the immune process which destroys the pancreatic β cells. While environmental 'antigens' will have some role, an inherent susceptibility to developing diabetes has been recognized for many years. Approximately 20% of first-degree relatives will have diabetes, and concordance in identical twins is around 50%: that it is not 100% adds weight to an environmental agent having a role in developing diabetes.

Different subtypes of the HLA cell membrane immune protection system (HLA-DR type) is associated with a high risk of diabetes, whereas other types (HLA-B2) appears to deliver protection against diabetes. The HLA system may just be a marker associated with susceptibility or indeed, as some have suggested, may be the molecular abnormality that allows an abnormal presentation of an antigen to the β cell membrane. Other immunological markers have been isolated, reflecting β cell damage, and these may be present for some considerable time before the presentation of clinical diabetes. In large epidemiological studies, immunological markers (islet cell antibodies, insulin autoantibodies, and glutamic acid decarboxylase (GAD) antibodies) have been found to be present in most teenagers developing diabetes for on average 2 years. The clinical picture of diabetes emerges when over 80% of pancreatic β cells have been destroyed.

How can it be prevented?

The autoimmune process of type I diabetes, with its long prodromal period before clinical presentation, appears to offer the possibility of immune modulation therapy, either to prevent the initiation of the immune process or retard its progress to full destruction of the β cell of the pancreas. Detection of first-degree relatives of index cases well before any clinical symptoms of hyperglycaemia is possible with a high degree of sensitivity and specificity of the tests: HLA typing and testing on routine basis for insulin autoantibodies, islet cell antibodies and GAD antibodies. Currently there are several worldwide multicentre studies investigating various agents or processes that may modify the immune process: nicotinamide (vitamin B_6 complex), low-dose oral insulin, and breast feeding. Results of these trials will be available early in the millennium. As yet, population screening at birth for high-risk patients using HLA typing lacks sufficient specificity to justify long-term 'antidiabetes' therapy, and lack of a specific antigen prevents 'diabetes vaccination programmes'.

---

circulating glucose concentration. The aim of treatment is by balancing the known insulin absorption pattern against the expected changes in circulating glucose following meals and exercise.

Insulin

Human soluble insulin is the basic preparation, which is now produced biosynthetically. Injected into the subcutaneous skin layer, it will begin to increase in blood concentration, reaching a peak within 30 min (newer insulin analogue preparations give even faster absorption properties). However, to match the requirement for a continual baseline concentration of insulin and high levels in the few hours after a meal, various insulin preparations have been developed with altered (delayed) absorption characteristics (isophane and lente insulin preparations). Most young children manage on a two injection per day regimen using a mixture of short and longer absorption insulin. As they approach the teenage years, some require more injections a day (i.e. a multiple-injection regimen) to maintain their blood glucose stable. Some paediatricians suggest that more intensive regimens should be applied straight from the onset of the diabetes, but this is controversial. Most clinicians agree that an individual insulin regimen should be constructed for each child.

Diet

To match the expected persisting high levels of insulin, carbohydrate intake is controlled both in quantity and time. The recommended diet is high in fibre and complex carbohydrate, low in simple sugars and low in saturated fats. Children are usually prescribed regular snacks, particularly if given two injections of insulin a day. On a multiple-injection regimen, snacks can be omitted.

Monitoring

The effectiveness of the diabetes regimen is monitored by the average level of blood glucose and the response of the glucose level to specific situations (exercise, social activities, meals etc.). The introduction, in the 1980s, of simple bedside methods for measuring the blood glucose concentration from capillary finger prick samples revolutionized the understanding of the ambient glycaemic control of diabetic patients. It was realized that therapy was suboptimal in relation to achieving normal glucose concentrations. Monitoring has been further improved with the introduction of glycated haemoglobin (Hb A) measurement, which gives a measure of the average glycaemic control over several weeks. A diabetic clinic has individuals with a range of glycated haemoglobin (usually the Hb A_{1c} fraction) from normal (around 6%) to above twice the expected. These data have forced centres to look at the effectiveness of their services and, in particular, the advice that they give to patients. Central to this has been the introduction of the specialist diabetes nurse, who visits the patients at home and helps them and their families to take on the management of the diabetes.

Complications

Acute

Hypoglycaemia (blood glucose level <3.5 mmol/l; see p. 173) is common but usually relatively mild. Severe hypoglycaemia (loss of consciousness, convulsions) is a frightening experience for both patients and families, and is a feared complication. Many diabetic patients who have had a severe 'hypo' will often choose to run their glucose levels higher than is desirable. While keeping tight glucose control (i.e. Hb A_{1c} in the normal range) increases the risk of hypoglycaemic episodes, near-normal stable control reduces the risk. Treatment is by initially correcting the hypoglycaemia by ingestion of simple sugar (glucose sweets or drinks, milk and biscuits) or anti-insulin measures (glucagon injection, special oral glucose solution) or glucose by intravenous infusion in hospital. Attention to the details of why a 'hypo' may have occurred (missing food; very energetic exercise without carbohydrate cover; vomiting; overdose of insulin) is essential with a view to prevention of further episodes.

Diabetic ketoacidosis

DKA usually occurs because of insulin omission in young people who are known to have diabetes. Whether deliberate or the result of a 'chaotic' lifestyle, DKA should be preventable by close attention to detail and continual support of the patient. If DKA does occur it is major emergency and requires intensive therapy in hospital: intravenous fluids for salt and water replacement, insulin infusion, and biochemical and physiological monitoring for several hours. Again, it is important to review the cause to prevent subsequent episodes.

Erratic control

Unfortunately, many diabetic patients have periods of 'swinging glucose levels' with frequent episodes of hypoglycaemic episodes and DKA. Brittle diabetes is the term given to patients at the extreme end of this spectrum. For most children and teenagers this represents not a physiological problem but emotional difficulties in adhering to the daily regimen of diabetes: an inability to cope with regular injections, frequent monitoring and special attention to their diet. Virtually all diabetics have difficulties at some point. While most come to terms with the disease, a small group have severe persisting difficulties in controlling their diabetes. Erratic control is usually related to personal, home and family problems: separating parents, school problems, difficulties in personal relationships, alcoholism or drugs. A major part of the diabetes service is to support families in these difficulties and manage their diabetes despite these problems.

Micro- and macrovascular disease:

After several years of diabetes, long-term poor glycaemic control puts patients at risk of microvascular damage to many organs (eyes, kidneys, small capillary blood vessels) as well as at a high risk of coronary artery disease and stroke in later life. This legacy of damage reveals itself clinically in the third and fourth decades of life, and is related to the duration of poor glycaemic

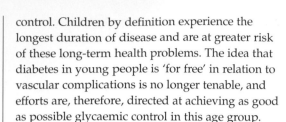

control. Children by definition experience the longest duration of disease and are at greater risk of these long-term health problems. The idea that diabetes in young people is 'for free' in relation to vascular complications is no longer tenable, and efforts are, therefore, directed at achieving as good as possible glycaemic control in this age group.

Patient support groups

An aspect of diabetes worth emphasizing is the efforts made by patients and young people themselves in managing and treating their own disease. Patient support groups have always been prominent, and the British Diabetic Association was formed over 60 years ago by physicians with an interest in diabetes and diabetic patients, notable amongst them H.G. Wells. Most countries have their own patients' organizations which are linked together through the International Diabetes Federation.

Thyroid disorders

Compared with adults, thyroid disorders in children have two important distinctions that influence their clinical presentation and management: (1) lack of the thyroid hormone in early infancy and childhood will have a devastating effect on brain development; (2) thyroid disease will effect growth and development.

Hypothyroidism

Aetiology

Congenital This is usually primary, i.e. the defect is in the thyroid gland. This can be an embryological development defect, leading to thyroid dysgenesis (60%), an ectopic thyroid (often sublingual) or an absent gland (25%). Thyroid hormone biosynthesis defects are much rarer (5%), and frequently have a strong family history, usually with an autosomal inheritance. Several specific enzymes deficiencies have been detected in the pathways incorporating iodine into the cell and in the organification processes for the production of the thyroid hormones triiodothyronine (T_3) and thyroxine (T_4).

Congenital secondary and tertiary disease is a deficiency in TSH secretion following congenital brain abnormalities affecting the pituitary gland (secondary, e.g. absence of the gland) and the hypothalamus (tertiary, e.g. septo-optic dysplasia).

Acquired Primary thyroid disease is either a delayed presentation of thyroid gland dysgenesis or the development of autoimmune hypothyroidism (Hashimoto's disease). Secondary and tertiary thyroid disease is caused by TSH deficiency consequent on pituitary disease (secondary, e.g. craniopharyngioma or trauma) or hypothalamic disease (tertiary, e.g. congenital brain abnormalities or radiation damage).

Clinical presentation

Neonatal period The classical presentation of 'cretinism' which should now be confined to history, is characterized by prolonged jaundice, poor feeding, constipation, excessive weight gain in relation to length, a floppy infant, umbilical hernia and obvious neurodevelopmental delay at 3–4 months of age. A low threshold to simple biochemical investigation for any of the above symptoms should prevent irreversible neurological damage. However, with the advent of neonatal screening, it was realized that many children with a less severe clinical presentation would slip through clinical surveillance programmes. The ideal target for the screening programme is to detect hypothyroid children and place them on thyroxine by 2 weeks of life. Leaving treatment until 3 months of age places the child at a high risk of neurological damage.

The older child An older child will present often with a long history of 'mild' symptoms: general malaise, poor school performance, poor growth, delayed puberty. A goitre maybe the only physical sign apart from short stature.

Thyroid function tests

Using direct and sensitive hormone assays the confirmation of thyroid disease has become relatively simple: low free T_4 and T_3 and elevated TSH levels. A delayed bone age confirms the effect on growth. Thyroid scanning in infancy may demonstrate an ectopic or absent gland.

Management

T_4 hormone replacement therapy should be started as soon as possible, particularly in the young, to prevent neurological damage. T_4 preparation (originally from desiccated gland tissue, and now a synthetic preparation) has been available for several decades. Given orally the dose is based on body size and titrated against thyroid function tests (normalization of T_4 and TSH levels), loss of clinical symptoms and improvement in growth.

Hyperthyroidism

Aetiology

Thyrotoxicosis in the young develops, as in adults, as part of the spectrum of autoimmune thyroid disease. The specific antigenic stimulus remains unknown: a strong family history is often seen with thyroid and other autoimmune diseases. Antibodies against thyroid cells induce a state of overproduction of thyroid hormone. Free T_4 and T_3 concentrations rise markedly and remain elevated. In some cases the initial autoimmune response changes and induces cell destruction and hypothyroidism: the picture of initial thyrotoxicosis followed by hypothyroidism is called 'Hashitoxicosis'. Although hyper-thyroidism usually occurs in young teenagers (girls > boys), it can present in the young child. Neonatal thyrotoxicosis may occur in babies born to mothers with autoimmune thyroid disease, secondary to the passage of antibodies across the placenta: this is usually temporary but may result in permanent cell damage.

Clinical presentation

The disease presents classically with general malaise and behavioural changes (anxiety, sleep disturbances), with the physical signs of goitre, tachycardia, weight loss, accelerated growth and exophthalmus. Left untreated this will progress, leading after several months to thyrotoxic crisis: severe tachycardia, high-output heart failure, skin changes, and severe weakness.

Management

Treatment is aimed initially at reducing the systemic effects of the thyroid hormones with a β blocker, usually propranolol, if appropriate. Carbimazole may be used subsequently to prevent further immune destruction of the thyroid gland. Long-term therapy is either by radioimmune therapy or thyroidectomy, which renders the patient hypothyroid, requiring life-long T_4 therapy.

GROWTH DISORDER

Children may grow abnormally slowly or rapidly, leading to short or tall stature, respectively. While in the majority of children the growth represents an extreme of the normal expected growth pattern or a response to an underlying organic disease (see Ch. 2), for some children a height outside of the normal range is secondary to an underlying endocrine disorder.

✳ KEY DIAGNOSIS

Short stature

The majority of children and teenagers presenting with short stature (height <3rd centile for age and sex or < −2 SD (standard deviations) of the reference population) have familial short stature (FSS), a constitutional delay in growth and puberty (CDGP) or a combination of both (see Ch. 2). While in clinical practice the majority of children presenting with concerns about growth (shortness and tallness) do not have any underlying pathology, diagnosis can be difficult at the extremes of normal variation. Irrespective of the underlying cause, the child or teenager may require behavioural and emotional support to cope with the concerns they have with their stature. In children presenting between −2 and −3 SD for their height, less than 10% will have an organic basis; this increases to 50% beyond −3 SD and risk of organic disease rises further as the shortness increases.

Aetiology

Short stature can be classified into idiopathic, primary and secondary.

Idiopathic

- FSS: height <3rd centile, short parents with height within the calculated target range, normal growth velocity, final height <3rd centile.
- CDGP: short stature in childhood which is below the expected parental height target range, retarded bone age, period of low growth velocity (<25th centile) which improves spontaneously during puberty, delayed onset of puberty, adult height within normal range and ultimately within parental target range.

Primary

Primary short stature is defined as an intrinsic disorder of the growth of cells and/or bone growth plates:

- Chromosome syndromes: Turner, Down, William and Prader–Willi syndromes.
- Dysmorphic syndromes with no current chromosome abnormality: Noonan and Russell–Silver syndromes.
- Intrauterine growth retardation (IUGR): birth weight <3rd centile, i.e. 2500 g. There may be known environmental causes (smoking, alcohol, drugs, malnutrition, placental dysfunction, congenital infection) or, as in 50% of cases, no obvious cause.
- Skeletal dysplasias: achondroplasia, spondyloepiphyseal dysplasia and osteogenesis imperfecta.
- Storage disorders: mucopolysaccharidosis and glycogen storage disease.

Secondary

Growth failure related to specific non-endocrine diseases All illness can give rise to growth failure. Indeed, intercurrent pyrexial illness will slow growth temporarily. The following are disease states where growth failure can be a primary symptom with major concerns for the patient and should be excluded in children with growth failure:

- Gastrointestinal disorders: inflammatory bowel disease (Crohn disease and ulcerative colitis); coeliac disease

- Renal failure
- Chronic anaemia; thalassaemia, parasitic infestation, iron deficiency anaemia
- Chronic infections: tuberculosis and HIV
- Poverty
- Psychosocial problems.

The last two are probably the commonest reasons for growth failure and short stature worldwide, including the UK. Growth failure has been recognized in severe child abuse, with dramatic responses in growth noted in removal from the abusive environment. Perhaps accepted less well in modern Britain has been the general negative effect on growth of poor social conditions.

Growth failure secondary to a specific endocrine disorder

- Thyroid disease (see above)
- Cushing syndrome
- Growth hormone deficiency.

Clinical presentation

Strict measurements of height and growth velocity are essential to define the problem (see Ch. 2).

Short stature can be part of a general presentation (as a secondary symptom) or the primary problem noted on clinical examination or during health surveillance. Severe pituitary problems with loss of hGH, TSH and ACTH production tend to present early in life with hypoglycaemia, prolonged jaundice and early growth failure; life-threatening infections and general malaise may also occur. Classically, the child with hGH insufficiency presents in midchildhood with minimal symptoms other than short stature; this is often noted around the age of 5 years when the child is compared with his or her new school friends.

Growth hormone (hGH) deficiency

Growth failure and short stature are secondary to hGH deficiency in the following:

- hGH gene deletion: this is extremely rare, occurring in families and characterized by extreme short stature and high antibodies to administered hGH.

- Pituitary abnormalities:
  - Primary hGH deficiency is caused either by congenital lesions of the brain (e.g. septo-optic dysplasia) or a developmental tumour classically a craniopharyngioma
  - Secondary causes are amongst the most common reasons for developing hGH deficiency, and are the result of damage to the pituitary gland or the hypothalamus of the brain, most frequently by radiotherapy given for leukaemia or brain tumours
- Idiopathic hGH insufficiency: this has been estimated to have a prevalence of 1 in 5000 of the population. However, difficulties arise in defining hGH insufficiency and separating a true physiological deficiency from a suppressed function. Poor health and social circumstances will reduce hGH secretion from the pituitary gland. The dynamic tests of hGH secretion appear to have low specificity and sensitivity, and the complete clinical picture should be taken into account when diagnosing hGH insufficiency:
  - Growth failure (height velocity <10th centile over 1 year)
  - Absence of general illness, including severe social difficulties
  - Increased body fat content
  - History of 'hypoglycaemic' episodes
  - Very low hGH and IGF-1 levels on testing
  - Possible pituitary abnormality on MRI examination.

Management

Few options exist for the treatment of idiopathic and primary causes of short stature. While hGH therapy will in some instances increase growth velocity, this is a temporary effect, and final height is not effected. Surgical procedures (limb lengthening) are offered to children and adults with bone dysplasias: this is a protracted and difficult treatment taking at least 1 year and requires a dedicated team offering continual support to the patient.

Growth improves in cases of short stature due to general illness with the successful treatment of the underlying cause. hGH replacement is very successful in definitive hGH deficiency. It has to be given by daily injections, with regular monitoring of growth. Growth hormone is species specific, and initially it was prepared from human cadavers. Tragically a small number of cases of Creutzfeldt–Jacob disease (CJD) have occurred in children given hGH; now all preparations are produced by biosynthetic methodology.

METABOLIC DISTURBANCE

＊ KEY DIAGNOSIS

Hypoglycaemia

Hypoglycaemia is one of the commonest features of metabolic disease. Any child who develops documented low blood glucose levels (<3.5 mmol/l) with symptoms requires investigation to exclude underlying pathology.

Aetiology

The commonest cause of hypoglycaemia is in type I diabetes (see above), and is the result of an inappropriately high insulin concentration and/or a deficiency in mobilization of glucose in time of excess body demand (fasting state, infection, trauma). Other causes are uncommon and related to metabolic defects in either glycogen breakdown or glucose neosynthesis.

Neonatal hypoglycaemia is seen frequently in low birth weight and premature infants. This is secondary to defective mobilization of fuel stores due to inefficient enzyme and hormone systems in babies that are frequently ill. Although transient, the hypoglycaemia is nevertheless dangerous to the baby (see Ch. 4). Persisting hypoglycaemia or low glucose concentrations in mature and or normal-weight infants is usually secondary to specific problems. The commonest is hypoglycaemia in infants of mothers with type I diabetes, who usually have had poorly controlled diabetes during pregnancy. In this situation, a persistently elevated maternal glucose concentration results in a greater than normal flux of glucose across the placenta which stimulates fetal insulin secretion. This hyperinsulinaemia results in fetal and neonatal excessive growth and immediately after birth, neonatal hypoglycaemia – both features are typical of the infant of a diabetic mother. The hypoglycaemia may take days to settle, and is often associated with other metabolic disturbances such as neonatal jaundice and neonatal hypocalcaemia. Specific metabolic or hormone syndromes causing hyperinsulinaemia are rare causes of neonatal hypoglycaemia: nesidioblastosis (a congenital developmental excess of disrupted islet cell tissue of the pancreas); Beckwith–Wiedemann syndrome (exomphalos, macroglossia, gigantism, hyperinsulinism, chromosome 11 abnormalities, risk of Wilm tumour).

Apart from type I diabetes, persistent and well-documented hypoglycaemia in infancy and childhood is usually caused by an underlying hormone or metabolic defect: hGH deficiency (see above); cortisol deficiency; fatty acid oxidation defects; urea cycle defects; glycogen storage defects.

Clinical presentation

In the infant and young child the symptoms will often progress rapidly to neuroglyopenic symptoms (p. 165). Associated metabolic findings will point to the diagnosis, which will require extensive and detailed radiological, endocrine and metabolic function tests, together with genotyping to confirm the exact diagnosis.

Other metabolic findings with the hypoglycaemia may suggest specific aetiologies:

- Ketosis and elevation of fatty acid levels: hGH deficiency and/or cortisol deficiency
- No ketosis and low fatty acid levels: hyperinsulinism
- No ketosis and raised fatty acids: fatty acid oxidation defects
- Raised lactate levels: inborn error of metabolism
- High insulin and low c-peptide levels: factitious use of insulin.

Vigilance at the time of the hypoglycaemic episode is vital, with blood and urine sampling immediately the hypoglycaemia is confirmed.

Management

The acute episode is treated as for type I diabetes. Correction of the underlying cause, if possible, is the best option for recurrent hypoglycaemic episodes. For example, surgery (95% pancreatectomy) for hyperinsulinaemic states, hGH and cortisol supplementation in pituitary deficiency, and specific metabolic therapy for inborn errors of metabolism.

Obesity

While obesity in general is not considered to be a metabolic disease, evidence is accumulating that underlying metabolic differences between individuals account for the variation in weight, despite apparently similar calorie intake (see Highlights and Hypotheses: obesity – a social disease or genetically determined?).

Obesity should be defined as a body mass index (BMI: weight (kg)/(height (m))^2) above the 97th centile for age and sex. However, with the concern of increasing obesity in the Western world, including the young, a BMI >85th centile is taken as overweight (and at risk for obesity), and obesity defined as a BMI > 97th centile for age and sex (BMI >30 kg/m^2 as an adult).

Aetiology

For most children and teenagers the cause of obesity is excessive calorie intake for their energy needs. While often disputed by the child and their parents, research has shown definitively this to be the case in 90–95% of children and teenagers with obesity (see Highlights and Hypotheses: obesity – social disease or genetically determined?). There are a small number of syndromes that may present with obesity:

- Prader–Willi syndrome: low birth weight, severe weight increase from age 2 years, short stature, hypotonia, almond-shaped eyes, high forehead, hypogonadism, behavioural problems including overeating and food scavenging, and partial deletion of long arm of paternal chromosome 15 or maternal disomy
- Cushing syndrome (usually secondary to administered steroids, very rarely due to adrenal or pituitary disease): short stature, abnormal excessive fat distribution (facial 'moon face', cervical 'buffalo hump'),

abdominal striae, capillary bleeding and hypertension
- hGH deficiency.

Clinical presentation

Nutritional excess characteristically presents with relatively tall stature (although weight is in excess of the height); this distinguishes simple obesity from the rare syndromes mentioned above with short stature and obesity. Early puberty and a similar family habitus are common features.

Management

This is has to be tackled on a personal and social level. Dietary advice has to be given together with behavioural support, not just focusing on healthy eating but also on social interactions and personal feelings. Specific programmes for overweight children have some success, but overall this has proved to be a difficult area. Drug therapy has limited use in the management of obesity in the young.

HIGHLIGHTS AND HYPOTHESES

OBESITY

Social disease or genetically determined?

The incidence of obesity in the Western world is rising, with 14% of adult men and 24% of adult women defined as overweight, and 15–20% of adolescents considered overweight. Of overweight children, 90% will become obese as adults. Obesity is a major risk factor in diabetes, cardiovascular disease, hypertension and strokes. Excessive calorie intake in relation to energy requirement is the fundamental cause of excessive body fat. The metabolic pathways are designed to accumulate body fat in the 'fortunate' biological state of food abundance where intake is above energy needs.

Patients are adamant, however, that their intake is not excessive – 'I eat the same as my friends'. This is apparently borne out if the patient's own recall of his or her food intake is used to calculate his or her eating pattern, and a genetically driven metabolic cause is then suggested – 'It's my metabolism, doctor'. This latter view has been dispelled using newer measurements of total energy intake and daily energy expenditure: by labelling oxygen and carbon with naturally occurring isotopes (^{18}O and ^{13}C), dilution experiments of doubly labelled water ($H_2^{18}O$) and carbon dioxide ($^{13}C^{18}O_2$) have revealed that obesity in adults is usually associated with significantly higher energy intake than the patients admit to.

However, recently the pendulum has swung back towards different metabolic rates determined by genetically derived cellular controlling systems and hormones. In particular, the hormone leptin has opened a whole new area of research. Leptin, which is produced in humans by white fat cells, was discovered in the genetically obese ob/ob mouse, which has a homozygous deletion of the leptin gene. Leptin is related to body fat content, and feeds back to the hypothalamus to signal satiety (i.e. to reduce appetite). When it is low or absent, satiety is reached at a higher than normal level of food intake, and obesity results. While leptin abnormalities appear to be only a very rare cause of obesity, its detection has linked, hormonally and metabolically, for the first time body size and the appetite centre.

While the major therapeutic option for correcting 'overeating' is a major social challenge, at the individual level the approach is behavioural. Research into leptin and related hormones may transform the pharmaceutical approach to the management of obesity in the future.

FURTHER READING

Brook C D G (ed) 1995 Clinical paediatric endocrinology, 3rd edn. Blackwell, Oxford
Court S, Lamb B (eds) 1997 Childhood and adolescent diabetes. Wiley, Chichester

Hughes I A 1989 Handbook of endocrine invesitgations in children. Wright, London
Wales J K H, Rogol A D, Wit J M 1996 Color atlas of pediatric endocrinology and growth. Mosby Wolfe, London

CHAPTER 10

The nervous system

D. F. Haddad

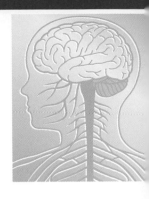

CORE PROBLEMS OF THE NERVOUS SYSTEM

CORE PROBLEM	KEY DIAGNOSIS	RELATED TOPICS
• Altered consciousness	Encephalopathy	Encephalitis Meningitis[14]
• Convulsions	Idiopathic epilepsy	Fever and fits
• Spasticity	Cerebral palsy	
• Hypotonia and weakness	Muscular dystrophy	
• Headache	Migraine	Brain tumours
• Abnormal head size or shape	Hydrocephalus	Microcephaly Craniosynostasis

Where the primary location of a topic is in another chapter, this is indicated by a superscript

ESSENTIAL BACKGROUND

INTRODUCTION

Neurological disorders in children pose special challenges and difficulties for the clinician. The accurate description of many of the symptoms related to disorders of the nervous system and the demonstration of unequivocal neurological signs are frequently not possible in children, since the required degrees of articulation and cooperation are not obtainable from the young. Instead, the clinician has frequently to rely on hints and clues that are more suggestive than definitive.

The nervous system is more vulnerable than any other system to a wide range of insults and injuries, whether occurring in utero at the early developmental stages, perinatally or later in life. Involvement of the nervous system manifesting itself as fits, altered consciousness or other neurological syndromes is frequently seen in children in the advanced stages of severe illness affecting other systems.

The imperative for early diagnosis in neurological disorders stems from the fact that, in many instances, the injury sustained by the nervous system can be limited and even reversed if the appropriate intervention is employed early enough. Furthermore, the course of many progressive neurological disorders can be slowed or halted by implementing appropriate measures. Even where there are established lesions of the nervous system, much of the deformity and functional impairment may be avoided by the early application of the right therapeutic strategies.

ANATOMY AND PHYSIOLOGY

The nervous system develops from the embryonic neural tube which originates from a groove in the dorsal ectoderm of the embryo (Fig. 10.1). At the anterior end a globular expansion appears which later splits into two lateral expansions. These represent the future cerebral hemispheres and lateral ventricles. The tissue around the ventricles is formed by migration of cells generated by the repeatedly dividing layer of cells of the

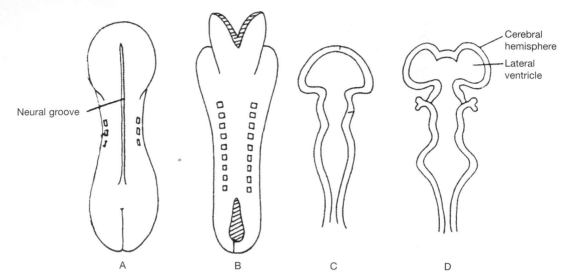

Figure 10.1 Schematic representation of the embryological development of the nervous system. (From Behrman R E et al 1995 Nelson textbook of pediatrics, 15th edn. W.B. Saunders)

ventricular walls. As these cells migrate outwards they retain their connections with their original positions through processes and projections.

At the end of this process the cellular grey matter occupies the outer part of the brain while the white matter, formed mainly from cellular projections and processes (neuronal dendrites and axons), is located underneath. At the innermost position lies the ventricular system, which is a modification of the original neural tube.

This process can go wrong at several points. Failure of closure of the original groove results in neural tube defects which may be at the cephalic end (encephalocele) or caudal end (spina bifida, meningomyelocele, see Ch. 16). Faults in cell migration result in distortion of the brain architecture which is associated with serious clinical consequences (cell migration disorders). If the ventricular system is narrowed or obstructed in any of its sections, the cerebrospinal fluid (CSF) circulation is impeded, and hydrocephalus may result.

The nerves and interneuronal connections are poorly myelinated in babies, resulting in delayed nerve conduction and poor cortical control of somatic innervation. During the first year of life, normal infants may display varying degrees of increased or decreased muscular tone (hypertonia

or hypotonia) and brisk tendon reflexes. The nature of the plantar responses in small infants is controversial (see p. 185).

Myelination of the intracranial nerves and connections is chiefly responsible for the accelerated rate of growth of the brain and thus the increase in the size of the head seen during infancy. As this process of myelinization and functional maturation progresses, muscular tone, tendon reflexes and the plantar responses assume the 'normal' pattern seen in older children and adults.

CSF circulation

The CSF is formed by a process of active secretion by the choroid plexus in the lateral ventricles, from where it flows via the foramina of Monroe to the third ventricle. From there, via the aqueduct of Sylvius, the CSF flows to the fourth ventricle and then to the spinal canal. In the fourth ventricle the CSF also gains access to the subarachnoid space through two foramina in its roof (the foramina of Luschka and Magendie). Thus, the CSF flows around the brain and spinal cord in the sub-arachnoid space as well as within the ventricular system and spinal canal. It is absorbed back into the blood in certain specialized areas of the subarachnoid space, the arachnoid villi (Fig. 10.2).

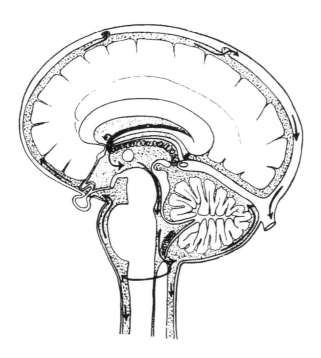

Figure 10.2 Schematic representation of the CSF circulation. (From Behrman R E et al 1995 Nelson textbook of pediatrics, 15th edn. W.B. Saunders)

Normal CSF values

Colour	: transparent, 'gin-clear'
Pressure	: 50–150 mmH$_2$O (higher in the flexed position)
Cells	: up to 5/mm^3; all lymphocytes (up to 15 in neonates)
Protein	: 100–400 mg/l (up to 1200 mg/l in neonates)
Sugar	: 60% of blood sugar (CSF sugar level of <2.0 mmol/l should suggest inflamed meninges regardless of the concurrent blood sugar value)
Organisms	: none, CSF is sterile

HISTORY, EXAMINATION AND INVESTIGATION

History taking

Symptoms of neurological disorders can be specific or non-specific. In either case, the presentation may be acute, subacute or chronic. The specific symptoms of neurological disorders in a child fall into one of the following categories:

- Fits, headaches and other paroxysmal events
- Altered consciousness
- Abnormal somatic function:
  - Sensation (including special senses)
  - Muscular power and tone
  - Balance and coordination
  - Abnormal movements
- Abnormal size or shape of the head and other visible abnormalities

Non-specific symptoms include:

- Concerns regarding development
- Changes in behaviour or performance
- Disturbances of other physiological functions, e.g. vomiting, incontinence, constipation, feeding and swallowing difficulties.

Two situations merit special attention, since they give rise to a constellation of symptoms (and signs) which allow a recognizable pattern to manifest. These are meningeal irritation (meningism) and elevated intracranial pressure.

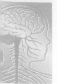

The specific symptoms and clinical problems relating to neurological disorders will be discussed in detail later in this chapter (see Core problems) under the appropriate headings. Meningeal signs are discussed in Chapter 14 on infectious disorders, while developmental delay and delayed walking are outlined in Chapter 3.

Although the general principles of paediatric history taking still apply, certain areas of the history require special attention and may have to be expanded when evaluating children with a suspected neurological disorder:

- *Presenting complaint*: the child and parents may have difficulty in providing accurate descriptions of the symptoms, and occasionally there may be an element of misinterpretation. Every effort should be made to obtain as much detail as possible, and to explore all the features that may help distinguish between the various possible explanations for a certain presentation (e.g. a fit versus breath holding). The child and parents should be guided as to the level of detail required.
- *Duration of the illness*: this may provide some insight into the nature of the pathological process and its aetiology. For example, a sudden appearance of symptoms and rapid progression may suggest trauma or infection. Such a course is unlikely to be due to a brain tumour, though exceptions do occur.
- *Past medical history:* this must be scrutinized with special attention to episodes of severe illness. Details of the pregnancy or labour and condition at birth should be obtained, as well as progress in the neonatal period. Any link between an untoward event and the appearance of symptoms should be noted, but care should be taken not to conclude a causal relationship solely on the basis of temporal links.
- *Developmental history*: this provides useful information about the integrity and functional capacity of the nervous system. A $2\frac{1}{2}$ year old toddler who is able to walk up stairs without holding on to the banister is unlikely to have a significant weakness of the lower limbs or pelvic girdle. However, such inference has its limitations, and subtle degrees of abnormality may not be picked up. On the other hand, if the history reveals that the child is unable to perform a certain age-appropriate skill, other possibilities should also be explored (see Ch. 3). Developmental arrest and regression refer to failure to progress following a period of normal development, and loss of previously acquired skills, respectively. Both patterns are suggestive of the presence of an underlying neurological disorder, although other mechanisms may occasionally be responsible. The timing of such an arrest or regression may also point to its cause.

- *Epidemiological history:* a contact's history and vaccination history are helpful when evaluating the possibility of infection. A recent vaccination raises the possibility of a vaccine reaction. Serious neurological sequelae resulting from the administration of the currently licensed childhood vaccines are extremely rare (see Ch. 17). Nevertheless, suspicions of such a reaction frequently arise, particularly when there is a temporal link between the discovery of a neurological abnormality and the administration of a vaccine. It is important to make sure that questioning about the vaccination history and any observed reactions does not leave the incorrect impression that a serious reaction to vaccination is a likely event.
- *Systemic review:* this provides some information about the autonomic functions of the nervous system. Thus, growth disturbances, excessive or absent sweating, vomiting, feeding and swallowing difficulties, constipation or soiling, urinary retention or incontinence may all signify a disturbed autonomic function rather than a localized cause. The presence of pathology affecting other systems may suggest a syndrome or a multisystem disorder.

In the course of a chronic neurological illness, changes in behaviour or personality and deterioration in mental functioning may be perceived by parents and other care-givers much earlier than any specific symptom. Such changes may be very significant but subtle and difficult to detect by a stranger.

The value of a good history in the diagnosis of neurological disorders cannot be overestimated. In certain situations, the diagnosis may be entirely dependent on the history (e.g. epilepsy, breath holding).

The neurological examination

The normal findings on neurological examination of children (Table 10.1) are age-dependent, and knowledge of the pattern accepted as normal for each age group is crucial for the correct interpretation of the elicited signs.

The techniques that can be utilized in the neurological examination of children vary according to age. In older children, a good degree of cooperation can be expected, and the neurological examination is conducted along the same lines as in adults. In babies and young infants, where no formal cooperation is possible but where resistance to the examination is minimal, the examiner aims to keep the disturbance of the infant to the minimum and relies heavily on observation of natural behaviour, as well as on the primitive involuntary reflexes and induced behaviours and movements.

The situation is particularly difficult in the case of older infants and toddlers; while an adequate degree of cooperation is still unlikely, this group of children tends to get upset easily. On the

slightest hint of being observed or assessed they frequently modify their natural activities and simply refuse to perform. Frequently they cut down on their active movements, resist passive movements, and deliberately suppress their reflexes by refusing to relax. The only hope is to make the examination as informal as possible, more like a game, involving the parent(s) and keeping the child comfortable for the length of the examination.

The technique of the neurological examination appropriate for toddlers is outlined in the next section. For the neurological examination of young infants (see Beyond core: notes on the neurological examination of infants).

Mental status

The neurological examination should begin by assessment of the mental status and level of consciousness: is the child alert, drowsy or comatose?

Within the alert state, variations include appropriate and inappropriate behaviours, irritability and confusion. A drowsy state is normally seen in children with lack of sleep and around their bedtime. A pathological nature is suggested when drowsiness seems inappropriate (the parents' account may be helpful in this). Sleep differs from coma by the ease of arousal and maintenance of the awake state afterwards. The depth of coma is also measured by arousability and responsiveness: responds to voice/commands, responds to pain, no response. The Glasgow Coma Scale (GCS) is a more detailed system used for grading the level of consciousness. A modified version is used for children.

Gait, balance and coordination

These are best assessed by observing the unaware child while at play and other natural activities. Building a tower by stacking 1 inch (2.5 cm) cubes on top of each other, working on a jigsaw or drawing are all suitable activities to gain information about coordination. Children should be able to walk and run smoothly by 2–3 years of age, but this is subject to variation. A limp is defined as the gait adopted when the body weight

---

Table 10.1   A general scheme for the neurological examination of children

- Assessment of mental state and level of consciousness
- Gait, balance and coordination
- Cranial nerves
- Motor system
    Tone and posture
    Bulk
    Power
    Reflexes
    Abnormal movements
- Sensation
- Autonomic function
- Meningeal signs
- General examination
    Skull shape and size, anterior fontanelle and sutures
    Dysmorphic features
    Skin signs
    Skeletal deformities
- Soft neurological signs

is not borne by the lower limbs symmetrically; this can be due to pain, shortening or weakness. Tiptoeing may be due to spasticity or shortening of the Achilles tendons. However, many normal children walk on their tiptoes intermittently without underlying pathology. Kicking a ball, walking upstairs and riding a tricycle are suitable activities to learn about balance as well as muscular power.

Children of 4–5 years of age can be asked to hop and skip and perform some simple manual skills. Older children can be expected to comply with the testing for 'cerebellar signs', and it is therefore possible to assess balance and coordination more formally.

Assessment of balance and coordination is an important part of the neurological examination of children since a proportion of the central nervous system (CNS) pathology in children mainly affects the infratentorial structures: the cerebellum and brain stem (certain brain tumours, some types of cerebral palsy).

Cranial nerves

The symmetry of the facial expression, particularly during laughter or crying, should be noted. Eye movements are tested by observing the child while visually following a moving object of interest. This is done while the mother/assistant gently holds the head to restrict its movement. Pupil size and reaction should be noted. Because of the possibility of causing distress, assessment of tongue and palate movements should be left to the end of the examination.

Ophthalmoscopy in children requires skill and patience. An assistant may be able to distract the attention of the child and stop him or her from looking constantly at the ophthalmoscope light. Frequently, pupillary dilatation is required.

Smell and taste are not tested routinely in children. Hearing and visual acuity are usually tested as part of health surveillance programmes (see Ch. 3).

Motor system
Tone
Information about muscular tone is gathered from observing posture and assessment of resistance to

passive movements. Bed-bound severely hypotonic children adopt a frog-like position: lying in the supine position with their hips abducted and knees flexed. Arching is the posture of marked hypertonia. Hyperextension of the head, extended hyperpronated upper limbs with fisting (clenched hands with the thumb held inside) and extended lower limbs that are adducted with plantar flexion of the feet are other typical postures of hypertonia. The legs tend to cross when these children are held vertically (scissoring – Fig. 10. 3).

The resistance to passive movements of the joints is best assessed in the unaware young child. While showing pictures in a book, or engaging the child in conversation or other activity, the

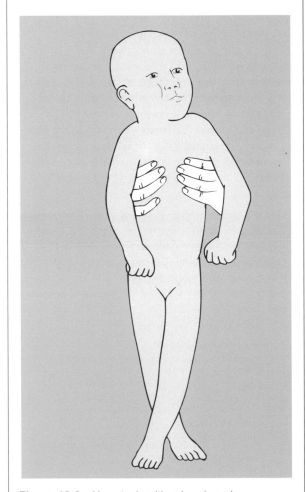

Figure 10.3 Hypertonia with scissoring – legs cross owing to adductor spasm, hands clenched

movements around the ankle, knees and hips and the tone of the upper limbs are assessed. In a similar way, distraction is used when testing the tendon reflexes. In older cooperative children, the resistance to passive movements is assessed in the usual manner.

Power

The symmetry of active movements should be noted. The ability to rise from the lying position, walking upstairs or pedalling a tricycle all indicate normal strength in the lower limbs and pelvic girdle. Allowing the child to pull on a string held by the examiner at the other end provides some information about strength in the upper limbs.

In older children, formal testing of power is usually possible. For the sake of comparison and follow-up, muscle strength is graded as follows:

0 = no power
1 = minimal movements present
2 = movements possible only horizontally (with gravity)
3 = movements against gravity are possible
4 = movements against resistance
5 = normal strength.

Reflexes

Deep tendon reflexes can be obtained from a toddler who is adequately distracted, otherwise any attempts at this are likely to be futile. The ankle and knee jerk in the legs and the biceps, triceps and pronater reflexes in the upper limbs are all obtainable. These are brisk in infants and anxious older children, but they are symmetrical. If pathologically exaggerated, the reflexogenic zone is increased and the reflex is obtained even when tapping away from the usual area for that particular reflex.

Clonus is a sign of an upper motor neuron lesion and is associated with hypertonia and exaggerated reflexes. It is best demonstrated in the ankle by sudden dorsiflexion of the foot while the leg is slightly flexed at the knee. A few beats of clonus may be normal in small infants. However, sustained clonus is significant, as is any asymmetry.

Muscle bulk

This is assessed by inspection and palpation. Muscular atrophy is marked in lower motor neuron lesions. Hypertrophy is seen in athletes. Pseudohypertrophy is the enlargement of weak muscles due to fatty infiltration (e.g. Duchenne muscular dystrophy).

Abnormal movements

Several types of involuntary movements in children are described:

- Intention tremor – one of the cerebellar signs
- Tics – can be transient or life-long (e.g. Gilles de la Tourette's syndrome)
- Chorea, athetosis and dystonia – abnormal movements seen in diseases of the basal ganglia.

Sensation

This is not routinely tested in children. When deemed necessary it may be tested in the cooperative child along the same lines as in adults. Grasp, rooting and sucking reflexes can be utilized for this purpose in babies.

Autonomic function

Pupil size and reactivity should be noted. Disturbances in heart rate, blood pressure or respiratory pattern may all result from abnormal autonomic innervation. Excessive or absent sweating and abnormal temperature control are other signs to look for. Disturbance of growth is one of the earliest signs of craniopharyngioma.

The meningeal signs

These are discussed under the heading Meningitis in Chapter 14.

General examination

The following parts of the general examination are particularly relevant:

- Measurement of the occipitofrontal circumference and plotting the results on a growth chart should routinely be performed in children younger than 2 years of age. Transillumination of the skull is helpful in the diagnosis of subdural effusion. Megalocephaly, hydrocephaly and microcephaly are discussed later in this chapter, as are abnormalities of skull shape and craniosynostosis.

- The anterior fontanelle should be examined in the non-crying baby held in the upright position. In this position, the skin overlying the anterior fontanelle is level with, or slightly below, the rest of the surface of the skull. A bulging tense fontanelle is a sign of increased intracranial pressure (see Fig. 14.1). In chronic cases, the size of the fontanelle may be enlarged and the cranial sutures separated. A significantly depressed anterior fontanelle is seen in dehydration.
- The presence of dysmorphic features may suggest a particular syndrome. However, this finding can be incidental.
- Because the skin and the nervous system both develop from ectoderm, a number of the neurological developmental abnormalities may have associated skin signs and stigmata (the neuroectodermal syndromes). Tuberous sclerosis, neurofibromatosis (see Fig. 16.8) and Sturge–Weber syndromes (see also Fig. 16.14) are important examples.
- Looking for any musculoskeletal deformities is an important part of the neurological examination of children with chronic neurological impairment, since much of the morbidity in such cases is due to the preventable musculoskeletal deformities that develop.
- Findings on examination of other systems may be of relevance. Thus, a purpuric rash supports (see Fig. 14.9) the diagnosis of meningitis, while hepatosplenomegaly in a child with abnormal muscle tone may suggest a metabolic storage disorder.
- The developmental examination is frequently carried out as part of the neurological examination as a screening for any underlying neurological impairment. It also provides a rough indicator to the normality or otherwise of mental functioning.

Soft neurological signs
This term refers to poor quality and precision of performance of certain tasks. Such poor performance may be accepted as normal at a younger age, but may correlate with learning difficulties and attention deficit disorder if it persists. The soft neurological signs do not signify a specific pathology. They include awkward and clumsy performance (sometimes with associated extraneous movements) on carrying out certain motor tasks, such as hopping, tandem walking, hand pats and repetitive and successive finger movements.

Investigation

In multisystem syndromes and disorders, the presence of haematological, biochemical, or chromosomal abnormalities may point to the diagnosis. Investigations specific to the nervous system include: lumbar puncture, electroencephalography, imaging, and electrophysiological studies.

Lumbar puncture
Examination of the CSF obtained by lumbar puncture is crucial for the diagnosis of bacterial meningitis (the CSF findings in different types of meningitis are discussed in Ch. 14).

CSF analysis for various bands of protein, lactate and other metabolites is also of diagnostic value in degenerative and metabolic disorders of the CNS. Examination of the CSF cells may also be of value in neoplastic infiltration of the meninges such as in leukaemia.

Lumbar puncture is a distressing and rather invasive procedure, and should only be done by a trained person. Adequate explanation of the procedure to the child and family is necessary, and sedation may occasionally be required. Lumbar puncture is contraindicated in the presence of:

- Signs of increased intracranial pressure
- Focal neurological signs
- Possibility of spinal cord compression
- Infection involving the skin overlying the space between L_3 and L_4 (the site for lumbar puncture)
- Any coagulation defect (should be corrected prior to the procedure).

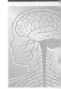

BEYOND CORE

NOTES ON THE NEUROLOGICAL EXAMINATION OF INFANTS

Clues to problems of balance and coordination in infants are: marked tremor, inability to reach and grasp objects beyond 5 month of age, and insecure sitting and standing. The presence of nystagmus and vomiting are also suggestive.

The posture in the full-term normal newborn is 'flexed' with flexed upper and lower limbs. Premature babies are normally hypotonic with a more extended posture.

In small babies, tone is also assessed by head lag, arm and leg recoil, the scarf sign and the popliteal angle. Head lag on dorsal and ventral suspension (poor head control) is a normal finding in neonates, particularly if premature. If head lag is marked or if it persists beyond the first few weeks, it may indicate weakness or hypotonia (see Fig. 3.1).

If the leg or arm of a baby is held flexed and then extended suddenly, it normally recoils to the flexed position, whereas it remains extended in hypotonia. If the flexed elbow is moved sideways across the body, it does not go beyond the midline in babies with normal tone. To measure the popliteal angle, with the knee flexed, the hip is flexed to bring the thigh and knee to the abdomen, then the knee is extended; in a normal newborn, 80° can be achieved.

A discrepancy between ventral and dorsal suspension may be seen transiently in normal babies before they develop full head control, but later may signify underlying spasticity such as that caused by cerebral palsy. Thus, there is marked head lag on dorsal suspension (pulling to sit, see Fig. 3.1) while on ventral suspension the head not only does not sag but is held above the plane of the body because of dominant extensor tone.

Mild and variable degrees of hypo- or hypertonia are normal in infants, including fisting.

However, within the first weeks of life the infant is expected to hold his or her hands open for longer periods, and for most of the time by 3 months of age.

In babies, active movements should also be noted. The Moro (see Fig. 3.2) and parachute reflexes provide valuable information on symmetry of movements. Babies with normal strength of the shoulder girdle will be able to support their weight when held from the axillae. They 'slip through' if weakness of this muscle group is present. Similarly, they will be able to weight bear on each of their extended legs with minimal help from the examiner when held in the upright position.

The plantar reflex is obtained by gentle stroking on the outer sole working from the heel and half the way to the toes. With the correct technique it is said that plantar flexion of the big toe is obtained even in newborns. Some people argue, however, that in early infancy the plantar responses are extensor and turn to flexor type only later. Whatever the truth of this, an extensor response is abnormal in an older infant, and asymmetry is always significant; the primitive reflexes are discussed in Chapter 3.

Imaging

Skull radiography is useful in detecting bony abnormalities, intracranial calcification and signs of long-standing increase in intracranial pressure. Calcification may be seen in intrauterine infections (toxoplasmosis and cytomegalovirus infections in particular), or at the site of an intracerebral tumour (a craniopharyngioma for example). Widening and erosion of the sella are other important signs of craniopharyngiomas.

Skull radiographs also provide useful information about the state of the cranial sutures. The value of skull radiography in evaluating children after head trauma is controversial.

Cranial ultrasound scans are possible in small children with open anterior fontanelles. This mode of imaging can be performed at the bedside with little disturbance to the child, and is very popular in the evaluation of sick neonates and infants because of its safety and convenience.

Ultrasound scans provide useful information about the size of the ventricles, intraventricular bleeds (see Fig. 4.4) or the presence of cerebral cysts. Their value is limited in assessing the architecture and structure of the brain substance itself.

Computerized tomography (CT) and magnetic resonance imaging (MRI) have dramatically improved our ability to diagnose intracranial pathology by non-invasive means. Information about the architecture of the brain, the character of grey and white matter, the cerebral vasculature, intracranial pressure and the ventricular system can all be obtained from these scans, as well as the presence of any intracranial lesions such as tumours (see Fig. 11.13), bleeds or haematomata (Fig. 10.4). They are an essential part of the patient work-up where neurosurgery is contemplated.

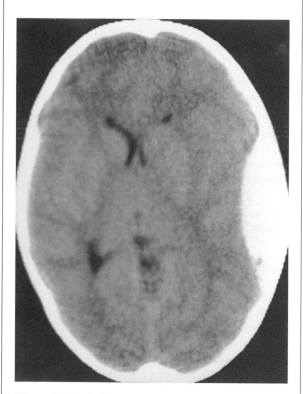

Figure 10.4 A CT scan of the brain of a 10 year old boy who sustained a head injury. Approximately 9 h later a lens-shaped density was seen over the left hemisphere with midline shift diagnostic of an extradural haematoma

Electroencephalography

Recording of the electrical activity of the brain allows some information to be obtained about the functional activity of the brain. It is of great value in confirming the presence of ongoing seizures if this diagnosis is not obvious from clinical observation (so-called electrical status). Electroencephalograms (EEGs) may also confirm the presence of a tendency toward recurrent convulsions (epilepsy), but the diagnosis of this condition remains largely clinical. Certain EEG patterns may be indicative of particular infectious, metabolic or degenerative pathology.

Electromyography and nerve conduction velocity

These techniques are valuable in the diagnosis of primary muscle and neurological disorders, and in making the distinction between these two pathological groups.

Other investigations

Muscle enzymes, nerve and muscle biopsies may also be obtained.

PATHOPHYSIOLOGY AND CLASSIFICATION

The multitude and diversity of causative factors underlying CNS pathology in children makes attempts at classification difficult. However, a general framework can be used to categorize most neurological disorders in children, and may aid their understanding (Table 10.2).

Neurological disorders can be congenital or acquired. Such division may not always be clear-cut. It is now widely believed that many of the disorders of the nervous system, as with diseases of other systems, may result from the interaction of a genetic predisposition with environmental (acquired) influences. Nevertheless, we shall retain this division since it is still useful in many cases.

Within each of the two categories it is usual to make a distinction between progressive and static disorders of the nervous system. Such categorization is more applicable to the nervous system than any other because of the limited

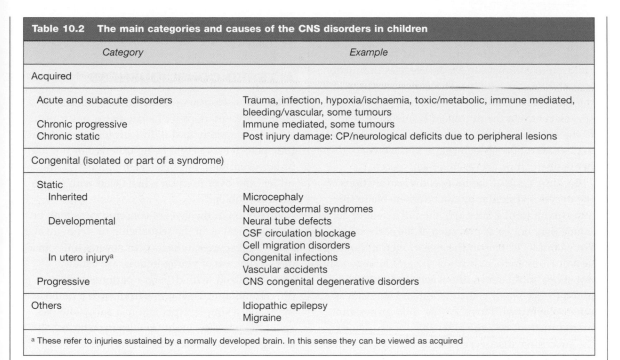

Table 10.2 The main categories and causes of the CNS disorders in children	
Category	*Example*
Acquired	
Acute and subacute disorders	Trauma, infection, hypoxia/ischaemia, toxic/metabolic, immune mediated, bleeding/vascular, some tumours
Chronic progressive	Immune mediated, some tumours
Chronic static	Post injury damage: CP/neurological deficits due to peripheral lesions
Congenital (isolated or part of a syndrome)	
Static	
Inherited	Microcephaly
	Neuroectodermal syndromes
Developmental	Neural tube defects
	CSF circulation blockage
	Cell migration disorders
In utero injury[a]	Congenital infections
	Vascular accidents
Progressive	CNS congenital degenerative disorders
Others	Idiopathic epilepsy
	Migraine

[a] These refer to injuries sustained by a normally developed brain. In this sense they can be viewed as acquired

ability of nervous tissue to regenerate. Thus, many of the CNS transient pathological processes (such as asphyxia, infection, trauma, etc.), if severe enough, may leave a long-lasting postevent effect.

Static brain lesions, whether they are part of a congenital disorder, faults in brain development or resulting from an injury sustained while the CNS is still in the developmental stage (whether in utero, at birth or in early childhood) can result in a posture and movement disorder referred to as cerebral palsy (CP).

Some of the disorders affecting the CNS can be viewed as pathological states that can arise from a number of 'primary' pathological processes. Examples are microcephaly and hydrocephalus; both can be determined genetically or arise from errors of development (at the stage of cell migration and the evolution of the ventricular system respectively). Alternatively, either can be acquired; microcephaly can be secondary to severe brain damage sustained at an early age (interfering with subsequent brain growth), while hydrocephalus may develop as a complication of obstruction to the outflow of the CSF from any

cause (e.g. postinfection, tumour). Either of these conditions may coexist with CP.

Prognosis

Concerns regarding prognosis and final outcome in children, whether presenting with an acute CNS injury or showing early signs of a chronic neurological disorder, frequently arise. Such concerns can add to the strains of the parent–doctor relationship, and should be addressed in a tactful but honest and direct manner. With the advances in brain-imaging techniques, the paediatric neurologist is better equipped to estimate the risk of chronic disability in many cases, but it is still far from being an exact science, and a number of factors continue to contribute to the inaccuracy of prognosis estimates in children with neurological disorders. One or more of these factors may, to a varying extent, exert influence in each individual case.

There is some, albeit limited, ability to regenerate, and affected areas of nervous tissue may show slow recovery. This may take weeks and even months. The extent of the residual brain lesion and neurological deficit may be overestimated in the early stages. There is also a special ability of some parts of the CNS in children to compensate for deficiencies in function of each other (plasticity). This is best illustrated by the example of children sustaining injury to the speech centre in the dominant hemisphere prior to the age of 7–8 years, who are subsequently able to develop a new speech centre in the other hemisphere, thus preserving their speech.

Because some of the more complex functions of the nervous system may not be amenable to the assessment until a later age, the full extent of an injury may not be appreciated at the early stages. For example, lesions in the area of motor planning sustained in utero, at birth or in early infancy may not show until later in life, when the toddler is noted to have poor coordination and clumsiness when playing with toys. As the child grows and more functions become amenable for assessment, the successive discovery of deficits may create the false impression of a progressive CNS disorder or worsening of the static condition.

Static lesions may give rise to progressive skeletal deformities, in the absence of the appropriate posturing and physiotherapy. On the other hand, adequate exercise and training of the relevant areas may strengthen the muscles, improve coordination, optimize the utilization of the remaining neurological function and may restore the use of the affected area to near-normal levels.

CORE PROBLEMS

The presenting features of neurological disorders in children, in most cases, fall within one of the following categories:

- Altered consciousness
- Convulsions
- Spasticity
- Hypotonia/weakness
- Headache
- Abnormal head size/shape
- (Developmental delay)
- (Delayed walking).

The topics in parentheses are discussed in Chapter 3.

ALTERED CONSCIOUSNESS

Altered consciousness is one of the most complex clinical presentations in the paediatric age group. Parents frequently find it difficult to express what they perceive as a child being different or not his or her usual self. Physicians are prone to both under- and over-reaction when faced with such a clinical problem.

Alteration in the level of consciousness may be physiological as in the sequencing of sleep/awake states. Such cycles, which occur several times in a day in the case of young infants, are usually individualized, with different patterns seen in different infants. Deviations from such a pattern may have a simple explanation: a baby who has spent the previous night up with earache or colic can be unusually sleepy or drowsy on the following day. Parents tend to volunteer such an explanation but, occasionally, have to be prompted.

History of administration of a medication such as an antihistamine or phenothiazine is also relevant. Such medications may be marketed as cough or vomiting medicines, and the parents may be unaware of their side-effects. The altered metabolism of these drugs in children means that drowsiness may ensue or persist for up to a few days.

Altered consciousness may, however, reflect a more sinister CNS pathology. Such pathology may originate within the CNS itself, or may reflect CNS involvement in pathology arising in other organ systems.

Altered consciousness is a central feature of many primary CNS disorders. Inflammation of the brain tissue, particularly due to infection whether viral or bacterial, is an important example of one such disorder (encephalitis). The term 'encephalopathy' is more generic, and denotes brain tissue injury and brain function disturbance regardless of aetiology.

Mechanisms for involvement of the CNS in pathological processes originating in other systems include:

- Abnormalities in gas exchange; brain hypoxia and/or carbon dioxide narcosis (respiratory failure)
- Abnormalities in brain perfusion, whether due to reduction in the hydrostatic pressure (such as in shock and hypotension due to severe dehydration or bleeding, etc.) or due to disturbances of the osmotic balance across the blood–brain barrier and brain oedema (as in water intoxication, hypo/hypernatraemia and their treatment, diabetic ketoacidosis and its treatment)
- Hypoglycaemia
- Accumulation of toxic substances affecting brain function and structure, metabolic disorders, renal or hepatic insufficiency, postasphyxial insults, overdose intoxication (accidental, deliberate, self-harm), etc.

The severity of the alteration in consciousness seen in these states varies from mild drowsiness to severe coma, depending on the severity of the underlying illness. Some of the conditions listed above are common and should be routinely checked for in any child with altered consciousness. This is particularly true of hypoglycaemia, hyponatraemia and abnormalities of gas exchange.

When the conditions underlying the alteration in consciousness are recognized early enough, their correction is usually all that is required to restore consciousness to normal. However, if the situation has already progressed and the pathophysiological sequence of events leading to encephalopathy has already been initiated, simple correction of the underlying mechanism may prove insufficient and further therapeutic and supportive measures may be needed.

✳ KEY DIAGNOSIS

Encephalopathy

Regardless of aetiology and whether it is due to a primary CNS disorder or the result of CNS involvement in pathology originating elsewhere, brain tissue injury sets in motion a sequence of pathophysiological processes that can lead to further brain tissue injury and perpetuate a cycle

that can operate independently of the underlying cause, augmenting the degree of such injury.

As in other organs and systems, tissue injury leads to inflammation, swelling and function impairment of the affected areas. In the brain, however, two additional factors characterize this response. Firstly, the brain is located in a rigid bony structure, the skull. Secondly, brain tissue responds to certain changes in its environment by abnormal electrical activity: seizure activity or fits.

Brain swelling within the confinements of the skull can result in dangerous elevation of the intracranial pressure and hence to a reduction in the perfusion pressure (brain perfusion pressure is equal to intravascular hydrostatic pressure minus intracranial pressure), with consequent ischaemia, while the increased metabolic demands imposed on brain tissue by prolonged fitting render it more vulnerable to injury and indeed may itself cause damage (particularly temporal lobe damage).

Figure 10.5 depicts the interaction between these factors.

Another mechanism that may augment brain tissue injury operates through the effect of brain function disturbances on the performance of other organ systems. Since the brain controls many of the body physiological functions, brain tissue injury may result in impairment of such control with consequent disruption of vital physiological functions. In turn, such disruption may lead to further brain tissue injury. For example, in a child who suffers an asphyxial insult (birth asphyxia, near-drowning) resulting in brain tissue damage, such damage (if in the right location) together with any resultant brain oedema and/or convulsions may impair the respiratory centre, leading to respiratory failure. The resultant hypoxia and hypercapnia can lead to further brain injury. Another self-perpetuating cycle of reciprocal injury and detriment ensues.

Clinical features

Two groups of symptoms and signs contribute to the clinical picture: general features related to the underlying process (constitutional symptoms: rashes, fever, etc.) and features related to the brain involvement itself (disturbances of function, brain oedema, seizure activity).

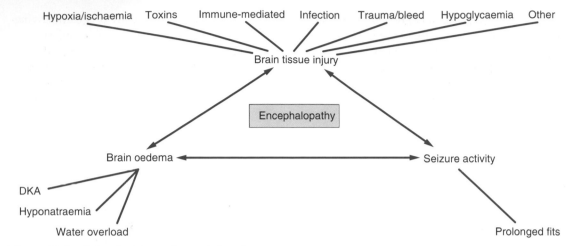

Figure 10.5 Pathophysiology of encephalopathy

General features
Features of generalized illness may include fever, a history of exposure and the presence of characteristic lesions (e.g. purpuric rash in the case of meningococcal infection), while hepatomegaly, haematuria or arthritis may point to liver disease, renal pathology or connective tissue disorder, respectively.

Disturbance of brain function
The diversified and varied functions of the brain can be categorized into autonomic, somatic, and higher functions (intellectual functions or cognition). Depending on the extent and severity of the brain involvement, impairment of these functions, singularly or in combination, may be present to a varying extent:

- Impaired cognition is a major feature of encephalopathy. Only subtle changes may be seen early, but these may progress to a state of confusion, deterioration of the level of consciousness and coma. Frequently there is a fluctuation in the level of consciousness and the impairment of mental functioning.
- Neurological signs such as muscle weakness and abnormalities of tone and reflexes are frequently present in encephalopathy. These tend to vary and shift during the course of the illness, reflecting the diffuse nature of brain involvement.
- Abnormalities of the heart rate, rhythm, vasomotor instability, abnormal breathing

patterns and disturbances of sphincter control all can occur.

Brain oedema
A degree of brain oedema is frequently present in encephalopathy. This may be aggravated by the syndrome of inappropriate antidiuretic hormone (ADH) secretion (see Ch. 14) frequently seen in children with cerebral pathology. Many of the features of brain oedema are thought to result from overstimulation of the parasympathetic centres in the brain as a consequence to the associated increase in intracranial pressure. These features include:

- Headaches
- Drowsiness
- Vomiting
- Seizures
- Bradycardia
- Hypertension
- Papilloedema.

Late signs that signify the development of life threatening complications, namely herniation of brain structures through the tentorium or the foramen magnum, include the sudden appearance of focal neurological signs, unequal pupils and abnormal breathing patterns.

Seizure activity
Fits with postictal phenomena and an alteration in consciousness are frequently present. Prolonged

seizures may also contribute to brain oedema and brain cell injury.

Fitting in a child who already suffers from impaired consciousness can be difficult to recognize. This is particularly true when the fitting does not involve a prominent clonic phase. Any paroxysmal phenomena in a child with altered consciousness should raise suspicion.

Diagnosis

This is a multilevel process:

1. The diagnosis of the presence of encephalopathy
2. The recognition of any accompanying fitting or brain oedema
3. Early recognition of the possible complications of encephalopathy which include disturbances to ventilation and perfusion as well as other physiological functions
4. The aetiological diagnosis to determine the precise pathophysiology underlying the encephalopathy.

Investigation

Investigations should be aimed at the 'levels of diagnosis' listed above:

1. Few tests are specific enough to be used to confirm or refute a diagnosis of encephalopathy. This diagnosis largely remains clinical. An EEG may show a generalized slow-wave pattern which is consistent with the presence of generalized brain pathology but is not diagnostic. Only certain patterns of EEG changes are specific for particular types of encephalopathy. An example is the EEG findings in herpes simplex encephalitis.
2. An important use of the EEG is to identify any ongoing seizure activity. CT and MRI (and ultrasound scanning in infants) are helpful in identifying brain oedema and other types of intracranial pathology. Low serum sodium levels, coupled with high osmolarity of the urine are consistent with the syndrome of inappropriate ADH secretion.
3. Frequent evaluation of blood gases, blood sugar, fluid and electrolyte balance and other indices of the vital physiological functions are important aspects of the investigations.
4. Investigations aimed at the aetiology of the encephalopathy should be planned according to the available clinical data. Screening for various types of infections and toxins, and liver and renal function testing, may all be relevant.

A special case is the performance of a lumbar puncture in a child with encephalopathy who is suspected of having meningoencephalitis as the underlying pathology. Unless the presence of increased intracranial pressure and/or focal intracranial pathology is reliably excluded, lumbar puncture is contraindicated. Frequently this means obtaining CT scans prior to the procedure.

Management

Monitoring and close observation are the mainstays of the management of children with encephalopathy. This should preferably be undertaken in an intensive care unit with adequate facilities. In certain cases, monitoring of intracranial pressure by means of a pressure transducer may be necessary.

Ventilatory and circulatory support should be provided as necessary. Maintenance of an adequate level of blood sugar is crucial, and careful attention should be paid to the fluid and electrolyte balance. Fluid restriction, to two-thirds of the usual maintenance, is the general rule to offset the risk of the inappropriate ADH secretion, but this should be reconciled with the need to achieve adequate perfusion. Fluid restriction can be relaxed or tightened in accordance to clinical and laboratory parameters of the hydration state.

Seizure activity should be controlled, as far as possible, with the use of anticonvulsants, and treatment aimed at the underlying aetiology should be instituted as necessary. Measures to control brain oedema include:

- Fluid management (fluid restriction, use of diuretics, osmotic diuresis by using mannitol)
- Hyperventilation to achieve a state of hypocapnia and cerebral vasoconstriction can

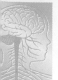

be employed in cases of significant rise in intracranial pressure which fail to respond to the less invasive measures.

- Steroids in certain cases.

CONVULSIONS

A convulsion can be defined as an involuntary paroxysmal event (motor, sensory, autonomic or psychological) that is related to an outburst of abnormal electrical neuronal discharge. The terms 'fit', 'seizure' and 'convulsion' are used interchangeably.

Convulsions should be differentiated from other similar phenomena which are not related to abnormal electrical discharges of the cerebral neurons. These include breath holding, migraine and, in neonates, jitteriness.

Convulsions are involuntary. They cannot be suppressed or provoked (with very few exceptions). Thus, convulsions usually do not happen in response to pain or anger. This is in sharp contrast to breath-holding attacks. Reflex anoxic seizures are similar to breath holding in that they occur in response to pain but they involve attacks of pallor and slow heart rate, probably related to stimulation of hypersensitive vagal receptors. They are not epileptic in origin (despite the use of the word 'seizures').

Convulsions are usually followed by a postictal period, which frequently involves deep sleep for a variable length of time and which may be followed for a few hours by headache, drowsiness or slurred speech.

Some varieties of migraine may have a dramatic onset, with alteration in perception and consciousness. The headache is usually prominent from the outset.

The recognition of convulsions in neonates is particularly difficult. Jitteriness, which involves rhythmic shaking of the extremities, may be seen in babies after difficult labours, and also with hypoglycaemia or hypocalcaemia. Sometimes, however, no obvious cause is found. Jitteriness can be induced by sudden movement of the limb, and if the extremity is held, the shaking stops. In this age group, however, convulsions may be very subtle, and sometimes the only manifestation of a convulsion is blinking or sucking movements or a change in respiratory pattern and apnoea.

Other events that may occasionally have to be considered in the differential diagnosis of convulsions include some types of cardiac arrhythmias, particularly those associated with sudden slowing of the heart rate or a pause in the cardiac activity (Stokes–Adams attacks). A prominent tonic phase and pallor characterize these attacks. Clonic movements and jerking may accompany severe bouts of coughing such as those seen in pertussis, or may be part of pseudoseizures which are psychological in origin.

It would be wrong to assume that certainty can always be attained in diagnosing fits. Not infrequently, episodes may continue to be of undetermined nature, and the decision to investigate, treat or to allow a period of observation has to be taken on the merits of each individual case.

There are several types of convulsion and different classifications. Knowledge of the particular type of convulsion is crucial, not only because of relevance for diagnosis but also because of implications for treatment and prognosis.

A simple working classification of convulsions is shown in Table 10.3.

An important clinical feature in the categorization of a convulsion is the state of consciousness. Consciousness is lost in generalized convulsions and preserved in the simple focal variety. In complex partial convulsions, consciousness is altered (adult patients with this type of convulsion frequently refer to their experience as 'a dreamy state').

The mechanism underlying convulsions is not completely understood. A convulsion is thought

Table 10.3	Classification of convulsions
Generalized	**Focal or partial**
Generalized tonic clonic	Simple focal
Absences	Complex partial
Atonic	
Myoclonic	
Infantile spasms	

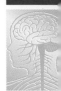

to represent a reaction of the brain to disturbances in its environment. Such disturbances may be due to local causes such as pressure, structural abnormalities and tumours or due to more generalized physiological disturbances such as hypoglycaemia, hypocalcaemia, etc. However, in a large proportion of children with single or recurrent fits, no abnormality can be detected, and these convulsions are referred to as idiopathic.

Fitting is one of the common presentations in children. Of all children, 5% experience at least one seizure during their childhood. The overwhelming majority of these children will have had febrile convulsions.

The cause of fitting in children generally falls into one of the following categories:

- Febrile convulsions
- Acute encephalopathy (CNS infections, hypoglycaemia, etc.)
- Epilepsy: idiopathic and secondary
- Unclassified.

✷ KEY DIAGNOSIS

Idiopathic epilepsy

A convulsion does not in itself constitute epilepsy. Epilepsy is a disorder that involves recurrent convulsions which are not associated with fever and not part of an acute illness.

Idiopathic epilepsy refers to the tendency of having recurrent convulsions with no identifiable cause. The prevalence of idiopathic epilepsy is 0.5% of the total population. Secondary epilepsy indicates the presence of an identifiable underlying cause for the recurrent fits. Such underlying cause may be congenital (tuberous sclerosis) or acquired, static (post-traumatic brain scarring) or progressive (brain tumour).

Children with either type of epilepsy may experience any of the different types of fits. One exception is typical absence attacks, which are almost always due to idiopathic epilepsy.

Clinical features

Absences refer to attacks of sudden, brief loss of consciousness with little or no accompanying features. Muscle tone is preserved and body posture is maintained. To an observer, the child looks vacant as if day dreaming. This type of seizure has a characteristic pattern on the EEG.

Generalized tonic–clonic convulsions involve loss of consciousness, a tonic phase when body musculature stiffens with cessation of breathing and cyanosis due to the involvement of the respiratory muscles. This is followed by a clonic phase when organized and selective contraction of muscles leads to rhythmic movements. These are the commonest type of convulsions, though they are rarely seen in young infants, reflecting the immature state of the intracerebral pathways at that stage. These convulsions can be due to epilepsy, febrile convulsions or other pathology.

Myoclonic convulsions are sudden shock-like contraction of the muscles. There is usually also a brief loss of consciousness. Several varieties of myoclonic convulsions are recognized, some of which are associated with poor prognosis. *Myoclonic convulsions* are more likely to occur in young children and infants, and may represent a type of generalized convulsion that an immature brain generates. Though this type of convulsion may be seen in certain forms of idiopathic epilepsy, it can also be associated with structural brain abnormalities and metabolic disturbances.

Atonic convulsions involve sudden loss of muscle tone as well as loss of consciousness.

Simple focal convulsions imply no loss of consciousness, with only localized (focal) involvement of the brain in the seizure activity. This may show itself as jerking, involving one group of muscles or abnormal sensory phenomena. A variety of simple focal epilepsy specific to children is benign rolandic epilepsy. These occur in otherwise normal children, usually around 7–9 years of age. They involve the face and tend to occur during sleep. The EEG shows an abnormal spike focus in the centrotemporal or rolandic area.

Complex partial convulsions are episodes of alteration in consciousness (frequently described as 'a dreamy state') associated with automatisms (stereotyped semipurposeful movements such as swallowing chewing movements) as well as autonomic features such as pallor, flushing, or dilatation of pupils, etc.

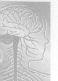

Infantile spasms, characterized by repeated clusters of brief contractions of the trunk and limbs resembling a startle reaction, usually begin in early infancy. They may be associated with structural and metabolic abnormalities which carry a poor prognosis.

Convulsions may be predated by a prodromal phase lasting a few hours or days, in which children may display changes in mood and behaviour, etc. These patterns may be recognized by parents, who with time are able to anticipate that a convulsion is likely to occur. In many cases an aura is also present, a sensory phenomenon perceived by the child immediately before the convulsion itself.

Occasionally a convulsion may not fall neatly within any of these categories, and mixed features may be present. Focal convulsions may develop into generalized ones (secondary generalized convulsions). Complex partial convulsions are usually the most difficult to categorize in children, who may find it difficult to describe their feelings.

In secondary epilepsy the clinical picture also reflects the underlying condition.

Diagnosis

Diagnosis almost entirely depends on the history. In certain cases, video recording of the events may be helpful. Rarely, an episode occurs during an EEG recording, and the findings may confirm or exclude the fact that the particular type of episode is due to a fit.

In certain cases, depending on the type of epilepsy involved, some clues in the EEG in the interictal period (period between fits) may point towards a tendency for a particular type of fit. This is probably the main reason why EEGs are requested in children with a history of fits. However, in certain types of epilepsy as many as one-third or more of the affected children may have normal EEGs in the interictal period. Likewise, some individuals without epilepsy may have changes on the EEG similar to those found in epilepsy.

The EEG yield may be enhanced by employing certain techniques, most commonly photostimulation, hyperventilation and sleep deprivation; 24 h recordings may also be useful.

Figure 10.6 depicts the patterns that may be seen in certain types of seizure.

The extent of the search for an underlying cause for idiopathic epilepsy is determined individually in the light of the historical, clinical and other data. As a minimum, the majority of children should have a full biochemical screen including blood sugar measurement. Ultrasound, CT and/or MRI may also be indicated, particularly in children with focal fits, frequent difficult to control fits and in those with other clinical features pointing to CNS pathology.

Children with epilepsy, particularly those who are mentally handicapped or with difficult to control fits, should be examined carefully for the presence of skin stigmata of the neuroectodermal syndromes (neurofibromatosis and tuberous sclerosis). Chromosomal analysis and genetic studies may also be helpful.

Treatment

There is still controversy as to when treatment with antiepileptic drugs should be started. Depending on the type and duration of the first fit, it is reasonable to withhold treatment in otherwise healthy children until after the second fit, since a large number of such children may never have a recurrence. Almost all drugs used in the treatment of epilepsy have significant side-effects. Table 10.4 outlines the main antiepileptics used in children and their main side-effects.

Newer drugs, the use of which is still being assessed in children, include lamotrigine and gabapentin. They look promising in terms of safety and efficacy. Vigabatrin is another anticonvulsant which has recently been used in children; it is useful in infantile spasms, but there are a number of side-effects, including visual disturbances, which limit its use in children.

The family should be informed about the diagnosis and its implications. Fears regarding normal development and mental functioning should be directly addressed. Withdrawal of treatment in idiopathic epilepsy can be attempted after achieving a period of 2 years free of fits.

The need for supervision of activities such as swimming should be explained to the family and school teachers. They can also be supplied with rectal diazepam to use if a convulsion goes on for

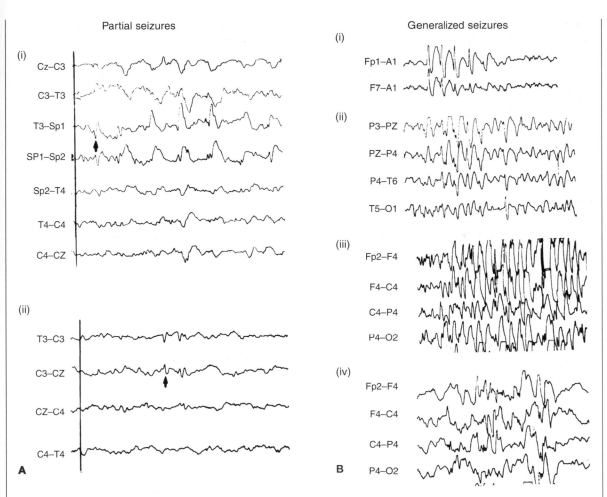

Figure 10.6 **A**, An EEG of partial seizures: (i) spike discharges from the left temporal lobe (*arrow*) in a patient with complex partial seizures, (ii) left parietal central spikes (*arrow*) characteristic of benign partial epilepsy with centro-parietal (rolandic) spikes. **B**, Representative EEGs of generalized seizures: (i) 3/sec spike and wave discharge of absence seizures with normal background activity, (ii) complex myoclonic epilepsy (Lennox–Gastaut syndrome) with interictal slow spike waves, (iii) juvenile myoclonic epilepsy showing 6/sec spike and waves enhanced by photic stimulation, and (iv) hypsarrhythmia with an irregular high-voltage spike and wave activity

more than 5 min. Guidelines and demonstration of its use should be made available.

In secondary epilepsies, attempts at treatment of the underlying cause should be undertaken if feasible.

Status epilepticus (prolonged fits)

One of the important aspects of treatment is how to manage an acute seizure episode. Generally speaking, the majority of children with fits, whether epileptic or non-epileptic in origin, stop

fitting spontaneously within a few minutes of the onset of the fit. The recommendation is to wait for 5 min before any action is taken. The child during this period should be removed from areas of danger and put in the recovery position.

For fitting that continues beyond 5 min, the following steps should be taken:

- Ensure adequate airway and breathing; apply suction and oxygen if necessary
- Give rectal or intravenous diazepam; can be repeated after 10 min if necessary

Table 10.4	Anticonvulsants		
Drug	Indication	Side-effects	Monitoring
Sodium valproate	Generalized tonic–clonic, absence, myoclonic and focal convulsions	Drowsiness, abnormal liver function, behavioural problems	Liver function tests
Carbamazepine	Generalized tonic–clonic and focal convulsions	Drowsiness, bone marrow suppression	Blood levels and full blood counts
Phenobarbitone	Neonatal convulsions	Drowsiness, interferes with learning abilities	Blood levels
Phenytoin	Effective in a wide range of seizure disorders	Drowsiness, liver enzyme inducer, rashes, bone marrow suppression, etc.	Used mainly in the management of status epilepticus

- Check blood sugar and gases, biochemical screen and anticonvulsant levels (if a known epileptic patient)
- Start intravenous fluids and ensure adequate perfusion; monitor blood pressure
- Give rectal paraldehyde if the fitting continues, together with an intravenous loading dose of phenytoin under electrocardiogram (ECG) control (possible arrhythmia)
- Admit to the intensive care unit for clonazepam infusion if still fitting; general anaesthesia may be required.

Fever and fits

Fitting in a pyrexial child is one of the most common presentations in paediatric practice. In the vast majority of cases, the convulsion represents a reaction to the fever and is not related to any other CNS pathology. These convulsions are called febrile convulsions. However, in a few cases this presentation may point to significant underlying pathology, whether primarily arising within or outside the CNS.

In the approach to the child presenting with fever and convulsions, three questions have to be answered; the first two pertain to the management in the acute stage while the third question is related to further follow-up management:

[1] Could the convulsion have been caused by a serious acute CNS pathology? CNS infections (meningitis/encephalitis) feature high on the list of possibilities, since they offer an explanation for both the fever and the convulsion. However, CNS involvement in other types of pathology should also be considered; hypoglycaemia and other metabolic encephalopathies are important examples. Furthermore, many metabolic disorders may be tipped into decompensation by intercurrent infections leading to metabolic/toxic encephalopathy.

[2] Is there an identifiable cause for the fever? Two objectives are served in looking for a source of the fever in a pyrexial child presenting with a fit. First, it may help in making a decision regarding the previous question since fever with no obvious cause is one of the recognized clinical presentations of intracranial infection (see Ch. 14). The other objective is to identify the underlying illness (e.g. tonsillitis or urinary tract infection), which will warrant attention on its own merits.

[3] If on careful assessment there is no indication of a serious acute or ongoing CNS pathology that could have caused the convulsion, it can be assumed that the convulsion has been triggered or caused by the fever itself. The question is now: Was this a febrile convulsion (convulsion caused by fever) or was it an epileptic convulsion simply triggered by the fever?

Table 10.5 lists the features which are helpful in reaching the diagnosis.

Table 10.5 The differential diagnosis of fits in febrile children[a]

Convulsions due to CNS infection/pathology	Febrile convulsions	Epileptic convulsion triggered by fever
Convulsions can be prolonged and may occur in succession	Convulsions are brief, usually <5 min	Convulsions may be prolonged, some lasting >15 min
Convulsions can be generalized or focal of any type	Convulsions are typically generalized, usually tonic–clonic, but 'atonic' types can occur	Convulsions can be generalized or focal of any type
Postictal period prolonged	Usually well and playful by the time seen in hospital	Postictal period prolonged
Any age	Unusual beyond the age range of 6 months to 5 years	Any age
More fits may occur in the same acute episode. Later recurrences if permanent damage occurs	Only rarely do more fits occur in the same febrile episode. 50% chance of later recurrences with fever	Recurrences
Absence of an identifiable focus of infection, or features of CNS infection are present	Frequently a focus of infection as a cause of fever is found	Frequently a focus of infection as a cause of fever is found
Generally unwell	Convulsions occur as the child's temperature rises to high levels. Otherwise well child	Convulsions during mild fever
Presence of other signs and symptoms of intracranial infection/encephalopathy	There may be a family history of febrile fits	History and examination reveal higher risk for epilepsy: developmental delay, chronic neurological disability, family history and/or dysmorphic features, etc

[a] It should be realized that all of these features are simply 'risk factors' that favour a certain diagnosis and are not diagnostic or exclusive of any of the possibilities. For example, children with urinary tract infection or non-specific viral illnesses may have a fever with no obvious cause but still have febrile fits, while children with meningitis may have another focus of simultaneous infection (e.g. otitis media)

Absence of the symptoms and signs of meningitis/encephalitis should be confirmed by careful questioning and detailed neurological assessment. Simple febrile convulsions are characterized by brief postictal drowsiness; any clouding of consciousness in a child with this presentation should raise suspicion.

Febrile fits require no treatment in the majority of cases. Only rarely is a febrile convulsion prolonged and treatment with rectal diazepam warranted. Similarly, no prevention is required in the majority of cases but may be considered if the convulsions are very frequent or prolonged.

The incidence of epilepsy in children with febrile fits is slightly increased above that of the general population. This may reflect the fact that some of these children have epileptic fits triggered by fever.

SPASTICITY

A mild, generalized increase in muscle tone does not always signify pathology. Normal full-term babies in early infancy display increased muscle tone intermittently, particularly when they are hungry, cold or crying. Babies with marked or persistent generalized increase in muscle tone, or with any asymmetry, should be evaluated further. Increased muscle tone is a sign of an upper motor neuron lesion. By far the commonest underlying condition of the persistent increase in muscle tone in children is CP.

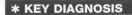
✳ KEY DIAGNOSIS

Cerebral palsy (see also Chs 3 and 17)

CP is best defined as the motor manifestation of non-progressive brain damage sustained during infancy and childhood. It is a movement and posture disorder that results from a static brain lesion. Such lesions may be genetically determined (inherited or familial forms of CP), developmental (CP resulting from brain structural defects) or may represent the aftermath or damage by an injury sustained by a structurally normal brain (congenital infections, birth asphyxia, neonatal jaundice or meningitis).

The hallmark of CP is increased muscle tone. However, there are different patterns of manifestation, and some may involve hypotonia. Both the pattern and severity may vary with age, and in many cases the tendency is towards amelioration of the condition with time. However, worsening of the condition may occur because of the progression of the skeletal and postural deformities which compound the neurological disability.

The lesions underlying CP may also result in impairment of other functions of the brain. The most important associations include mental handicap, epilepsy, and impaired vision and hearing.

Occasionally the impact of these associations on the life of the child and the family may prove more disabling than the difficulties in movement and balance resulting from the CP, particularly if the latter is mild.

The prevalence of CP is estimated at 2 per 1000 of the population. When the condition was first described it was suggested that the primary causes were birth trauma and asphyxia, and it was held that improvements in obstetric care would reduce the incidence. However, over the subsequent 30 years there has been a significant improvement in obstetric and antenatal care but the expected reduction in the incidence of CP has not materialized. The present view is that congenital brain defects, as well as congenital abnormalities of other systems that may interfere with the normal process of birth and lead to birth trauma and asphyxia (regardless of the quality of obstetric care), may account for a substantial number of children who develop CP.

Anatomically, the major motor centres in the brain are the motor cortex, basal ganglia and cerebellum. The clinical effects of involvement of any of these centres may dominate the picture, and hence the following varieties of cerebral palsy are recognized: spastic, choreoathetoid, ataxic and mixed.

Clinical features

These depend on the pattern of CP and also vary with age:

- *Spastic CP.* This is the commonest form. It may be severe, affecting the four limbs (quadriplegia), and then it is usually associated with epilepsy and mental retardation as well as other disabilities. When there is paralysis in the lower limbs while the upper limb involvement is mild, the condition is referred to as spastic diplegia. Children with this type of CP frequently have a history of prematurity. Hemiplegia and monoplegias can also occur.
- *Choreoathetoid (extrapyramidal) CP.* The main feature here is dystonia and choreoathetoid movements. In the 'old days' this type of CP used to be most commonly caused by kernicterus due to severe unconjugated neonatal hyperbilirubinaemia in haemolytic disease of the newborn resulting from rhesus incompatibility.
- *Ataxic CP.* This is an uncommon type of CP, and impairment of balance and coordination is the central feature.

Some of the children who later develop spastic types of CP may in infancy have unusually low tone. However, the exaggerated tendon reflexes serve to differentiate this from other types of hypotonia. Children with cerebellar ataxia are usually hypotonic.

The signs of CP may be subtle early in life. Certain manifestations in infancy may point towards a high risk of developing CP later in life. These include:

- Persistence of primitive reflexes
- Persistent abnormal muscle tone

- Delay in gross motor development
- Asymmetry in the use of the two sides of the body.

Depending on the severity and extent of the brain lesion, there may be feeding difficulties, recurrent aspiration and chest infections. Lack of mobility and abnormal function of striated and smooth muscles may lead to reflux oesophagitis, urinary retention and incontinence, recurrent urinary tract infections and renal failure, constipation or faecal incontinence. Microcephaly may also be associated, as well as mental handicap, blindness and other disabilities.

At the other end of the spectrum, children with mild monoplegia or hemiplegia may have no signs apart from a minor deficiency in the use of the affected side. Sometimes the manifestations are limited to upward plantar reflexes, exaggerated reflexes or clonus on the affected side.

Diagnosis

The diagnosis is clinical, and based on the history, physical examination and exclusion of progressive disorders. Depending on nature and severity of the brain lesion, brain imaging may show minimal changes or it may show brain atrophy with cavity formation or other structural defects.

Management

A multidisciplinary approach is required. One of the main goals of the management of children with CP is the prevention of skeletal deformities that would otherwise develop because of unbalanced posturing, muscle power and tone. Regular physiotherapy and physical exercise should be provided. Frequently, the parents will be able to do this with appropriate training and education.

A 'statement of needs' should be prepared as early as possible, and appropriate placement in a school with the facilities to look after the child's needs is mandatory. Some children may benefit from attendance at specialized nurseries and schools.

In severe cases, modification of the child's home to suit the use of wheelchairs and other appliances is important. The use of various mounts and sitting, standing and walking aids may help in maintaining the correct posture and mobility. The use of various modern technological appliances may help circumvent disability and help overcome handicap.

The family of a child with severe CP needs a great deal of support. It is important to offer an honest and comprehensive explanation of the possible causes, the risk of recurrence and the possible prognosis. Genetic counselling should be offered in appropriate cases.

The approach to, and management of, children with CP should serve as an example of the management of children with chronic disability of any kind. What sets aside children with CP is not the nature of the brain lesion but the fact that this is a condition with physical disability that is established early in life and which interferes with the motor development of the child. Thus, children who sustain brain damage as a result of head trauma or car accidents in childhood may develop with neurological and physical disabilities that should be managed along the same lines as children who are born with defective brains or who suffer neonatal brain injury.

When learning difficulties are associated with CP, the approach to this should be along the lines discussed in Chapter 3. Epilepsy should be controlled with the appropriate medication (see Table 10.4).

HYPOTONIA AND WEAKNESS

Decreased muscle tone is a normal finding in premature babies. In full-term neonates, intermittent mild generalized hypotonia is seen after feeds and during sleep.

Generalized hypotonia is one of the non-specific signs of severe systemic illness including shock, septicaemia and severe dehydration. In the case of the neonate, birth asphyxia is frequently followed by hypotonia, and the duration of the latter may correspond to the severity of the asphyxial injury.

Though hypotonia is one of the characteristic signs of a lower motor neuron lesion, it can arise from lesions anywhere on the motor pathway. Table 10.6 lists some of the more important

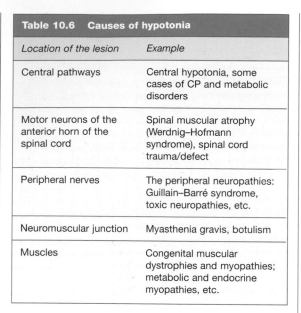

Table 10.6   Causes of hypotonia

Location of the lesion	Example
Central pathways	Central hypotonia, some cases of CP and metabolic disorders
Motor neurons of the anterior horn of the spinal cord	Spinal muscular atrophy (Werdnig–Hofmann syndrome), spinal cord trauma/defect
Peripheral nerves	The peripheral neuropathies: Guillain–Barré syndrome, toxic neuropathies, etc.
Neuromuscular junction	Myasthenia gravis, botulism
Muscles	Congenital muscular dystrophies and myopathies; metabolic and endocrine myopathies, etc.

examples of hypotonia, and relates them to the location of the lesion.

When hypotonia is the result of a lower motor neuron lesion it is usually associated with hyporeflexia. Muscular atrophy is also seen in chronic cases.

✳ KEY DIAGNOSIS

Muscular dystrophy

Muscular dystrophies are a group of inherited disorders that are determined by different genetic traits; they vary in their severity from the severe cases that lead to death in the neonatal period to ones that cause only minor disability.

The term 'muscular dystrophy' implies a disease of muscle which is both inherited and progressive, and in which degeneration of the muscle fibres is a feature. In the past there was some confusion about the different types of muscular dystrophy, their inheritance and their relationships to each other. However, with the progress in molecular genetics, the nature of the genetic defect provides a basis for defining these entities.

Duchenne's muscular dystrophy is one of the most common serious congenital disorders. The incidence is 1 in 3600 live born male infants. It

follows an X-linked recessive inheritance. Becker's muscular dystrophy is probably the same disease with the same locus and gene being involved but to a lesser degree; consequently it follows a milder course.

Aetiology and genetics

The gene of Duchenne's muscular dystrophy is one of the best studied (see Ch. 16). It is located at locus 21 of the short arm of the X chromosomes (Xp21), and codes for a protein, dystrophin, which is vital for the metabolism of muscle fibres. It is present in skeletal muscle, smooth muscle and heart muscle. Abnormalities in this protein are thought to account for the clinical manifestations of Duchenne's muscular dystrophy.

The absence or reduction of dystrophin interferes with the metabolic activities of muscle fibres and renders them more susceptible to necrosis. Depending on the nature and severity of the genetic defect, dystrophin may be absent, reduced or present in normal amounts but defective in function. The weakness and other manifestations vary from severe to mild according to the functional capacity of the dystrophin produced.

The necrotic muscle fibres release their enzymes into the surrounding fluids and plasma. This accounts for the elevated enzyme creatinine kinase (CK) level which, in severe cases, may be 1000 times the normal value. In mild cases and in carriers (mothers and sisters of affected children), the elevation of the CK level is moderate. Females, however, may get the disease through the Lyon phenomenon (random inactivation of one of the X chromosomes, leading in some carriers to the inactivation of more X chromosomes bearing the normal gene than those bearing the abnormal gene).

Clinical manifestations

Male affected babies are usually normal at birth. A few may have delayed gross motor development. The majority, however, achieve the early milestones at the expected ages, although careful attention may show subtle signs of weakness, particularly in the limb girdle muscles in infants and toddlers.

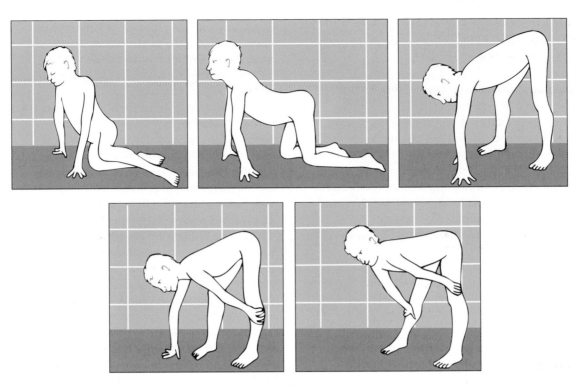

Figure 10.7 Gower sign: 'climbing up the legs' in muscular dystrophy

The classic Gower sign can be elicited in the majority of affected children by 5–6 years of age (Fig. 10.7). When asked to rise from the supine position, the child will do so by first turning into the prone position and then lifting his body on to all fours and before adopting the vertical position by 'climbing up the legs'. This manoeuvre is characteristic of Duchenne's muscular dystrophy, but is seen in cases of weakness of the pelvic girdle muscles of any type. Other characteristic signs include the enlargement of the calves (pseudohypertrophy due to infiltration by fat), which contrasts with the wasting of the thigh muscles and winging of the scapulae (see Fig. 16.9).

The weakness is progressive, and the proximal muscles are worst affected. Functions such as handwriting and the use of cutlery may be preserved until late. With time, the respiratory muscles are involved, with weak cough and shallow breathing leading to frequent chest infections and respiratory failure. Involvement of the pharyngeal muscles leads to frequent choking and aspiration. Urinary and faecal incontinence are late signs. Cardiomyopathy is also part of the disease, and is one of the main causes of death. Intellectual impairment occurs in all patients, but the degree of severity is variable.

Diagnosis

The CK level is greatly elevated from birth, with the serum concentration rising to tens of thousands international units (IU) per litre (normal is less than 155 IU/l). A normal CK level rules out the diagnosis. Evidence of cardiomyopathy may be seen on the ECG, which shows characteristic myopathic features. Normal motor and sensory conduction studies differentiate this condition from neurological causes of muscular weakness.

The diagnosis can be confirmed by genetic studies, which can be performed on cells obtained from samples of blood, muscle cells or chorionic villi (in the case of prenatal diagnosis, as early as 12 weeks of gestation) using Southern blotting or the polymerase chain reaction (PCR). The diagnosis can also be established through the analysis of muscle biopsy tissue for dystrophin, using immunochemical methods.

Treatment

There is no known medical intervention that slows the relentless progression of the disease. However, the complications can be treated and the quality of life improved for these unfortunate children. The use of physiotherapy to avoid and treat skeletal deformities and contractures and to preserve strength as long as possible is a central strategy of management. Treatment of heart failure and chest infections should be provided as needed.

Depending on the course of the disease, some children are confined to a wheelchair by 7 years of age. Others will continue to be ambulatory until 10 years of age or beyond. It is important to preserve ambulation as long as possible with interventions such as physiotherapy, orthotic devices and even surgery if required (some patients may require Achilles tendon lengthening), since skeletal deformities such as scoliosis, which is a major complication because of its effect on respiratory function, are less likely to occur if the child is not confined to a wheelchair or bed.

Good nutrition is important. However, care must be taken to avoid obesity to which these children are predisposed because of depression and lack of activity. Some studies have indicated a role for steroids, but this is still controversial. The family requires a great deal of professional help and support, and genetic counselling should be offered in all cases.

The cloning of the gene encoding dystrophin opens up the possibility of gene therapy utilizing such techniques as the introduction of the normal gene into the affected muscles through direct injection or using certain viruses as vectors. Investigation of these exciting possibilities is still in its early stages.

HEADACHE

Probably all children experience a few episodes of sporadic headache. Headaches frequently accompany colds, flu illnesses and fever from other causes. As long as the headaches are infrequent, short lived and mild, they should cause no concern, and parents rarely seek medical advice with this complaint.

Long-lasting and/or severe headaches can be a feature of many serious disorders including meningitis, encephalopathy, head trauma and other conditions associated with raised intracranial pressure. Headaches are a prominent feature in pneumonia, particularly the so-called atypical pneumonia. These pathologies are discussed in the relevant sections and chapters of this book.

It is estimated that 10% of all children suffer from recurrent headaches at some stage in the first 10 years of life. The most common cause of recurrent headache is migraine. Other types of functional (non-organic) headaches, such as stress or tension headaches, are also common. Several organic causes need also to be considered, including chronic sinusitis, malocclusion disorders and refraction errors of the eye (eye strain). Most notably (but rarely) recurrent headaches may be the presenting feature of slowly rising intracranial pressure, and in the paediatric age group this raises the possibility of an intracranial tumour.

Headaches due to chronic sinusitis tend to occur late in the morning. The location depends on the sinuses involved, but headaches due to sinusitis are generally frontal, and may be described as arising from the face. Nasal stuffiness may result in a nasal type of speech and mouth breathing. Snoring at night and waking up with dry cracked lips are frequent consequences, and tenderness over the maxillary and frontal bones may be present.

Abnormal bite and malocclusion may result in unequal distribution of force during chewing, giving rise to muscle strain and headaches. Refraction errors may also strain the eye and accommodation muscles and result in headaches. Both conditions are rare causes of recurrent headaches, but a check by a dentist and optometrist may be required in the evaluation of some children with recurrent headaches.

The most reliable way to confirm or refute the presence of an intracranial pathology is brain imaging. CT and MRI can demonstrate the vast majority of such lesions. Nevertheless it is expensive and impractical to subject a large number of children presenting with recurrent headaches to a brain scan in the hope of picking up the occasional child whose recurrent headaches are caused by an intracranial pathology. It is therefore necessary to use clinical judgement to select the high-risk patients in whom such an investigation is warranted. The following features are risk factors for intracranial space-occupying lesions:

- Early morning headache
- Vomiting characteristically unassociated with nausea
- Progressive course with the headaches initially sporadic then more frequent
- The presence of focal neurological signs
- Changes in behaviour, personality and intellectual functioning and performance
- Associated fits
- Worsening of the headache on straining and bending (these activities further increase intracranial pressure).

Any child with recurrent headaches associated with one or more of these features qualifies for brain imaging (see Fig. 11.13). MRI has the advantage of being able to detect lesions in the posterior fossa and also changes in the texture of the brain substance itself.

Functional or tension headaches may be related to anxiety and stress. They are the second most common cause of headaches in children following migraine, with which they may coexist in the same child. They usually occur in spells of several days and are not associated with nausea or vomiting. Functional headaches are usually mild to moderate in severity and rarely interfere with daily activities. All of these features help make the distinction from migraine

✳ KEY DIAGNOSIS

Migraine

Migraine is thought to be related to an imbalance in the levels of circulating serotonin and other vascular dilating peptides, resulting in dilatation of the cranial and facial vessels. The exact mechanisms are unknown, but hormonal changes, food allergies, genetic factors, personality traits and stress may interact to trigger an attack in a susceptible person. The relative significance of these factors varies in different individuals.

In 90% of cases the family history is positive, usually on the mother's side, and the diagnosis should be doubted if the family history is negative. However, it is important to note that some mothers may not consider mild recurrent headache as being due to migraine.

Migraine is the commonest cause of recurrent headache in children. Its incidence is estimated at around 5% among school children, and the majority of adults suffering from migraine have a history of headaches dating from childhood. Migraine can affect even young children (the youngest child in the literature in whom the diagnosis has been made was 1 year of age). Many cases have been diagnosed as infantile colic. Irritability of unknown cause or cyclic vomiting may be migraine which goes unrecognized because of the child's difficulties in communicating his or her symptoms.

Migraine is not necessarily a lifelong disorder. Spontaneous remissions may occur during the second decade.

Clinical features

Migraine is a clinical diagnosis. It should be suspected when there is a history of recurrent headache with symptom-free intervals. In addition, the diagnostic criteria require at least three of the following:

- Nausea or vomiting
- Unilateral location
- Abdominal pain
- Associated aura
- Relief following sleep
- Positive family history.

There are several variants of migraine. By far the commonest in children is the common migraine type in which there is no aura proceeding the attack. Although unilateral headache is one of the diagnostic criteria, in most children the headaches are bilateral. The headache is usually throbbing in quality and lasts for several hours, sometimes longer. In children it is frequently associated with nausea and vomiting; it may also be accompanied by fever and abdominal pain.

In the classical migraine variant, an aura in the form of flashing lights, blurred vision, etc., precedes the attack. Sometimes this takes the form of confusion and distortion of body image ('Alice in Wonderland experience' – it is interesting to note that Lewis Carroll was a migraine sufferer).

Other variants include cyclical vomiting, acute confusional states and complicated migraine. The last refers to a migraine variant in which focal neurological signs such as hemiplegia, ophthalmoplegia, reduced vision, or changes in the level of consciousness accompany the attack. Such presentations are difficult to distinguish from syndromes related to focal intracranial pathology, and deserve full investigation.

In many cases, migraine may be triggered by increased levels of stress at home or at school. This may be related to academic performance or other aspects of school life, and these issues should be discussed in detail, preferably involving the teachers as well.

There are no tests to confirm the diagnosis of migraine. However, investigations may occasionally be indicated to rule out other possibilities. The extent of such investigations are dictated by the mode of presentation. Usually the main issue is to differentiate headaches due to migraine from those due to increased intracranial pressure because of a mass lesion; scanning is then the investigation of choice.

Treatment

Although a large number of possible triggers have been identified in children, their relevance in each individual case varies. Missing a meal, oversleeping or undersleeping, getting excited or worried or even laughing excessively have all been implicated, as have chocolate, cheese, fizzy drinks, colourings, flavourings and preservative agents. Rather than complete avoidance, a sensible approach is to restrict only those factors which trigger headaches in the individual child.

Most migraine attacks are mild and respond to paracetamol. In some cases, because of the associated nausea and vomiting or because of the associated intestinal motility disturbances, oral medication may not be effective. This is the basis for the widely available combination of paracetamol with an antiemetic or other drug which affects gastrointestinal motility. Such combinations are frequently effective. Only rarely is an acute attack of migraine severe enough to warrant further treatment. In these cases, the ergotamine preparations can be used in older children provided their migraine variant does not involve focal signs. Sumatriptan, a selective 5-HT receptor agonist, is an effective treatment in adults, but not licensed for children.

In severe migraine with headaches that are frequent and severe enough to cause significant disruption to the child's everyday life (e.g. school attendance), pharmacological prophylaxis may be indicated. In the UK, two main drugs are used. Pizitofen, with its antiserotonin and antihistamine activity has the side-effects of drowsiness, impaired learning and increased appetite. The β blocker propranolol is effective because it prevents the vasoconstriction phase that is thought to usher in the vasodilatation. It is used in severe cases, where other measures have failed or where features of anxiety coexist (e.g. palpitations). It, of course, is contraindicated in asthma and diabetes.

ABNORMAL HEAD SIZE OR SHAPE

Measurement of the occipitofrontal head circumference is an integral part of the physical examination of young children. The mean occipitofrontal circumference of male full-term babies is around 35 cm (the measurement immediately after birth may be inaccurate because of associated oedema of the scalp, haematomata or overriding of skull bones). The rate of growth of the brain is, proportionately, the fastest of the parameters of physical growth. During the first year the head circumference increases by 12 cm whereas during the second year, it increases by 2 cm. The skull size approaches its adult value at around 7 years of age.

Three types of skull abnormalities are recognized: increased size, small size and abnormal shape. There is a spectrum of severity for each of these abnormalities, and mild cases can be regarded as being variations of normal.

Increased head size may be due to hydrocephalus, subdural effusion or megalocephaly.

Subdural effusion results in expansion of the subdural space. It may be postinfective or due to haematoma (see Fig. 10.4) resulting from accidental or non-accidental injury or a bleeding tendency. Characteristically, there is prominence of the parietal areas of the skull, in contrast to the frontal bossing frequently seen in hydrocephalus. Transillumination of the skull in a dark room can demonstrate effusions in young infants.

Megalocephaly, an increase in the brain mass itself, is a rare condition which may be familial or be part of certain syndromes.

Like other anthropometric measurements, head size is subject to normal variation. There is an area of overlap between normal children with small heads and those whose head size is pathologically small. Microcephaly refers to a head circumference that is more than 3 SD below the mean (between the 0.1 and 0.2 centiles on growth charts).

Craniosynostosis is another condition that may also, albeit rarely, result in a small head size (see Beyond core: craniosynostosis).

✱ KEY DIAGNOSIS

Hydrocephalus

Hydrocephalus refers to a state of increased pressure within the ventricular system. It results from an imbalance between production and absorption of the CSF. Apart from rare cases of increased production of the CSF by a papilloma, by far the most common cause is impaired absorption. CSF absorption may be impaired because of obstruction to its flow within the ventricular system (obstructive hydrocephalus) or because of impaired absorption in the subarachnoid space (communicating, non-obstructive hydrocephalus).

The increased pressure within the ventricular system is transmitted to the inside of the skull. In infants with open sutures, this leads to separation of the sutures, expansion of the skull and a visible increase in the size of the head. In older children and adults with rigid bony skulls, little or no expansion is possible, and a build-up in pressure quickly leads to signs of raised intracranial pressure. In both groups, the increased pressure within the ventricular system may reach a point where it overcomes the impedance to absorption and/or slows secretion of the CSF, and a new steady state between production and absorption of CSF is achieved (arrested hydrocephalus). Brain damage may occur if the build up in pressure within the ventricular system continues untreated.

Clinical manifestations

The clinical picture of hydrocephalus may vary widely depending on the underlying cause and whether the condition is acquired or congenital, and whether the skull sutures are still open or not. Thus, hydrocephalus may produce only subtle symptoms and signs that are limited to excessive increase in the head circumference, or it may present the severe picture associated with increased intracranial pressure (see p. 190).

In the infant with open cranial sutures and the potential for skull expansion, excessive enlargement of the head is the most important sign. In the rare untreated case, the anterior fontanelle is wide and bulging and frequently there is prominence of the forehead. Paralysis of upward gaze may lead to downward deviation of the eyes, the so-called 'setting sun' sign. Upper motor neuron signs may be present, particularly in the lower limbs.

In older children with little potential for skull expansion, the signs are those of increased intracranial pressure. There is irritability, lethargy and vomiting. These signs also appear in infants when the expansion of the skull no longer keeps pace with the increase in the intraventricular pressure. Subtle changes in behaviour and personality and deterioration in academic performance may be the only appreciable features of slowly progressive hydrocephalus.

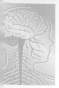

Percussion of a skull may produce a 'cracked pot' effect. Paralysis of the sixth cranial nerve may also be present.

Investigations

Skull radiography may show separation of the sutures and also a 'copper-beating' or increased 'thumb printing' (convolutional markings on the skull). Calcification may point to an underlying cause such as congenital infections. Ultrasound is a safe, convenient and effective mode of investigation of hydrocephalus. Measurement of the ventricular diameter allows the progression of hydrocephalus to be followed. CT scans and MRI are frequently undertaken in children with a closed fontanelle in order to outline the anatomical relationships and to look for the underlying cause of the hydrocephalus. Aqueduct stenosis, whether congenital or acquired, is one of the commonest causes of obstructive hydrocephalus. Communicating, non-obstructive hydrocephalus is usually the result of a previous episode of meningitis or subarachnoid haemorrhage.

Treatment

A trial of medical treatment may be warranted in certain cases. This includes the use of diuretics (e.g. acetazolamide), which provide temporary relief by reducing the rate of CSF production. However, in most cases surgical intervention is required, with insertion of a ventriculoperitoneal shunt. Possible complications of this procedure are blockage and infection.

Microcephaly

Microcephaly implies failure of normal brain growth. It can be primary, i.e. genetically determined (inherited or as a result of chromosomal aberrations and other mutations), and can be isolated or part of a syndrome. Microcephaly also results when the brain, with genetic coding for normal development, suffers an injury during the period of its most rapid development and growth, particularly in the prenatal period and the first 2 years of life. Table 10.7 lists some of these causes.

A small head circumference is evident at birth in primary microcephaly as well as in some of those cases of secondary microcephaly in which the insult to the brain was sustained prenatally. In other cases, an arrest or slowing of brain growth is noted on serial head circumference measurement. Other features are related to the associated deficiencies in brain function as determined by the underlying causes such as CP, epilepsy and mental handicap. Features of involvement of other systems will be seen in cases of multisystem syndromes.

The autosomal recessive form is the commonest inherited form of microcephaly, and tends to be severe. Associated features are backward sloping of the forehead and large ears. These infants may have normal motor development, but the majority end up with a severe degree of mental handicap.

Investigations

All the causes listed in Table 10.7 should be considered. However, the extent and order of the investigations should be determined by the historical data and findings on physical examination.

Chromosomal analysis and a TORCH (toxoplasma, (others), rubella, cytomegalovirus, herpes) screen may be indicated if there is evidence of a syndrome or congenital infection. Maternal phenylalanine levels should be determined in all cases with no obvious cause. Brain imaging may help to determine the aetiology (calcification in cases of congenital infections, atrophy and cavity formation in post-traumatic microcephaly) and also outline the extent of the underlying architectural derangement.

Treatment

Microcephaly is untreatable. However, the associated mental handicap, epilepsy or CP requires careful attention and treatment. The management of these conditions has been discussed under the appropriate headings.

BEYOND CORE

CRANIOSYNOSTOSIS

The growth of the skull follows that of the brain. This is only possible because the individual bones making up the skull remain separate during infancy, eventually fusing at the sutures, after which point no further growth is possible. Premature fusion is prevented by the continuous growth of the brain, which exerts pressure to promote skull expansion. It is therefore to be expected that premature fusion of the skull sutures occurs in microcephaly. However, premature fusion of the skull sutures may occur as a primary process because of abnormal development of the skull bones; this is referred to as craniosynostosis. The precise aetiology is not completely understood, and the condition can be isolated or part of a syndrome.

If premature fusion affects only one or a few sutures the consequences are mainly cosmetic:

- Fusion of the sagittal suture results in a long and narrow skull: scaphocephaly.
- Frontal and occipital plagiocephaly result from unilateral fusion of the coronal or lambdiod sutures, respectively. This results in unilateral flattening of the forehead or occiput.

- Bilateral fusion of the coronal sutures results in brachycephaly, a skull compressed from back to front.

There are several other deformities which result from isolated premature fusion of the various sutures.

Rarely, in addition to the cosmetic effects, partial fusion of sutures may result in a neurological deficit. Most notably, severe cases of premature fusion of the coronal sutures may result in shallow orbits, pressure on the eyeball and optic nerve entrapment. Abnormal nasal development may also be present in certain cases (e.g. Crouzon's syndrome).

When multiple or generalized premature fusion of the sutures occurs, the unyielding skull compresses the brain, and increased intracranial pressure results. In these cases, surgical intervention is necessary to create artificial sutures and thus allow brain growth. This is a traumatic procedure, and requires careful follow-up. Rarely, in cases of premature fusion of isolated sutures, surgical intervention is required for cosmetic reasons

Table 10.7	Causes of microcephaly		
Genetic	*In utero injury*	*Peri- and postnatal*	

Isolated
  Autosomal recessive
  Autosomal dominant
	Congenital infections: toxoplasmosis, rubella and cytomegalovirus	Birth trauma: hypoxic–ischaemic encephalopathy	

Part of a syndrome (chromosomal defects)
  Trisomy 21
  Trisomy 18
	In utero insults
	  Alcohol (fetal alcohol syndrome)
	  Maternal phenylketonuria
		Meningitis/encephalitis
		
		Head trauma
		Toxic/metabolic injury	

Other syndromes		Severe malnutrition	

FURTHER READING

Behrman R E, Kliegman R M, Arvin A M (eds) 1996 Nelson textbook of pediatrics, 15th edn. Saunders, London

Campbell A G M, McIntosh N 1997 Forfar and Arneil's Textbook of pediatrics, 5th edn. Churchill Livingstone, Edinburgh
Illingworth R S 1991 The normal child: some problems of the early years and their treatment, 10th edn. Churchill Livingstone, Edinburgh

CHAPTER 11

Haematology and oncology

D. F. Haddad

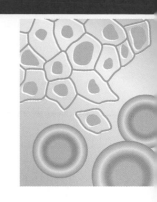

CORE PROBLEMS IN HAEMATOLOGY

CORE PROBLEM	KEY DIAGNOSIS	RELATED TOPICS
• Pallor	Iron deficiency anaemia	Physiological anaemia Haemolytic anaemia Acute lympho-blastic leukaemia Neuroblastoma
• Excessive bruising	Idiopathic thrombo-cytopenic purpura	Non-accidental injury[15] Henoch–Schönlein purpura[12] Acute lymphoblastic leukaemia Haemophilia A
• Fever[14]	Neutrophil disorder[14]	Infection[14]

Where the primary location of a topic is in another chapter, this is indicated by a superscript

CORE PROBLEMS IN ONCOLOGY

CORE PROBLEM	KEY DIAGNOSIS	RELATED TOPICS
• Malignancies	Acute lymphoblastic leukaemia Neuroblastoma Brain tumour	Neuroblastoma Retinoblastoma

ESSENTIAL BACKGROUND (HAEMATOLOGY)

ANATOMY AND PHYSIOLOGY

The fetal environment is characterized by relative hypoxia and a high rate of cellular division. This creates requirements of the blood and haemopoietic tissue of the fetus which are different from those in postnatal life. Furthermore, since the fetal environment is sterile, the demands on the white blood cells to police the environment against microorganisms are also different from those in postnatal life.

The first evidence of haemopoiesis can be seen in the yolk sac in the third week of gestation. By the sixth week of gestation the main haemopoietic activity is located in the liver. The bone marrow becomes the principal site for haemopoiesis in the last trimester of pregnancy.

Haemopoiesis begins with the production of pluripotent stem cells capable of differentiation into the three blood cell lineages (erythropoiesis thrombopoiesis and granulocytopoiesis). A number of mediators and growth factors influence the differentiation of the pluripotent stem cell and its future cell lineage.

Erythropoiesis

Because of the radically different oxygen supply system in the fetus and the relative hypoxia of fetal tissues, different types of haemoglobin are produced at different stages of pregnancy and in postnatal life. Although several types of haemoglobin are present both pre- and postnatally, by far the dominant haemoglobin in prenatal life is fetal haemoglobin (Hb F), while postnatally the 'adult' haemoglobin (Hb A) is predominant.

Hb F contains two pairs of polypeptide chains: two alpha chains and two gamma chains ($\alpha_2\gamma_2$) and constitutes more than 90% of the total haemoglobin in the fetus at midgestation. Levels gradually decline, and at birth Hb F makes up around 70% of the total.

Adult haemoglobin is composed of two pairs of polypeptide chains, two alpha and two beta chains ($\alpha_2\beta_2$). The production of Hb A starts early in the embryo, and significant amounts are found by 16 to 20 weeks of gestation. At term, adult haemoglobin Hb A constitutes around 30% of the total.

Postnatally there is a gradual decline in the amount of Hb F and a rise in Hb A, so that by 2 months of age the relationship between the two haemoglobins is reversed (see Table 11.1). At around 6–12 months of age postnatally, the adult pattern is attained in which Hb A is the dominant haemoglobin while the concentration of Hb F is less than 2%.

Another type of haemoglobin is Hb A_2, which consists of two alpha chains and two delta chains ($\alpha_2\delta_2$). Its concentration ranges between 2 and 3.4% by 1 year of age.

Compared to Hb A, the main differences exhibited by Hb F are:

- A different electrophoretic mobility
- Resistance to denaturation by alkali
- Oxygen dissociation curve shifted to the left, i.e. it has a higher affinity for oxygen, such that it is able to extract and hold on to the oxygen in a relatively hypoxic environment and is thus suited for the fetal conditions.

The pattern of relationship between the various haemoglobins can be altered in different situations:

- If the synthesis of a certain chain is inadequate. For example, in β thalassaemia major, the synthesis of the β chain is grossly reduced, and Hb F persists at high levels in these children.

- There is some elevation of Hb F levels under conditions in which there is bone marrow stress such as haemolytic anaemia, leukaemia and aplastic anaemia.
- There is some elevation in Hb F levels under conditions in which there is production of haemoglobin with an altered β chain such as in sickle cell disease (Hb S).

The levels of Hb F and Hb A_2 are also elevated in the thalassemia trait.

An understanding of the physiology of haemoglobin production is important for the correct interpretation of results of haemoglobin electrophoresis, which can be of great diagnostic value. Moreover, the ability to influence the various mechanisms regulating the switch-over between the different types of haemoglobin production may have therapeutic implications in those hereditary anaemias in which the production of a certain chain type is defective.

Granulocytopoiesis

The number of neutrophils continues to be small up to 24 weeks of gestation. This is mainly due to lack of stimulation of the white cell synthesis by the granulocyte colony-stimulating factor (G-CSF). However, at birth the leucocyte count rises (Table 11.1).

Thrombopoiesis

This is regulated by erythropoietin and a related protein called thrombopoietin. A number of other mediators are also involved. The platelet concentration attains its postnatal level from mid-gestation.

Normal values

The process of adaptation to extrauterine life is followed by ongoing physical growth and functional maturation. The blood and its constituents are in a dynamic state of continual change and adaptation to meet the ever-changing demands. Thus, since blood values change with age, a knowledge of the normal range for each

Table 11.1 Normal blood values in infants[a]

Age	Hb (g/dl)	Hb F (%)	Hb A (%)	Leucocytes (10^9/l)	Neutrophils (%)	Lymphocytes (%)
At birth	14–20	70	30	9–30	60	30
2–3 months	9.5–14	30	70	6–18	30	60
>6 months	11–14	<3	>95	6–15	45	45

[a] The figures here have been 'rounded' and are only approximate; race, geographic location and altitude above sea level are some of the factors that may influence the 'normal range'; the local laboratory reference values should always be consulted

age group is necessary for the correct interpretation of laboratory investigations (Table 11.1).

HISTORY AND EXAMINATION

History taking

Areas in history taking that require highlighting and expansion will depend on the nature of the presenting problem. Thus, a careful family and genetic history is required on suspicion of congenital anaemia. Dietary intake is crucial for the diagnosis of certain types of acquired anaemia. A history of jaundice, bleeding or dark discoloration of the urine (haemoglobinuria) may also be relevant in cases of haemolysis. A history of exposure to toxic substances or radiation is pertinent in cases of aplastic anaemia and malignancy as is a family history of malignant disorders.

Since disorders of platelets and white blood cells can also be congenital or acquired, both environmental influences and the genetic history should be explored carefully if such a disorder is suspected. A history of bruising, skin marks, haemoarthrosis, or nose or gum bleeds in the subject or family members is relevant in dealing with a potential genetic bleeding disorder. Disorders of the leucocytes may result in immunodeficiency with increased susceptibility to certain types of infection.

Physical examination

Pallor is best assessed from the colour of the lips and conjunctivae. The skin of some children may appear pale because of their complexion or vasoconstriction such as that seen in a cold environment. Jaundice is best assessed from the colour of the sclera. Petechiae, purpura, bruises and ecchymoses all describe lesions due to bleeding into the skin. These tend to change colour with the passage of time from red to blue, green and brown, as they fade away.

Lymphadenopathy is frequently overdiagnosed in children. The growth of the lymphoid tissue follows a different pattern from that of other physical parameters, and it is said that the lymphoid tissue reaches its maximal size around the age of 10 years. Lymph nodes are thus disproportionately large in normal children. This, together with the relative lack of subcutaneous tissue, means that they can be easily felt and sometimes are even visible in certain positions, and hence may cause undue concern for the parents. Transient increases in the size of lymph glands, particularly those in the neck, are also frequently seen in children, and this reflects the relatively increased frequency of ear, nose and throat and upper respiratory tract infections. The lymph node size, shape, consistency and mobility in relation to overlying skin and neighbouring tissues should be noted.

Palpation of the liver and spleen is an integral part of the assessment of a child with a possible haematological disorder. The liver is palpable up to 2 cm below the costal margin in normal children under the age of 2 years. The edge is usually smooth and sharp, and the consistency is soft. An irregular, round or hard liver edge is abnormal.

The spleen should not be palpable beyond infancy. However, in cases of lung overinflation, such as during an asthmatic attack or bronchiolitis, it may become palpable as it is displaced downwards by the diaphragm. It may also enlarge and become palpable transiently in the course of many bacterial and viral infections. A hard spleen is abnormal, and persistence of splenomegaly on repeated examination also warrants further assessment. In children, unlike adults, the edge of the enlarged spleen moves towards the pelvis rather than the umbilicus.

CLASSIFICATION OF COMMON DISORDERS

There is no one classification framework that can suitably apply to all the various pathologies of the blood and blood-forming tissue. However, a degree of uniformity can be achieved in utilizing a single classification system for the main pathologies affecting this organ system. The majority of haematological disorders can be characterized in terms of an increase or decrease in one or more of the values of the blood constituents detectable on the full blood count (FBC).

Anaemia, thrombocytopenia and neutropenia, whether occurring separately or in combination, can be explained on the basis of underproduction or increased loss of the corresponding cells (red blood cells (RBCs), platelets, neutrophils). Figure 11.1 illustrates the most important pathologies underlying anaemia which is defined as a haemoglobin concentration below the lower limit for age.

The anaemias can also be categorized according to the morphology of the RBCs (Fig. 11.2). Polycythaemia (haemoglobin concentration > upper limit of the normal range for age) in children beyond the neonatal period is relatively rare, and is most likely to be secondary to cyanotic heart disease.

The classification of neutropenias is illustrated in Figure 11.3.

Neutrophilia (absolute neutrophil count > upper limit for age) can occur in response to stress, including physical exercise and panic reactions. It is also a feature of many types of infection, both bacterial and viral. Whereas the

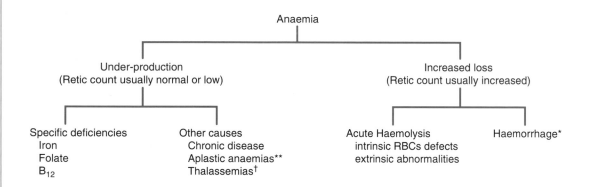

*In chronic haemorrhage, increased bone marrow activity may compensate for the ongoing loss. However, the loss of iron usually proves rate-limiting and anaemia of the iron deficiency type results, at which point the reticulocyte count may be normal or low.

**Reduced erythropoiesis due to infiltration of the bone marrow by malignant cells (e.g. leukaemia), or due to the effect of toxins is included in this category.

†In the thalassemias, there is an increased activity of the bone marrow but with intramedullary destruction of the red cells which do contain unbalanced amounts of the β and α chains.

Figure 11.1 Causes of anaemia

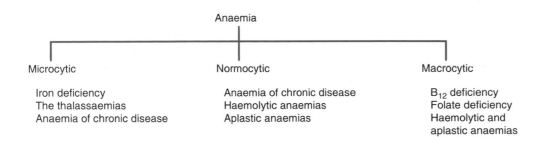

Figure 11.2 Classification of anaemia by RBC morphology

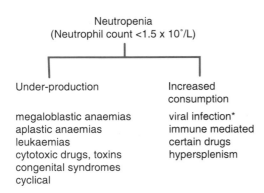

*These are the commonest underlying cause of neutropenia in children. The decrease in the neutrophil count lasts only a few days and is thought to be related to migration of the neutrophils out from the circulation to other sites, including the virus infected tissues. Some bacterial infections including severe sepsis, brucellosis and typhoid may also be associated with neutropenia.

Figure 11.3 Causes of neutropenia

elevation of neutrophil count is usually sustained in bacterial infections, in the majority of viral infections the neutrophilia is brief and frequently is superseded by a more sustained neutropenia after several days. Thrombocytosis (platelet count $>750 \times 10^9/l$) is most frequently encountered as a reaction to infection. It may also be found in iron deficiency anaemia, and is a feature of some relatively rare inflammatory disorders of children such as the vasculitis of Kawasaki's disease (see Ch. 12).

Disorders of the blood and blood-forming tissue can occur without appreciable quantitative changes of the three major cell types. Some malignancies, haemoglobin abnormalities, coagulopathies and functional defects of platelets and neutrophils belong to this category. Their diagnosis involves morphological studies of the blood film and other more specialized tests (these conditions will not be discussed in this section).

Haematological disorders can produce a large number of varied clinical features. However, the principal presentations of these disorders in children are:

- Pallor
- Excessive bruising and purpura
- Recurrent infections and fever.

Pallor, excessive bruising and purpura, and malignancy are discussed later. Recurrent infections/fever may reflect the immunodeficiency state which results from disorders of granulocytes. Derangements of other parts of the immune system (lymphocytes, complement etc.) may result in similar manifestations, and they are usually considered together. An outline of some of the immune disorders in children is provided in Chapter 14, and will not be discussed here.

CORE PROBLEMS (HAEMATOLOGY)

PALLOR

Generalized pallor of the mucous membranes reflects a reduced haemoglobin content of the tissues. This may result from decreased delivery of

body iron stores. Assuring adequacy of diet is important to prevent recurrences.

Physiological anaemia

The hypoxic conditions of intrauterine life requires a large RBC mass for effective oxygen delivery, and normal newborn babies are born with a haemoglobin level which is higher than that of older children. However, postnatally, there is a gradual drop in the haemoglobin level that begins at birth with the level reaching a nadir of around 9.5 g/dl (less in premature babies) between 6 and 12 weeks of age (Table 11.1). Several factors are involved in this physiological drop of haemoglobin levels in infants:

- There is a significant increase in tissue oxygen tension resulting from the switch of the oxygen supply from the placenta to the lung at birth, together with the increased levels of adult-type haemoglobin. This obviates the need for the intensive erythropoiesis seen in the fetus; erythropoietin levels in the small infant are low.
- Fetal RBCs have a reduced life span.
- The rapid increase in body weight and size of early infancy is associated with a relatively large expansion of the plasma volume, which overtakes the ability of the bone marrow to manufacture RBCs; there is thus a progressive 'dilution' of RBC mass and haemoglobin.

As the haemoglobin level reaches its nadir, erythropoietic activity is restored to a level appropriate to the body's needs.

The various haematological abnormalities resulting from the different pathological states that perturb erythropoiesis impinge on this pattern of physiological anaemia. Thus, haemolytic disease of the newborn and some nutritional deficiencies (e.g. of folate) may exaggerate the picture, while congenital cyanotic heart disease may blunt the fall in haemoglobin.

Haemolytic anaemia

The classification of haemolytic anaemias is given in Figure 11.4. Occasionally the genetic expression of more than one RBC defect can occur in the same individual, thus altering the phenotype.

Haemoglobinopathies

Haemoglobin is composed of two α globin chains and two non-α chains (β, γ, δ). Chain structure is determined by a pair of autosomal genes, and thus each haemoglobinopathy can exist in the heterozygous (mild) or homozygous (severe) state (e.g. sickle cell trait/sick cell disease, β thalassaemia major/β thalassaemia minor), and mixed haemolobinopathies can occur (e.g. sickle cell–thalassaemia).

The *thalassaemias* are a group of hereditary anaemias prevalent in certain areas of the world such as the Mediterranean basin, Middle East, Africa and South-East Asia. The underlying defect is due to deletions in either the α- or β-globin chain genes, resulting in a decrease or absence of mRNA for that particular chain and overproduction of those chains which are unaffected by the deletions. Since α chains are a

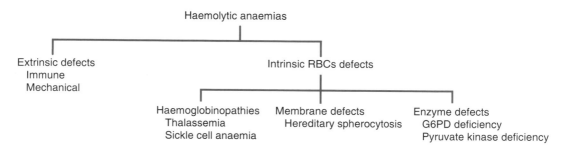

Figure 11.4 Classification of haemolytic anaemia

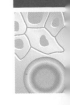

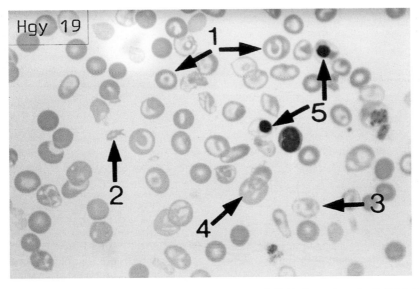

Figure 11.5 Cells marked 1 are target cells. Cell 2 is a poikilocyte. Cell 3 is hypochromic. Cell 4 is large and polychromatic. Cell 5 is a normoblast. These findings are typical of β thalassaemia. (Reproduced by courtesy of TALC)

component of fetal haemoglobin ($\alpha_2\gamma_2$), α chain mutations may be symptomatic in utero. Thus, infants with the homozygous form of α thalassaemia develop hydrops fetalis due to cardiac failure. Abnormalities in both β chains result in a severe chronic anaemia, β thalassaemia major, which presents once fetal haemoglobin production reduces; it is characterized by iron overload, transfusion dependence and growth failure. Treatment is by regular blood transfusion and iron chelation. The anaemia (Fig. 11.5) reflects both underproduction (due to increased intramedullary destruction of RBC precursors 'ineffective erythropoiesis') and a shortened life span of the RBCs. There is expansion of bone marrow cavities of all bones and extramedullary haematopoiesis in liver and spleen, resulting in hepatosplenomegaly.

Sickle cell anaemia is due to substitution of glutamic acid by valine in the sixth position of the β chain. The resulting haemoglobin polymerizes and aggregates in the deoxygenated state. The RBCs bearing such haemoglobin assume an elongated shape which is 'sickle-like' (Fig. 11.6). These RBCs have a shortened life span and tend to clump together and occlude capillaries, thus

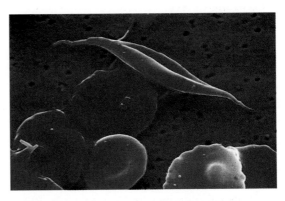

Figure 11.6 Electron micrograph showing the classical deformity of sickle cell anaemia. (Reproduced by courtesy of the Wellcome Trust Photographic Library)

interfering with the blood supply of tissues. Clinically this manifests itself by vaso-occlusive episodes, leading to infarction, which particularly involve the long bones but also abdominal organs and spleen; central nervous system infarction (stroke) may also occur. Repeated episodes of infarction of splenic tissue during early childhood results in autosplenectomy, and as a consequence susceptibility to infection with capsulated bacteria

SICKLE CELLS

Why do sickle cells sickle?

RBC volume is regulated by three membrane transport pathways. One of them, the KCl cotransporter, mediates KCl efflux to which water is linked osmotically – thus causing cell shrinkage. In normal RBC, the KCl cotransporter is switched off by low P_{O_2} and is refractory to the usual stimuli which activate it: hydrogen ions and urea. These stimuli are present in regions of the circulation, such as the renal medulla and active muscle, where the P_{O_2} is usually low. Recent research has shown that in sickle cell disease, the cotransporter remains active at low P_{O_2}. Thus RBCs in sickle cell disease are prone to shrinkage when exposed to hypoxia and this in turn initiates a cascade of events: raised intracellular haemoglobin concentration, polymerization of the abnormal haemoglobin (Hb S), sickling and vascular occlusion. If the hypothesis that this pathway is important in the pathogenesis of sickling crises is correct, it follows that agents which restore the normal relationship between P_{O_2} and cotransport activity may have a therapeutic role in sickle cell disease.

---

such as *Streptococcus pneumoniae*. Other acute episodes include aplastic, haemolytic and, in early childhood when the spleen is still typically large, sequestration crises. Treatment includes transfusion, oxygen, intravenous fluids, antibiotics and analgesia.

Membrane defect

In *hereditary spherocytosis*, the commonest hereditary haemolytic anaemia is in Caucasians, there is an autosomal dominant defect of a structural protein, spectrin, in the RBC membrane, resulting in RBCs that are spherical in shape (rather than biconcave). Such RBCs lose their deformability and are susceptible to damage in their passage through capillaries, particularly in the tortuous microcirculation of the spleen. The condition has a variable expression, and may present at any age from infancy to adulthood with jaundice and splenomegaly. Diagnosis is by RBC morphology (densely stained small erythrocytes) and by an increased rate of erythrocyte rupture during incubation with hypotonic saline (the red cell osmotic fragility test).

Enzyme defect

Deficiency of glucose-6-phosphate dehydrogenase results in an inability of RBCs to generate sufficient NADPH to maintain the necessary levels of reduced glutathione necessary to protect erythrocytes against the action of oxidants. The oxidative stress associated with infection, certain drugs and foods is the basis of episodic haemolysis in this X-linked inherited condition. It is rare in northern Europeans, more common in Mediterranean populations, and affects up to 10% of Afro-Caribbeans. Because only supportive care is possible during haemolytic crises, avoidance of precipitant drugs and chemicals is necessary. Exchange blood transfusion may be required in an affected neonate.

Normal RBCs can have a shortened life span because of the presence of abnormal antibodies directed against one of their component antigens. *Haemolytic disease of the newborn* and *autoimmune haemolytic anaemias*, whether idiopathic or part of generalized disease such as systemic lupus erythematosus, are examples. Haemolysis following transfusion of mismatched blood also belongs to this category.

EXCESSIVE BRUISING

A bruise is the result of bleeding into the skin. Petechiae, purpura, bruises and ecchymoses all describe skin bleeds that are of varying size and depth. The most useful clinical sign that distinguishes this type of skin lesion from others is the fact that they do not blanch on pressure. Other skin lesions such as macules, papules or urticaria are caused by varying degrees of vascular dilatation, and blanch on applying pressure.

Accidental trauma is the commonest cause of bruising in children. This is particularly true for younger children and toddlers. These 'run of the mill' bruises usually have a characteristic distribution (e.g. shins), and frequently the history confirms their origin.

Pathological or excessive bruising should be suspected whenever the size or amount of bruising (or other types of skin bleeds) seems to be disproportionate to the implicated trauma. In more severe cases such bruising may be spontaneous. However, unexplained bruising and bruising involving the head, trunk and proximal parts of the limbs, should also raise concern about the possibility of non-accidental injury (NAI, see Ch. 15). In the absence of NAI, excessive bruising suggests abnormality in the haemostatic mechanisms, i.e.:

- The vascular component, e.g. septicaemia, Henoch–Schönlein purpura (HSP)
- The formation of a platelet plug, e.g. thrombocytopenia
- The coagulation pathways, e.g. haemophilia
- The presence of an abnormal anticoagulant, e.g. systemic lupus erythematosus or anticoagulant therapy.

Bruising may be part of the skin lesions produced by septicaemias, particularly meningococcaemia and other conditions associated with disseminated intravascular coagulation (DIC). In these cases the pathogenesis involves vasculitis as well as thrombocytopenia secondary to DIC (septicaemia is discussed in more detail in Ch. 14).

In a relatively well child, purpuric rash and excessive bruising are most frequently caused either by Henoch–Schönlein purpura, a vasculitic disorder (see Ch. 12), or idiopathic thrombocytopenic purpura (ITP).

✳ KEY DIAGNOSIS

Idiopathic thrombocytopenic purpura

The hallmark of ITP is the striking reduction in the number of circulating platelets in the face of normal or even increased production by the bone marrow. ITP is the most common underlying cause of profound deficiency of platelets and associated mucocutaneous bleeding in children.

Aetiology

There is usually a history of viral infection in the preceding 2 weeks. Only in a minority of cases can antiplatelet antibodies be detected in the serum. Nevertheless, it is believed that an immune mechanism is the basis of the thrombocytopenia. The consensus model is that viral infection somehow stimulates the immune system to produce antiplatelet antibodies, either by altering the antigenic structure of the platelets or by the adsorption of viral antigens on to the platelets. The antibody-coated platelets are then removed from the circulation by the reticuloendothelial system, in particular the spleen.

Clinical manifestations

Mucocutaneous haemorrhages usually appear over a period of a few days (Fig. 11.7). These are of various sizes, ranging from petechiae to large

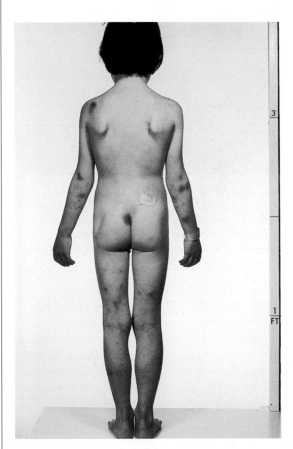

Figure 11.7 A child with extensive bruising (pinpoint petechiae to large bruising and ecchymosis) due to ITP. (Reproduced by courtesy of the Wellcome Trust Photographic Library)

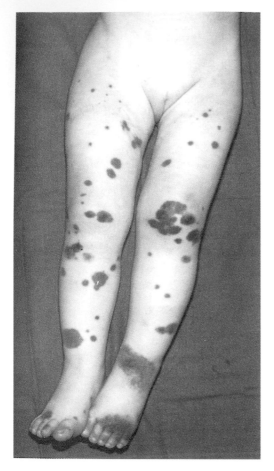

Figure 11.8 Raised extensive purpuric lesions together with swollen limb joints, especially of left ankle and knee, consistent with acute vasculitic rash of Henoch–Schönlein purpura. (Reproduced by courtesy of the Wellcome Trust Photographic Library)

bruises of asymmetric distribution. Unlike Henoch–Schönlein purpura (see Ch. 12 and Fig. 11.8), in which the purpuric lesions are predominantly located in the lower extremities, in ITP they are generalized. Nose bleeds are also frequent, but serious bleeding, such as intracranial haemorrhage, is rare and occurs in less than 1% of cases. Apart from the bleeding, the child is otherwise well in contrast to other conditions with thrombocytopenia (leukaemia, septicaemia, etc.). Splenomegaly and lymphoadenopathy are usually absent.

Although the onset of the skin bleeds is acute, ITP tends to follow a subacute course.

Spontaneous bleeding occurs in the first 1–2 weeks, and subsides thereafter; this applies equally to mucocutaneous bleeds and serious types of bleeding such as intracranial haemorrhage. Within 3 months the majority of patients recover completely, and in 90% of cases the platelet count will have returned to normal by 9–12 months from onset. Relapses are unusual. Cases in which thrombocytopenia persists beyond a year are classified as chronic. The differential diagnosis of bruising and purpura is given in Fig. 11.9.

Investigations

The platelet count is usually reduced to below $20 \times 10^9 /l$. Coagulation tests dependant on platelet function, such as bleeding time, are abnormal (this test yields no additional information, and is unnecessary in the presence of a low platelet count), while those independent of platelet function, such as prothrombin time (PT), partial thromboplastin time (PTT) and coagulation times, are normal. The white cell count and haemoglobin level are normal except in cases complicated by serious bleeding. Bone marrow aspiration reveals normal production of the three blood cell lines but megakaryocyte numbers are usually increased.

As yet there is no specific tests to confirm ITP. The differential diagnosis of conditions associated with purpuric rashes and excessive bruising can be divided into two main groups: those associated with thrombocytopenia and those which are not (thrombocytopenic and non-thrombocytopenic purpuras). A simple platelet count will allow the distinction between these two groups (Fig. 11.10).

Frequently, the crucial question is to distinguish between ITP and conditions with underproduction of platelets such as leukaemia and aplastic anaemia. The absence of other haematological abnormalities on the blood film, the good general condition of the child, absence of other signs (e.g. pallor, lymphadenopathy, splenomegaly) are in favour of ITP. However, if there is any doubt, a bone marrow aspiration should be carried out.

Treatment

ITP has an excellent prognosis, and spontaneous recovery over a period of several weeks is the

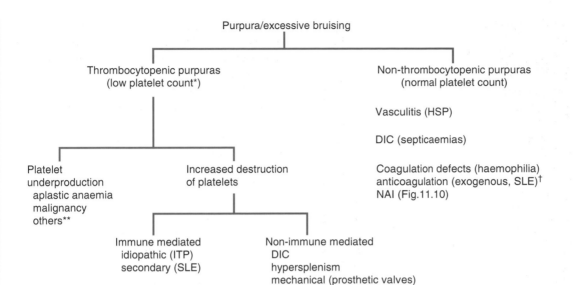

Purpura/excessive bruising

Thrombocytopenic purpuras
(low platelet count*)

Non-thrombocytopenic purpuras
(normal platelet count)

Vasculitis (HSP)

DIC (septicaemias)

Platelet
underproduction
 aplastic anaemia
 malignancy
 others**

Increased destruction
of platelets

Coagulation defects (haemophilia)
anticoagulation (exogenous, SLE)†
NAI (Fig.11.10)

Immune mediated
 idiopathic (ITP)
 secondary (SLE)

Non-immune mediated
 DIC
 hypersplenism
 mechanical (prosthetic valves)

* Many viral infections are associated with a transient decrease in the platelet count, whether
 due to underproduction or increased loss of platelets. The ingestion of certain drugs can
 also be followed by thrombocytopenia; the mechanisms involved are not always clear

**A number of congenital syndromes are associated with platelet underproduction.

† Therapeutic or accidental ingestion of anticoagulants. Anti-coagulant antibody in SLE.

Figure 11.9 Differential diagnosis of bruising/purpura

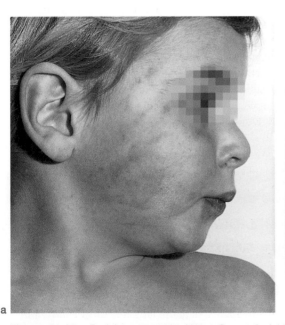
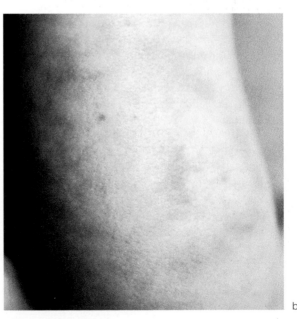

a

b

Figure 11.10 Bruising caused by NAI. **a** Severe facial bruising with the imprint of a human hand. **b** Bruising
delineating a human bite on the arm of a small child

rule. Severe spontaneous haemorrhages including intracranial bleeding occur in less than 1% of patients and are rare beyond the initial phase of the illness. Platelet transfusions are of transient benefit as their life in the circulation is short. However, they do have a place if life-threatening haemorrhage is suspected (e.g. an intracranial bleed). γ-globulin intravenous infusion and corticosteroid therapy have both been shown to be effective in reducing the severity of thrombocytopenia and shortening the duration of the initial phase. There is still no consensus as to whether this usually self-limiting condition should be managed with no therapy, with intravenous γ-globulin or corticosteroids. Avoidance of drugs which interfere with coagulation, such as aspirin, is wise, and reasonable efforts at protecting the child from trauma are recommended. In chronic cases (>12 months) splenectomy is of benefit.

Haemophilia A

The coagulation pathway is involved in a number of other physiological responses such as inflammation and tissue regeneration. Almost at each step of this complicated process, a defect of some kind or another has been described. Many of these defects result in excessive bleeding, but others may not have appreciable effects on haemostasis. Rarely such defects result in a tendency to thrombosis.

The haemophilias are a group of genetically determined coagulation defects which include factor VIII, vW factor and factor IX deficiencies (haemophilia A, von Willibrand's disease and haemophilia B, respectively).

Haemophilia A is probably the best known hereditary coagulation defect. It results from a deficiency in factor VIII of the coagulation pathway, leading to a bleeding tendency of variable severity depending on the degree of the deficiency. It is inherited as an X-linked disorder, and presents in early childhood. The hallmark of haemophilia is haemarthrosis, and life-threatening bleeding may follow trauma or surgery. Treatment is by infusion of purified factor VIII or, in those parts of the world where purified factor VIII is unavailable, the plasma fractions containing it.

ESSENTIAL BACKGROUND (ONCOLOGY)

Malignancy is relatively rare in childhood, with an incidence of around 2% of that in the adult population, but seems to be on the increase. Although improved anticancer treatment has transformed the scene, and a diagnosis of malignancy in a child is no longer the death sentence it used to be, childhood cancer continues to be a leading cause of protracted morbidity and death in children.

Many types of cancer are amenable to treatment, with long-term survival and cure being realistic aims. The chances of achieving a cure depend on type and aggressiveness of the tumour and, almost universally, early diagnosis and institution of appropriate treatment.

There are few specific clinical features for cancer. Rather, malignancies frequently masquerade behind non-specific symptoms. However, the unusual course of the illness, the degree of systemic upset and/or the poor response to treatment of an erroneously diagnosed non-malignant condition are features that point to the possibility of malignancy.

Although knowledge of the clinical features, methods for diagnosis and treatment of childhood malignancies is not expected from the non-specialist, it is necessary for all medical practitioners providing health care for children to be able to recognize the features that should raise suspicion of the possibility of malignancy (Tables 11.2 and 11.3).

CORE PROBLEMS (ONCOLOGY)

MALIGNANCIES

✱ KEY DIAGNOSIS

Acute lymphoblastic leukaemia (ALL)

The incidence of acute leukaemias in children in the UK is around 35 new cases per one million

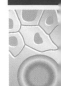

Table 11.2 Common clinical presentations in children and features suggestive of possible malignancy

Presentation Possible malignancy (italics)	Features pointing to possible malignant aetiology	Other non-malignant possible conditions
Flu illness/sore throat *Leukaemia* *Neuroblastoma*	No response to antibiotic treatment. Course prolonged. Associated systemic upset (pallor, poor appetite, weight loss)	Glandular fever, other specific infections
Headaches *Brain tumours*	Progressive course, features of increased intracranial pressure	Conditions with 'mass effect' (e.g. haematoma)
Lymphadenopathy *Lymphoma*	Progressive enlargement, usually painless, firm/hard in consistency may be attached to surrounding structures	Reactive, pyogenic, tuberculous and atypical mycobacteria lymphadenitis. Glandular fever
Diarrhoea *Neuroblastoma*	Severe chronic watery diarrhoea. Diarrhoea persists even when on nil by mouth. Low serum Cl^- and K^+	Other conditions with secretory-type diarrhoea (e.g. certain *Escherichia coli* infections)
Anaemia, neutropenia, thrombocytopenia *Leukaemia* *Neuroblastoma*	Combination of any two of these	Aplastic anaemia, folate or vitamin B_{12} deficiency, postinfective (viral)
Lumps *Soft tissue/bone tumours*	Not resolving in the expected time limit, even if associated with trauma	Chronic infections, bleeding disorders, connective tissue disorders
Chronic ear discharge/nasal obstruction *Rhabdomyosarcoma*	Evidence of infection is lacking and/or poor response to therapy	Foreign bodies, allergic conditions
Chronic wheeze/stridor *Lymphomata*	Persistent symptoms, diminished response to bronchodilators	External pressure from vascular rings or other structural

Table 11.3 The relative incidence of childhood cancers

Malignancy	Relative incidence (%)
Leukaemias	33.6
Brain and spinal tumours	23.5
Lymphomas	10.4
Neuroblastomas	6.8
Nephroblastomas	5.2
Bone tumours	7
Retinoblastomas	2.7

children per year. ALL constitutes about 75% of all cases, and is thus by far the commonest malignancy of childhood.

The definitive diagnosis of ALL is based on examination of the bone marrow. ALL is classified according to immunological and cytogenetic features of the leukaemic cells which indicate whether the malignant cells originate from a T or B cell lineage. The commonest form and best prognosis is associated with those cases of ALL in which the leukaemic cells are positive for early B cell markers.

ALL involves infiltration of the bone marrow by uncontrolled multiplication of the precursors of lymphocytes. As the disease advances, there is bone marrow failure and dissemination to other organs and tissues, giving rise to the main features of the disease. Although, in the majority of cases at diagnosis the malignant cell mass has 'spilled over' to the bloodstream and hence can be shown on a routine blood film, in some cases there are few or no malignant blast cells in the peripheral blood ('aleukaemic leukaemia'). A bone marrow examination should always be obtained if the condition is clinically suspected.

Clinical features

There is usually a few weeks' history of non-specific features such as poor appetite, irritability and lethargy, possibly associated with non-resolving sore throat or flu-like illness. The more specific features of bone marrow failure, the triad of pallor, bleeding and fever (reflecting anaemia, thrombocytopenia and neutropenia) follow. These features usually serve to raise the suspicion regarding the possibility of the diagnosis. Lymphadenopathy and hepatosplenomegaly are common but are not present in all patients at the time of diagnosis.

Investigations

A full blood count will reveal anaemia and thrombocytopenia in the majority of cases. The white cell count might be extremely high, low or normal. Blast cells usually can be seen on the peripheral blood film. Further investigations are designed to assess the extent of the involvement of various tissues and to obtain a more specific identification of the malignant cells.

Treatment

Cases will vary according to the risk group. There are four main phases of treatment:

1. The induction phase which is designed to induce remission by intensive chemotherapy with a combination of cytotoxic drugs.
2. Intensification blocks; it is the current recommendation that blocks of further intensive treatment are administered at certain intervals to ensure eradication of any leukaemic cells that have escaped the induction phase.
3. Central nervous system prophylaxis; certain areas in the body are relatively protected from the effect of cytotoxic treatment by virtue of the impermeability of the local capillary network. If the malignant cells manage to reach these areas, there is a chance they will escape the action of the standard therapy. Two such sites are the central

nervous system and, in boys, the testicles. A cytotoxic drug (methotrexate) and/or cranial irradiation are given to protect the central nervous system, since a relapse at this site is difficult to detect and treat.

4. Continuation therapy; most programmes will involve maintenance treatment for a period of 2 years.

Almost all cytotoxic drugs results in varying degrees of suppression of the bone marrow, and careful monitoring is required. Most of the success that has been achieved in the treatment of this previously uniformly fatal disease has been attributed to the scientific approach to evaluation of the various therapy regimens. The best possible outcome for a child with leukaemia can be achieved by enrolling in one of the treatment projects that are collectively run by the major paediatric haematology centres. In the UK, these treatment regimens are named UKALL protocols, and are designed to answer specific questions as to how to further perfect the treatment for this illness.

Prognosis

This depends on the risk group. Good prognostic features are: age at onset 2–5 years, white cell count less than $20 \times 10^9/l$, absence of central nervous system involvement, common (B cell lineage) leukaemic cell type, and presence or absence of certain chromosomal aberrations in the malignant cells. With the present treatment regimens, over 97% of patients achieve remission within the first 4 weeks of treatment. All children surviving from leukaemia require long-term follow-up to deal with the various physiological and psychological sequelae of the illness and its treatment. There is a continued risk of relapse for the first 8 years, and the possibility of a second cancer is also increased as a result of the treatment given.

✴ KEY DIAGNOSIS

Neuroblastoma

Neuroblastomas are the commonest solid tumours of infancy. Clusters of neuroblasts are seen in many aborted fetuses and in 1 in 200 of neonates dying from other causes. This frequency

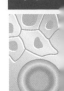

is far above the incidence of clinical neuroblastoma, and it is believed that these 'neuroblastoma in situ' undergo spontaneous regression. Spontaneous regression is seen in some cases of neuroblastoma diagnosed in infancy. Thus, neuroblastomas may represent a tumour that arises from clusters of neuroblasts normally present at a certain stage of development and which usually regress as maturation progresses. It is this lack of regression that results in disease.

Neuroblastomas arise from the neural crest cells of the sympathetic nervous system, and can originate anywhere from the posterior cranial fossa to the coccyx. However, more than half the cases originate in the adrenal glands, and three-quarters in the abdomen. At the time of diagnosis, almost three-quarters of children have metastases. Frequently the liver, bone and bone marrow are the sites for such metastases. The tumour cells are metabolically active and secrete a number of substances, including catecholamines.

Clinical features

Neuroblastoma can be responsible for a wide range of clinical features in children, and thus is included in the differential diagnosis of many childhood illnesses. Non-specific features include systemic illness with irritability and pallor. The latter is present even without bone marrow failure, and sometimes sudden bleeding into a large tumour mass may occur.

There are three groups of clinical features:

1. *Features related to the growth of the primary tumour.* These are frequently asymptomatic; a painless abdominal mass may be noted in the course of a physical examination conducted for another reason. In the chest the mass may be noted on chest radiography. However, sometimes signs due to local pressure may appear, such as Horner's syndrome from lesions in the cervical and upper thoracic region, nasal obstruction from tumours in the nasopharynx and problems of urination or defecation from tumours in the pelvis.

2. *Features related to the metastases.* Metastases in the liver results in hepatomegaly, while those in the orbit may cause proptosis and periorbital bruising. Bone metastases may result in bone pain and in bone marrow failure. Such cases of neuroblastoma need to be differentiated from leukaemia.

3. *Features related to the metabolic activity of the tumour.* An encephalopathy with cerebellar signs that include abnormal movements of the head, myoclonic jerks and random eye movement may occur in some patients. Severe diarrhoea of the secretory type, characterized by severe hypokalaemia, can also result. Rarely, the excess of catecholamines results in hypertension.

Blood chemistry and a full blood count reflect the involvement of the liver, kidneys and bone marrow. Measurement of urinary catecholamine metabolites (vanillylmandelic acid and homovanillic acid) are useful in diagnosis and monitoring of tumour response to treatment. Various techniques including computerized tomography (CT) and magnetic resonance imaging (MRI) and ultrasound scanning can all be used to define the primary tumour and metastases. Radioisotope scanning (Fig. 11.11), chest radiography and plain bone radiography are also useful. Methyliodobenzylguanine (MIBG) is an analogue of the catecholamine precursors, and is taken up by the tumour cells; scanning with technetium-labelled MIBG can thus be helpful in detecting metastases.

Management and prognosis

Depending on the age of the child and the stage of the tumour, surgical resection, chemotherapy and radiotherapy are employed to treat the disease. The survival rate in infants under 1 year of age with localized disease exceeds 90%. Neuroblastoma can be viewed as a congenital tumour, and thus the older the patient is, the more advanced is the disease and the poorer the prognosis.

✳ KEY DIAGNOSIS

Brain tumour

Brain tumours are the most common solid tumours of childhood and the second most

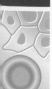

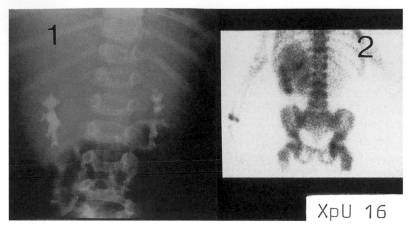

Figure 11.11 **1** An intravenous urogram showing a rotated right kidney with slightly dilated renal pelvis. The left kidney is normal. **2** The isotope scan shows a large black shadow in the lower part of the right hemithorax that is a suprarenal tumour – a neuroblastoma. (Reproduced by courtesy of TALC)

common malignancy in children after leukaemia. They can present at any age including during infancy.

Histologically, there are several types of brain tumours reflecting different types of cells present in brain tissue. However, the two most important histological types of brain tumours in children are astrocytomas, which arise from glial cells, and medulloblastomas, which are of primitive neuroectodermal origin. Gliomas and craniopharyngeomas are other examples of brain tumours in children.

Accurate identification of the histological type of brain tumour is not always possible in children and various immunological and histochemical methods are employed. In terms of location, brain tumours fall into two categories: infratentorial (posterior fossa tumours, usually medulloblastomas located in the cerebellum and sometimes encroaching on the brain stem) and supratentorial (usually astrocytomas, located in the cerebral hemispheres). Infratentorial tumours are more common in younger children.

Clinical features

The principal features of brain tumours in children are those related to increased intracranial pressure and the presence of focal neurological signs. Infratentorial tumours tend to cause a significant increase in intracranial pressure at a

relatively early stage because of obstruction of the cerebrospinal fluid circulation; if involving the brain stem there may, however, be long tract and cranial nerve signs. On the other hand, supratentorial tumours usually present with focal (long tract) neurological signs, and a significant increase in intracranial pressure usually occurs late in their course. The precise nature of the focal neurological signs produced by a brain tumour depends on its location.

Headaches are important features of brain tumours, but they are unlikely to be the sole manifestation of this pathology; they characteristically occur in the early morning, sometimes associated with vomiting. Brain tumours are also one of the causes of fits (secondary epilepsy), particularly of the focal type (see Ch. 10 for the clinical features of increased intracranial pressure and for the differential diagnosis of headaches and epilepsy).

Personality changes and deterioration in mental and academic performance as well as changes in behaviour are frequently the first symptoms of brain tumours. These may predate other more specific features by weeks or months. Such features are difficult to recognize by the examiner, and specific questioning of the parents and other adults involved in the care of the child (e.g. teachers) may help in obtaining this information. Poor coordination and loss of balance skills with ataxia and other cerebral signs are associated with posterior fossa tumours.

In advanced cases, there can be rapid progressive increase in the intracranial pressure, and 'herniation' of the brain stem through the foramen magnum may result. The rapid appearance of successive focal neurological signs, an abnormal pattern of breathing, unequal pupils or other signs of brain stem dysfunction are ominous signs of this life-threatening complication.

Management

If a brain tumour is suspected, lumbar puncture is categorically contraindicated. Brain imaging is crucial for the diagnosis. MRI is preferable to CT (Fig. 11.12) because of its ability to delineate the structures of the posterior fossa. The treatment of brain tumours should be undertaken by a team

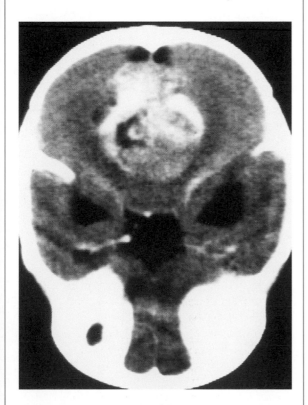

Figure 11.12 A CT scan of the brain with intravenous contrast showing a midline posterior fossa mass causing obstructive hydrocephalus and distorting the fourth ventricle. At operation the mass was confirmed as a posterior fossa primitive neuroectodermal tumour (medulloblastoma)

comprising the paediatric oncologist, neurologist and neurosurgeon. The prognosis depends on the type and location of the tumour. Multimodal therapy (chemotherapy, radiotherapy and surgery) is frequently required for the more aggressive types such as medulloblastomas, while low-grade astrocytomas are more likely to be curable by surgery alone.

Nephroblastoma (Wilms' tumour)

Nephroblastoma arises from the kidney, and should be included in the differential diagnosis of abdominal mass in a child. Hypertension and haematuria (microscopic or macroscopic) are associated findings in many cases. The incidence of nephroblastoma is increased in children with varioius congenital abnormalities and syndromes. Important associations include malformations of the genitourinary tract, hemihypertrophy and aniridia (bilateral hypoplasia of the iris).

Retinoblastoma

Retinoblastoma is a malignant tumour arising from the retina, and is associated with abnormalities of the long arm of chromosome 13. The predisposition for this tumour can be inherited in an autosomal fashion, and the tumour can be bilateral. The cardinal sign is leukocoria, which is a white reflex visible through the pupils and is caused by the tumour behind the lens. The diagnosis is confirmed on careful fundoscopic examination, usually under anaesthesia. MRI/CT scanning of the orbit may be undertaken to delineate the extent of the tumour and the degree of involvement of the optic nerve.

Enucleation of the eye is the standard treatment for unilateral disease, while in bilateral cases, radiotherapy may be used in an attempt to salvage vision of at least one of the eyes.

FURTHER READING

Behrman R E, Kiliegman R M, Arvin A M 1996 Nelson textbook of pediatrics, 15th edn. Churchill Livingstone, Edinburgh

Campbell A G M, McIntosh N 1997 Forfar and Arneil's textbook of pediatrics, 5th edn. Churchill Livingstone, Edinburgh

CHAPTER 12

Joint and bone disease

R. E. Olver

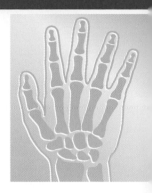

CORE PROBLEMS IN JOINT AND BONE DISEASE

CORE PROBLEMS	KEY DIAGNOSIS	RELATED TOPICS
• Painful/ swollen joints	Juvenile idiopathic arthritis	Reactive arthritis Henoch–Schönlein purpura Idiopathic pain
• Limp	Transient synovitis	Congenital dislocation of hip Perthes' disease Slipped femoral epiphysis
• Painful limb	Osteomyelitis	Septic arthritis Fracture[8]
• Curvature of the spine	Idiopathic scoliosis	Postural scoliosis
• Deformed foot[16]	Talipes[16]	Forefoot adduction Flat feet

Where the primary location of a topic is in another chapter, this is indicated by a superscript

ESSENTIAL BACKGROUND

INTRODUCTION

This chapter will focus principally on disorders presenting with musculoskeletal pain, disordered growth of the axial skeleton and conditions which are normal variants of growth and development of the limbs. Together they make up the bulk of locomotor problems in childhood.

ANATOMY AND PHYSIOLOGY

The anatomy of the long bone is shown in Figure 12.1. In infancy and childhood, increase in length and diameter of the bone takes place at the growth plate. This is a region of mechanical weakness through which separation of the epiphysis can take place as a result of trauma or chronic shear stress (e.g. slipped capital femoral epiphysis, see p. 243 and Fig. 12.6).

In the first year of life, the blood supply to the epiphysis is from the metaphysis via the growth plate. Hence trauma or bone infection during infancy may cause serious damage to the growth cartilage of the epiphysis with resultant deformity and loss of growth potential. However, in other circumstances such as chronic joint inflammation, there may be stimulation of the cartilage of the growth plate with excessive bone lengthening and resultant limb inequality.

The direct vascular communication across the growth plate of the infant (Fig. 12.1) allows direct spread of infection from the metaphysis to the epiphysis, and from there into the joint.

However, beyond the age of about a year, the blood supply to the epiphysis is routed via vessels in the joint capsule and joint ligaments with the vessels supplying the metaphysis becoming end arteries which coil sharply to end in venous sinusoids, causing relative stasis. This arrangement explains the predilection for osteomyelitis to occur in the metaphyseal region.

Infancy

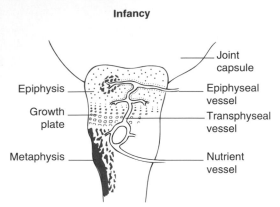

Childhood

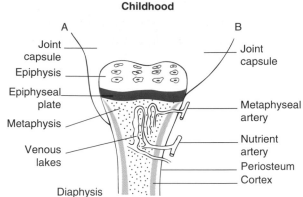

Figure 12.1   Anatomy of the long bone

After the first year of life, direct communication (and hence the potential for direct spread of infection) between the metaphysis and joint space occurs only where the distal insertion of the joint capsule incorporates part of the metaphysis within the joint, as occurs in the hip and shoulder (see p. 244).

The blood supply to bone beyond infancy is generally precarious, and because of rapid growth in relation to their blood supply, the secondary ossification centres of the epiphysis are subject to avascular necrosis (see Perthes' disease, p. 242).

Normal variants of limb growth and development

Growth and development of the child as he or she adopts an upright posture and learns to walk is associated with a number of normal variants in musculoskeletal anatomy and physiology. Understanding these normal variations in early childhood will allow appropriate reassurance to be given to parents and will avoid unnecessary investigations and interventions. The most common of these are: in-toeing, out-toeing, flat feet, forefoot adduction, toe walking, bow legs and knock knees.

Normal variants of long bone development

In-toeing due to internal tibial torsion is a normal phenomenon in 6–18 month old children as they begin to walk. Characteristically, the in-toeing

appears worse when the child is in shoes and he or she may stumble more than is usual. Beyond 2–3 years of age it is usually the result of femoral internal torsion involving the whole length of the shaft. There is a progressive natural correction towards the neutral position by 8 years, and a slower change thereafter. Tibial and femoral internal torsion can be differentiated by the alignment of the patellae, which point straight ahead in internal tibial torsion but point inwards (convergent 'squint') in cases of internal femoral torsion (Fig. 12.2).

Bow legs (genu varum) in infancy, often accompanied by internal tibial torsion which accentuates the bowed appearance, is physiological. It normally self-corrects by the age of 2 years, commonly converting to mild knock knee (genu valgum), which in turn resolves spontaneously by 5–8 years of age. Causes of persistent bowing include rickets, obesity and, rarely, metaphyseal dysplasia.

Normal variants of foot development

In forefoot adduction (metatarsus varus, Fig. 12.2), the forefoot turns inward in relation to the long axis of the heel. It is the result of intrauterine compression and, if flexible, usually self-corrects. Serial casts or an orthotic device may be necessary if the deformity is fixed.

Flat feet are the norm in the infant and toddler. Body weight is sufficient to flatten the arch, which reappears when the child is in a non-weight-bearing position.

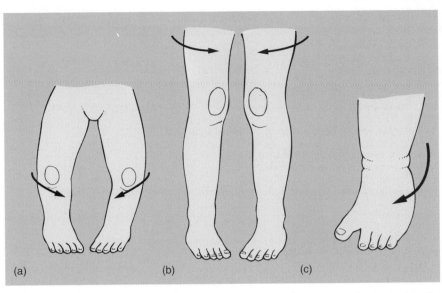

Figure 12.2 Causes of intoeing: **a** internal tibial torsion; **b** internal femoral torsion; **c** forefoot adduction (metatarsus varus)

Although toe walking is most commonly the result of excessive gastrocnemius muscle tone in children with cerebral palsy, it can be a normal variant in the early months of walking before the normal heel–toe gait develops.

HISTORY AND EXAMINATION

Much of the diagnostic difficulty relating to disorders of the musculoskeletal system centres on the differentiation between the many causes of pain in bone and joint (Table 12.1). As with pain in any system, it is important to start by obtaining a full description of the nature of the pain as well as its location, precipitating and relieving factors, duration, intensity and diurnal variation. Particularly important is the question as to whether the pain is aggravated by immobility, as in juvenile idiopathic arthritis (JIA) and related conditions, or by movement and activity, as in most other causes of musculoskeletal pain. The possibility of trauma, including child abuse, should be explored. Questions about general health, appetite, activity and mood may help differentiate between systemic and local pathologies. It is important to take a full psychosocial history; disordered

family dynamics or evidence of stress at home or at school may suggest a psychosomatic aetiology. Taken together, this information will very often allow an initial categorization of the symptoms as being mechanical, inflammatory (acute or chronic) or idiopathic (psychosomatic).

Examination of the child with musculoskeletal symptoms must include a search for associated features of systemic disease: pallor, generalized lymphadenopathy, hepatosplenomegaly, fever, rashes, inflammation of mucous membranes, and nail pitting. Examination of the musculoskeletal system should begin with an observation of gait, and must include an assessment of muscle power. It is important to determine the exact point of limb pain. The essential features of examination of the joints are set out in Table 12.2. Because of its deep location and relative inaccessibility, the assessment of the hip is necessarily more restricted than of other joints. Important aspects of hip examination include observation of leg length and resting position, palpation for tenderness and assessment of movement (including gait, Ortolani's test (see Fig. 4.1) and Trendelenburg's test (see p. 241) as appropriate).

Table 12.1 Differential diagnosis of musculoskeletal pain in children [a]

Avascular necrosis and degenerative disorders:
   Perthes' and other osteochondroses
   Slipped capital femoral epiphysis
   Chondromalacia patellae
   Hypermobility
Reactive arthritis: post-streptococcal, post-enteric, post-viral
Trauma (see Table 12.3)
Haematological: leukaemia, lymphoma, haemophilia, sickle cell anaemia
Rickets
Infection: septic arthritis, osteomyelitis, Lyme disease
Tumours: of cartilage, bone, muscle; neuroblastoma
Idiopathic pain syndromes
Systemic connective tissue disease: JIA, systemic lupus erythematosus, dermatomyositis; vasculitis

[a]Notes:
1. Arthritis may be a feature of inflammatory bowel disease and cystic fibrosis
2. Pain in the knee may be referred from the hip
3. JIA is a diagnosis of exclusion

Table 12.2 Joint examination

Inspection
1. Skin colour
2. Bony landmarks
3. Muscle bulk
4. Limb length
5. Resting position
6. Site of maximum pain

Palpation
1. Skin warmth over joint
2. Joint swelling: soft tissue, bony enlargement, intra-articular effusion
3. Site of maximal tenderness: joint margin, soft tissue, bony tenderness

Movement
1. Active movement: range, quality, compensatory use of other joints or recruitment of other muscle groups
2. Passive movement: range, guarding, pain

CORE PROBLEMS

PAINFUL/SWOLLEN JOINTS

Musculoskeletal pain is common in childhood and up to 30% of school children may be affected at some time. However, the presence of joint pain does not necessarily indicate arthritis. Conversely children, particularly young children, may not complain of pain but may nevertheless display obvious discomfort. The major causes of musculoskeletal pain are covered by the mnemonic 'arthritis' (Table 12.1).

Pain of *mechanical origin* is more common in older children and adolescents, and is almost always related to physical activity. Trauma is the single most frequent cause (Table 12.3), with the knee and ankle most commonly affected by strains and sprains of ligaments and tendons. These injuries may become chronic if not managed appropriately. Recurrent and minor trauma due to overuse may cause stress fractures or inflammation of periarticular tissues (tenosynovitis), as occurs in various sports and activities (e.g. tennis elbow, dancer's feet). Knee pain of mechanical but non-traumatic origin frequently originates from the patella; the most common cause being chondromalacia patellae, in which the posterior face of the patella is inflamed, sometimes in association with fragmentation of the articular cartilage. An intra-articular loose body can cause the affected joint to lock; alternatively, it may give way as sudden pain causes reflex inhibition of muscular contraction. Typically the pain of mechanical origin gives rise to a persistent ache with accentuated pain during and after physical activity, with symptoms increasing as the day wears on. Other causes of pain of mechanical origin include slipped upper

Table 12.3 Traumatic causes of musculoskeletal pain
Soft tissue Stretching of ligaments Stretching of muscles/tendons Compression (contusion) Overuse syndromes
Bone Fractures Stress fracture Greenstick fracture Epiphyseal separations
Joint dislocations/subluxations Radial head Patella (recurrent)

femoral epiphysis (see p. 243) and avascular necrosis (e.g. Perthes' disease).

Duration of symptoms and signs is of considerable help in differentiating between the possible causes of joint inflammation. Thus, infections, other than postinfectious (reactive) arthritis and Lyme disease (see Highlights and Hypotheses: Lyme disease), are generally short-lived (days or weeks), and the pain, like that of mechanical origin, is aggravated by movement. However, unlike the symptoms of mechanical aetiology and acute inflammation, those due to chronic inflammation follow periods of immobility. Thus, pain and stiffness are characteristically worse first thing in the morning or after prolonged sitting.

Chronic arthritis, lasting several months, is much more suggestive of juvenile idiopathic arthritis or possibly, systemic connective tissue disorder. Moodiness and irritability, together with other extra-articular manifestations such as fever, anorexia, weight loss or poor growth tend to correlate with the severity of the inflammatory process. Extra-articular signs, such as rash (e.g. psoriasis, systemic lupus erythematosus (SLE), dermatomyositis), mucositis (Kawasaki's disease, see Ch. 14) or muscle weakness (dermatomyositis), may be features of systemic connective tissue disease. Abdominal pain and bloody diarrhoea may indicate associated inflammatory bowel disease.

Idiopathic/psychosomatic pain is the most common form of chronic musculoskeletal pain. The symptoms, which can be dramatic, may be associated with non-specific features such as easy but variable fatiguability and poor school attendance. Pain may be persistent, diurnal or nocturnal. The confirmation of prominent symptoms with few or no objective signs and normal investigations (acute phase reactants: C-reactive (CRP) protein levels and erythrocyte sedimentation rate (ESR) are particularly useful in this respect) point to an idiopathic/psychosomatic disorder.

✳ KEY DIAGNOSIS

Juvenile idiopathic arthritis

JIA is a term used to identify a clinically heterogeneous group of disorders in children under 16 years of age characterized by arthritis of more than 3 months duration. The incidence of new cases of JIA in the child population is approximately 1 in 10 000, and the prevalence is about 1 in 1000.

JIA is an autoimmune disease in which genetic and environmental factors contribute to the pathogenesis. Thus, there are clear genetic associations between major histocompatibility complex (HLA) proteins and particular clinical JIA subgroups, particularly DR alleles (oligo- and polyarticular arthritis) and B27 (enthesitis arthritis). In genetically susceptible individuals there is evidence that infections may act as a trigger, stimulating the synthesis of proinflammatory cytokines by T cell clones cross-reacting with synovial collagen protein. Consistent with this view is the histopathology of JIA in which there is hyperplasia of the synovium with infiltrating activated T cells.

The classification of JIA has been an evolutionary process, reflecting the acquisition of knowledge about the pathogenesis and natural history of the different subgroups. A simplified version of the classification adopted by the International League against Rheumatism (1997) is as follows: systemic arthritis, oligoarthritis, polyarticular arthritis, enthesitis arthritis and psoriatic arthritis.

Clinical features

Oligoarthritis

Accounting for more than 60% of cases, oligoarthritis is the most common form of JIA. The criterion for inclusion in this subgroup is involvement of four or fewer joints at presentation, with further refinement of the diagnosis depending on the subsequent course of the disease.

In *persistent oligoarthritis*, the number of joints involved, principally the wrists, knees and ankles, does not increase beyond four. It affects young girls predominantly with a peak age of 3 years. Antinuclear antibodies are a marker for chronic anterior uveitis, which is common, and children in this group in particular need regular screening by slit-lamp examination. Constitutional symptoms are usually absent, but growth anomalies are frequently seen, with leg overgrowth due to unilateral knee involvement being typical. The prognosis is good, with remission in 4–5 years being the norm. Functional outcome depends on good management.

As the name suggests, *extended oligoarthritis* refers to JIA in those children who present with four joints or fewer affected and in whom the disease then extends to involve more joints, usually within the first year. The disease tends to be chronic and may be characterized by stiffness rather than hot swollen joints. Functional disabilities develop after a few years.

Polyarticular arthritis

About 15% of JIA cases fall into this category, of which a minority (less than 20%) are rheumatoid factor (RF)-positive. Mainly girls are affected, with the age of onset in late childhood/early adolescence. The clinical pattern of the RF-negative arthritis is similar to that of extended oligoarthritis, with stiffness a prominent feature. The disease begins in the large joints, particularly the wrists, knees and ankles, before involving the small joints of the hands (Fig. 12.3). Temporomandibular joint inflammation may be a feature. In the small number with RF-positive JIA (normally teenage girls) the disease tends to be very aggressive, and many patients require replacement of major joints in their 20s and 30s.

Enthesitis, systemic and psoriatic arthritis

Although individually uncommon, together these forms of arthritis account for the 25% of cases of JIA which are neither oligo- nor polyarticular.

Enthesitis arthritis is a disorder affecting predominantly boys in late childhood and early adolescence. It is thought to represent the childhood equivalent of ankylosing spondylitis, but peripheral arthritis and enthesitis (inflammation of tendons and ligaments close to their bony insertions) tend to predominate rather than sacroiliitis. The HLA-B27 phenotype and acute anterior uveitis are associated features. The disease tends towards chronicity, with up to 60% of those affected developing spondylitis. The arthritis of inflammatory bowel disease and postenteric infection may also present in this way.

The presentation of *systemic JIA* (the disease which Frederick Still described) is dominated by constitutional symptoms and signs with high fever, maculopapular rash, hepatosplenomegaly, lymphadenopathy and serositis. The peak age of onset is 2 years. Polyarthritis becomes prominent as the systemic features regress, usually after a period of weeks or months. In roughly half of cases the disease remits within 3–5 years but the remainder have a persistent polyarthritis and are subject to relapses of systemic symptoms – often triggered by minor infections. In the latter group, amyloidosis may develop, and the long-term prognosis for joint function is poor.

The presentation of *psoriatic arthritis* is usually oligoarticular with progression to polyarticular disease. In the not uncommon situation in which arthritis precedes the skin rash, helpful diagnostic features include pitting of the nails, dactylitis and a family history of psoriasis. The arthritis can be highly erosive.

Investigation

Investigation of a child with suspected JIA will include a full blood count, measurement of antinuclear antibody (ANA) and IgM RF, HLA typing (e.g. B27 in older boys), CRP or ESR as a measure of the degree of inflammation, and radiography of affected joints to assess the degree of erosion and demineralization. Magnetic resonance imaging (MRI) allows early detection of cartilage destruction. Additional investigations will

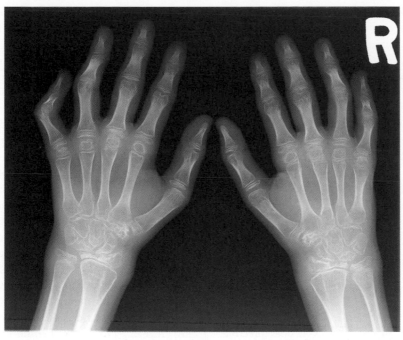

Figure 12.3　A radiograph of a young child with polyarticular JIA. Marked deformity of the carpal and metacarpal bones with generalized reduction in bone density can be seen. There is florid destructive arthritic change and a reduction in the joint spaces

be undertaken according to the likely differential diagnosis: anti-double-stranded DNA (SLE), C3 and C4 (SLE nephritis), creatine kinase (dermatomyositis), *Borrelia burgdorferi* antibody titre (Lyme disease) and bone scans (tumour, infection).

Treatment and outcome

Irrespective of the precise disease type, children with JIA require a multidisciplinary approach to management, involving not only doctors but also physiotherapists, occupational therapists and social workers. The parents and child need to be educated about the disease, and will require long-term support – over half of JIA patients continue to have the disease and pain after 15 years. Chronic illness as well as school absence holds back emotional and cognitive development, and as a result many experience feelings of depression and isolation. Employment prospects are poor for those with chronic disability, even where academic achievement is satisfactory.

NSAIDs

There is no cure for JIA. The aim of treatment is to control symptoms while maintaining function and

encouraging normal physical emotional and social growth. The use of non-steroidal anti-inflammatory drugs (NSAIDs), such as ibuprofen, naproxen and indomethacin (in ascending order of potency), together with physiotherapy is the mainstay of treatment of joint inflammation. NSAIDs have an immediate analgesic action but the full anti-inflammatory effects take 6–8 weeks to develop. Splinting, both to protect acutely inflamed joints at night and to maintain good functional position (e.g. working splints for the wrists) during the day, can have an important role.

Clinical response to drug therapy is assessed by improvement in mood, reduction in joint pain and inflammation together with improvement in function. CRP or ESR can be useful for monitoring disease activity, and serial radiography of affected joints will demonstrate the rate of progression of erosions and development of arthrodesis (Fig. 12.3).

Disease-modifying drugs

In those children with oligo- or polyarticular arthritis who fail to respond to NSAIDs after at least two 6 week trials of different drugs at maximal dosage, oral methotrexate may be very effective. Short courses of steroid may be helpful to overcome acute flare-ups but, other than for NSAID-unresponsive systemic JIA, long-term use should be avoided because of the dangers of growth suppression and bone demineralization. Monoarthritis, particularly involving large joints such as the knee or shoulder, may respond well to intra-articular steroid injection and prolonged remissions may be achieved.

Enthesitis arthritis is a specific indication for the use of sulphasalazine, while the disease-modifying drugs used in adult rheumatoid arthritis, penicillamine and gold, are reserved for RF-positive polyarticular JIA.

Reactive arthritis

The term 'reactive arthritis' refers to a heterogeneous group of short-lived post infective arthropathies: post-streptococcal, postviral (and presumed postviral where no infectious agent is identified) and postenteric. Although considered as separately defined entities, Henoch–Schönlein purpura and transient synovitis are reactive in as much as they frequently follow viral illnesses.

Rheumatic fever, which is now a rare condition in the developed world, is a post-streptococcal disorder characterized by a migratory transient arthritis associated with a variety of clinical features on which the diagnosis is based (see Beyond core: the diagnosis of rheumatic fever). The most important of these, in terms of morbidity, is carditis. Even in endemic areas, rheumatic fever is rare under the age of 5 years.

Postenteric arthritis is typically associated with *Salmonella*, *Shigella* and *Yersinia* infections but has also been reported in association with *Campylobacter* and *Giardia*. The majority of patients are HLA-B27-positive and enthesitis is common. A

HIGHLIGHTS AND HYPOTHESES

LYME DISEASE

Chance often plays a part in the process of discovery, but the dictum 'chance favours the prepared mind' is as relevant in clinical medicine as in other fields. The remarkable story of the discovery of Lyme disease demonstrates that, in addition to preparedness, intellectual curiosity and determination are essential attributes when it comes to turning clinical observations into clinical advances.

The story began in October 1974 in Old Lyme, Connecticut, when 8 year old Anne Mensch developed a sterile arthritis of both knees and was diagnosed as suffering from juvenile rheumatoid arthritis (as JIA used to be called before it was realized that chronic arthritis in childhood was, for the most part, unrelated to adult rheumatoid arthritis). At the time, her mother personally knew of five other cases of juvenile rheumatoid arthritis in

her small New England town, four of whom lived in the same street. She thought it very odd that, if this was such a common condition, she had not known a single case in New York where she had grown up. However, her general practitioner, paediatrician and orthopaedic surgeon saw nothing unusual in this clustering of cases when Mrs Mensch pointed it out to them. As she wrote later, 'everyone listened to me but no one heard me' (there is surely an important lesson here for all clinicians). However, Mrs Mensch was not easily deflected from her purpose, and was eventually referred to a Dr Allen Steere at Yale Medical School who was at the time a postdoctoral fellow working on white cell function in rheumatic disease. 'To my astonishment, Dr Steere was very receptive. He listened and heard me. He asked that I contact the people I knew and asked them to call him. He arranged a meeting

at the Old Lyme Town Hall to gather their histories.'

By careful questioning, the Yale group discovered that one patient remembered being bitten by a tick at the site of a skin lesion. The clustering of cases suggested an infectious cause and the observation that treatment with penicillin or tetracycline prevented the development of arthritis pointed towards a non-viral cause. The tick was identified as *Ixodes dammini* and the causative spirochaete, later named *Borrelia burgdorferi*, was isolated from the tick. Thus, in the span of 12 years, the cause of Lyme disease and Lyme arthritis had been discovered and a cure found. All as the result of the unique partnership between the patient's mother, who made the initial observation, and the clinical scientist who had the expertise and the intellectual curiosity to follow it up.

family history of spondyloarthropathy may be elicited.

Specific viruses associated with *postviral arthropathy* include: rubella, adenovirus, parvovirus, Epstein–Barr and cytomegalovirus. Although the initial presentation may be similar to that of JCA, the arthritis is typically short lived, lasting no more than a few weeks.

Henoch–Schönlein purpura

Henoch–Schönlein purpura is a common vasculitis of early (preschool) childhood and may follow a viral or streptococcal infection.

Clinical features

The most consistent features are non-thrombocytopenic palpable purpura, abdominal pain and arthritis. The purpura occurs in crops, and is distributed predominantly over the lower limbs and buttocks (see Fig. 11.8), although the whole body may be involved. Joint involvement is present in some two-thirds of cases, is highly variable and may take the form of an arthritis or arthralgia affecting predominantly large joints. It is often migratory. Abdominal pain is the result of bleeding into the gut wall and may be associated with intussusception. Renal involvement, with microscopic haematuria, may occur in up to 50% of cases but proteinuria and other features on nephritis are uncommon (<5%). Painful swelling of the testis may occur, mimicking torsion of the testicle.

Investigation and treatment

There are no specific laboratory findings. However, a full blood count should be carried out in order to exclude a blood dyscrasia and the urine tested for haematuria and proteinuria. Treatment is symptomatic (e.g. NSAIDs for joint pain), although there is some evidence that corticosteroids may reduce the duration of abdominal pain. Children with proteinuria and other features of nephritis (but not haematuria alone) require long-term renal follow-up.

BEYOND CORE

THE DIAGNOSIS OF RHEUMATIC FEVER

Major manifestations	Minor manifestations	Supporting evidence of streptococcal infection
Polyarthritis	Clinical	Increased titre of antistreptococcal (ASO) antibodies
Carditis	Previous rheumatic fever	
Chorea	or rheumatic heart disease	Positive throat culture for group A streptococcus
Erythema marginatum	Arthralgia	
Subcutaneous nodules	Fever	Recent scarlet fever
	Laboratory	
	Acute phase reactants:	
	ESR/CRP	
	Leucocytosis	
	Prolonged P–R interval	

Note: the diagnosis of rheumatic fever requires two major, or one major and two minor manifestations, plus evidence of streptococcal infection. Neither arthralgia nor a prolonged P–R interval can be used as minor criteria if polyarthritis or carditis are major criteria. Only one non-specific manifestation of inflammation can be used as a minor criterion (e.g. fever/ESR/CRP/leucocytosis)

Idiopathic musculoskeletal pain

This group of conditions is characterized by limb or joint pain in the absence of objective clinical signs of pathology. There may be evidence of psychosomatic disorder. Together, the idiopathic pain syndromes are probably more common than all the various categories of inflammatory joint disease.

Growing pains

Recurrent pains involving the knee, shin and calf may affect 10–20% of school-age children. The aetiology is unknown. Symptoms are predominantly nocturnal and frequently follow strenuous physical activity. The pain is often relieved by vigorous massage, and nocturnal analgesia with paracetamol or NSAIDs may be beneficial. The condition is benign and self-limiting.

Fibromyalgia

This condition has been said to account for up to one-third of adolescents referred for rheumato-logical evaluation. It occurs predominantly in otherwise healthy teenage girls, often high achievers, and is characterized by non-specific muscular aches and pains in the absence of signs of synovitis (although swelling may be reported by the family).

Symptoms overlap with the chronic fatigue syndrome and indeed, chronic fatigue and non-restorative sleep are often features of the disorder; other symptoms include headache and anxiety. Treatment involves reassurance, acceptance by the medical team that the symptoms are real, and graded physiotherapy. Low-dose antidepressant medication is used in some centres.

Hysterical conversion disorder

Limb dysfunction, with or without pain, may be a mode of presentation of children with psychological disorder. The patient may appear to be quite unconcerned by the degree of disability and signs may fluctuate. Lack of acceptance by the parents of a non-organic diagnosis may prolong the disability. Treatment consists of psychological

intervention, with physiotherapy to provide a focus for improvement.

LIMP

A useful way to approach the diagnostic problem of a child with a limp is to consider the causes according to the following groupings: musculoskeletal, with pain (see Table 12.1), musculoskeletal, without pain (leg length inequality, congenital dislocation of the hip, in and out-toeing), neuromuscular causes (e.g. cerebral palsy, myopathy).

Pain commonly accompanies limp in childhood. If it is of recent onset and the symptoms are worsening, the likely causes are trauma, infection, transient synovitis or slipped capital femoral epiphysis (Fig. 12.6). A limp that is at its worst first thing in the morning may be due to inflammatory joint disease. The origin of the pain may be the soft tissues, bone or joint.

✱ KEY DIAGNOSIS

Transient synovitis

Transient synovitis, or irritable hip, is the most common cause of inflammatory arthritis in childhood, accounting for up to 50% of cases of acute arthritis in some series; it is also the most common cause of limp associated with hip pain (Table 12.4). Boys are affected more commonly than girls. The onset is sudden and may follow an upper respiratory tract infection.

Clinical features

There is marked limitation of movement, particularly internal rotation, and the initial presentation may be difficult to differentiate from septic arthritis. However, lack of systemic features, such as toxicity and high fever, mitigate against a diagnosis of sepsis even though acute phase reactants and the white cell count may be minimally raised. The younger age of onset, typically 3–4 years, and usually short duration help differentiate transient synovitis from Perthes' disease (4–8 years of age) and slipped capital

Table 12.4 Common causes of hip pain
Transient synovitis of the hip/irritable hip
Perthes' disease
Slipped femoral capital epiphysis
Septic arthritis/osteomyelitis
JIA
Referred pain
to inner thigh, knee
from lumbar spine, sacro-iliac joint

femoral epiphysis which characteristically affects obese boys during adolescence. Most forms of JIA can be discounted since they rarely start in the hip.

Investigation and treatment

Ultrasound or radiography will usually demonstrate an effusion. Joint aspiration for culture should be undertaken if there is any doubt about the diagnosis, and may sometimes reduce the pain.

Treatment consists of bed rest and NSAIDs. There is no evidence that traction, which is traditional in orthopaedic wards, has any effect on outcome; indeed, heavy traction in extension may increase the tamponade effect of the effusion on the blood supply and predispose to avascular necrosis.

Congenital dislocation of the hip (CDH)

CDH occurs with a frequency of approximately 1 in 1000 live births, and presents with a limp in those children in whom the diagnosis is not made until the start of walking.

More appropriately termed developmental dysplasia of the hip, there is no actual dislocation at birth but rather a lack of normal development of the acetabulum and head of the femur. The condition is fully reversible only if corrected within the first few weeks of life, hence the importance of early diagnosis.

Clinical features

Diagnosis in the newborn period (see Ch. 4) is dependent on demonstrating instability of the hip joint by means of Ortolani's (see Fig. 4.1) and Barlow's tests. After the first month or two of life,

contractures begin to develop around the dislocated hip joint, tending to stabilize the joint but at the same time limiting abduction (normally 90°). Although not diagnostic, unilateral limitation of abduction is an important indicator for further investigation. Once the infant begins to walk there is a painless limp and lurch to the affected side, giving a swaying gait. When the child stands on the affected leg, the pelvis dips towards the opposite side due to weakness of the gluteal muscles (Trendelenburg's sign). The skin creases are frequently asymmetrical (see Fig. 16.11). Bilateral dislocation gives rise to a waddling gait.

Investigation and treatment

Radiography of the hip is unreliable in the newborn period but thereafter may show lateral displacement of the femoral head (Fig. 12.4), which also becomes displaced upward's once the child starts to walk. Ultrasound has the advantage of being able to demonstrate dynamic instability during manipulation of the hip and may be particularly useful in the newborn period.

Where dislocation is picked up early (preferably within the first 6 weeks), treatment consists of splinting the hips in 90° flexion and 50–60° adduction for 8–12 weeks, with follow-up for at least a year. Avascular necrosis is a complication of forced reduction of the dislocated hip or splints that are too tight.

Treatment of the child in whom the diagnosis has been missed is much more difficult and may involve surgical reduction and correction.

Perthes' disease

Osteochondrosis due to vascular insufficiency may affect a number of ossification centres, of which the capital femoral epiphysis (Perthes' disease) is the most important.

Clinical features

Typically this condition presents in boys of between 4–8 years in age with insidious pain in the hip and limb. Occasionally it may have an acute onset mimicking synovitis (see above). Pain

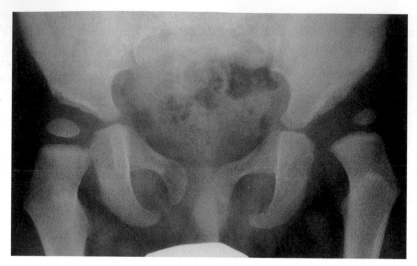

Figure 12.4 An anterior posterior view of the hips showing delayed ossification of the left femoral capital epiphysis associated with congenital dislocation of the hip and acetabular dysplasia

and discomfort may sometimes be referred to the thigh and knee. There may be few signs initially, but in established cases there is loss of internal rotation which may be associated with muscle wasting and limb shortening.

Investigation and treatment

Whereas plain radiography may initially be normal or show only a widening of the joint space, technetium bone scanning will provide evidence of complete or partial avascularity of the head of the femur with 'cold' areas of diminished uptake. Thereafter, radiography changes correlate with the progression of the disease. Decreased bone density in and around the joint is apparent after a few weeks and is followed by collapse and fragmentation of the femoral head (Fig. 12.5). Eventually the entire epiphysis is replaced by new bone producing a flattened sclerotic head. The shape of the femoral head will depend on the extent of necrosis, the anatomical and functional prognosis being best in those at the younger end of the age range with partial necrosis. Premature closure of the growth plate may occur with shortening of the leg.

The aims of treatment are to protect the head and keep it in the acetabulum. There is little evidence that interventional treatment is of value but, in the more severe cases, the hip can be braced in abduction and internal rotation or a femoral osteotomy performed.

Slipped capital femoral epiphysis

This condition is the result of separation of the proximal femoral epiphysis through the growth plate, and occurs typically in obese males during early adolescence. It is bilateral in approximately 20–25% of cases. Symptoms are usually insidious in onset but may be acute following a minor twisting injury. Limp is associated with hip pain, but in some cases pain may be referred to the thigh or medial side of the knee. The diagnosis is confirmed by radiography (Fig. 12.6), which must always include a lateral view of the hip. Treatment is by pinning the head, but there is a significant risk of avascular necrosis (20–30%) and a high incidence of early onset degenerative arthritis. Prophylactic pinning of the contralateral side should be considered.

LIMB PAIN OF ACUTE ONSET

The principal diagnoses relating to acute onset of pain in a leg or arm associated with fever are osteomyelitis and septic arthritis. However, sickle cell anaemia and malignancy can also present in

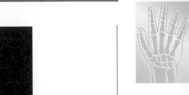

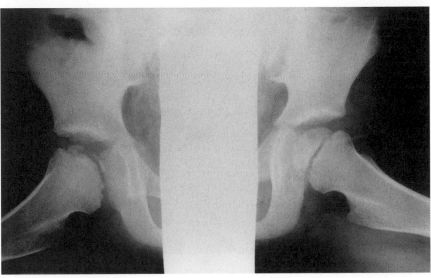

Figure 12.5   A frog-leg lateral view of the hips showing near complete collapse of the right femoral epiphysis in keeping with avascular necrosis (Perthes' disease)

this fashion. JIA and other connective tissue disorders may present initially with a monoarthropathy (not usually the hip), but post-infectious arthritis and other forms of reactive arthritis usually involve multiple joints from the outset. Trauma and most of the other conditions listed in Table 12.1 are not usually associated with fever.

Osteomyelitis

Bony infection may occur as a result of direct invasion via a penetrating wound or open fracture, but haematogenous spread from a distant site (usually not identifiable) is much more common. Beyond the neonatal period (see Ch. 4), *Staphylococcus aureus* accounts for at least 80% of infections, with the remainder caused by a heterogeneous selection of bacteria including *Streptococcus pyogenes*. *Salmonella* osteomyelitis is a particular risk in children with sickle cell anaemia. Since the introduction of routine HIB vaccination, *Haemophilus influenzae* has become uncommon.

Although almost any bone can be infected, it is the long bones that are usually involved with abscess formation, beginning in the metaphysis where, beyond infancy, the nutrient arteries end (see Fig. 12.1). Under a year of age, osteomyelitis may be multifocal and, since the nutrient arteries traverse the growth plate, direct infection of the epiphysis and adjacent joint may take place. Beyond infancy the growth plate is an effective barrier, preventing direct spread of infection into the joint. Nevertheless the joint may become infected if the metaphysis is intracapsular (e.g. hip and shoulder). At any age, the infection may spread from the primary focus in the metaphysis to the medullary cavity, or to the subperiosteal region, where abscess formation may take place.

Clinical features

Presentation varies according to age. In infancy, the clinical features may be subtle and non-specific, with irritability, failure to feed and normal or low temperature. Nevertheless, handling of the affected limb is resented and pseudoparalysis may be present. In the older child, the presentation is acute, with pain, severe local tenderness over the metaphysis and high fever. If untreated, swelling and erythema develop over the affected area.

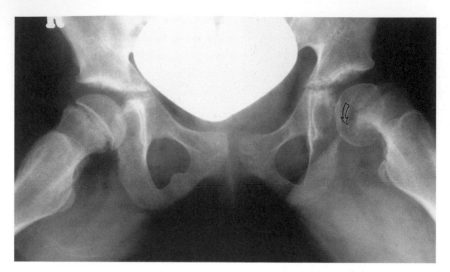

Figure 12.6 A frog-leg lateral view of the hips showing displacement of the left femoral capital epiphysis

Investigation and treatment

Culture of blood, together with subperiosteal and, where appropriate, joint aspiration allow positive microbial identification in 50–60% of cases and should be undertaken before treatment is started. Levels of acute phase reactants (CRP, ESR) and the white cell count will be raised, although the neutrophil response in infants may be weak. Technetium bone scanning provides early and accurate localization of infection while radiological changes generally require 10–11 days to develop (but less in infants). The earliest bony radiographic change is an area of rarefaction at the site of infection, followed by elevation of the periosteum (Fig. 12.7). Later, bone destruction and sequestrum formation become evident.

A satisfactory outcome depends on early and effective antibiotic treatment. Intravenous flucloxacillin and fusidic acid in high dosage provide effective antistaphylococcal cover. Initially they can be combined with an aminoglycoside such as gentamicin to provide cover for Gram-negative organisms, a particularly important consideration in the newborn period. Parenteral therapy should continue for at least 48 h beyond the point at which the child becomes afebrile, after which oral therapy for 4–6 weeks is necessary to ensure eradication of infection. Surgical intervention in the acute phase is usually only indicated to drain a collection of pus.

Septic arthritis

Joint infection is usually the result of haematogenous spread, except in infancy where direct spread from the adjacent metaphysis can occur. The majority of cases occur in the preschool age group. *Staph. aureus* is the most common causative organism at all ages, with the addition of group B streptococcus and Gram-negative organisms under 4 months of age, and *Strep. pyogenes* in older children.

Clinical features

In infancy there is typically pseudoparalysis with rigid guarding of the affected limb. At all ages the joint is swollen, tender and hot to touch. There is intense pain on even the slightest movement whereas usually, some movement can be elicited in osteomyelitis if undertaken gently. The hip is typically held flexed and abducted.

Investigation and treatment

The approach to investigation and treatment is as for osteomyelitis. Early in the course of the disease, radiography or ultrasound may show

also have a therapeutic effect. Open surgical drainage may sometimes be required where there is poor response to antibiotic therapy.

Prognosis can be good if treatment is instituted promptly. However, sequelae are common, particularly in the weight-bearing joints of young infants. In these cases, with premature closure of epiphyses, ischaemic necrosis of bone and disruption of the joint due to dislocation or subluxation may occur. Long-term follow-up is essential.

CURVATURE OF THE SPINE

✳ KEY DIAGNOSIS

Idiopathic scoliosis

Scoliosis is defined as lateral curvature of the spine. It may be structural or postural.

Clinical features

Although associated with a number of conditions (e.g. cerebral palsy, neurofibromatosis, Marfan's syndrome), over 80% of cases of *structural scoliosis*

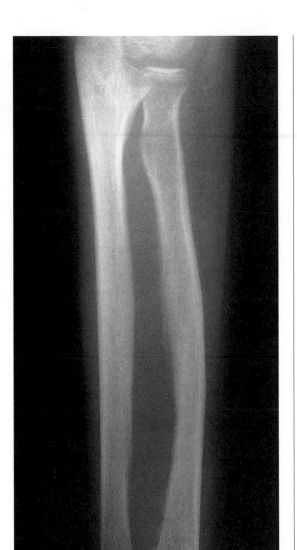

Figure 12.7 A radiograph of the left forearm showing periosteal new bone formation on the distal left radius associated with loss of bone density in the distal radial metaphysis in keeping with osteomyelitis

widening of the joint space while later radiography may show evidence of coexisting osteomyelitis. Joint aspiration for microbiological diagnosis must be undertaken in all cases; it may

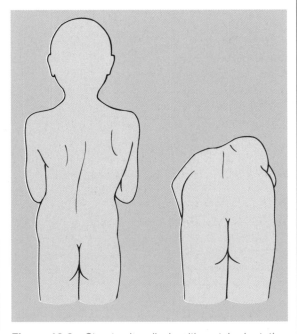

Figure 12.8 Structural scoliosis with vertebral rotation demonstrated by a rib hump on bending forwards

243

are idiopathic. There is a strong genetic component, with a positive family history in 30% of cases and a 3–4-fold preponderance of females. Examination of the siblings as well as the index case should always be undertaken. On examination, asymmetry of the waistline may be noted, and a rib hump may become obvious when the patient is asked to bend forwards (Fig. 12.8).

Investigation and treatment

The disorder is usually asymptomatic and is commonly picked up during adolescence. Curvature involves the midthoracic spine, and has a marked tendency to progress.

Progression is monitored by means of serial radiography. Bracing is required for curves of 20–40°, and beyond 40° spinal fusion may be indicated to stabilize the spine. Curves greater than 60° are associated with significant impairment of pulmonary function.

Postural scoliosis is most common in the lumbar spine as compensation for leg shortening. It disappears on sitting and is readily correctable with a shoe lift.

FURTHER READING

Milles M L 1995 Pediatric rheumatology. The Pediatric Clinics of North America 42: 5

Woo P, Wedderburn L R 1998 Juvenile chronic arthritis; seminar. Lancet 351: 969–73

CHAPTER 13

The special senses

D. F. Haddad

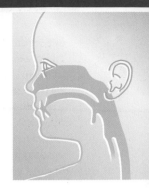

CORE PROBLEMS OF THE SPECIAL SENSES

CORE PROBLEM	KEY DIAGNOSIS	RELATED TOPICS
• Squint	Amblyopia	Cataract
• Red eye	Conjunctivitis	Periorbital cellulitis Ophthalmia neonatorum Stye
• Runny nose	Allergic rhinitis	
• Painful ear	Acute otitis media	Chronic serous otitis media
• Recurrent sore throat	Chronic tonsillitis	Adenoidal hypertrophy Tonsillar hypertrophy Obstructive sleep apnoea
• Skin inflammation	Eczema	Seborrhoeic dermatitis Irritant/contact dermatitis
• Skin infection	Impetigo	Herpes simplex[14] Scalded skin syndrome Scabies Headlice

Where the primary location of a topic is in another chapter, this is indicated by a superscript

ESSENTIAL BACKGROUND

The topics discussed in this chapter relate to some of the most common clinical conditions in the paediatric age group. These conditions are a major cause of distress for the children and their families, and contribute significantly to the demands imposed on the health services.

Involvement of the organs of special senses in systemic disease is discussed in the relevant chapters. Acute infections of the ear, nose and throat are discussed in the chapter on respiratory disorders (Ch. 6), and skin rashes in the chapter on infections and immune disorders (Ch. 14).

CORE PROBLEMS (EYES)

AMBLYOPIA

Aetiology and pathogenesis

The formation of a clear retinal image is necessary to provide adequate stimulation for the development of visual function. Conditions that interfere with the production of a clear retinal image in early childhood result in understimulation of the central visual pathways and poor development of vision in the affected eye or eyes. This state of affairs is referred to as amblyopia. Visual potential is completely achieved by 9 years of age, and defects occurring prior to this age are capable of producing a degree of amblyopia. However, it is in the first few months of life when the risk of amblyopia is greatest.

Examples of conditions which impair the retinal image are severe refraction errors and congenital cataracts affecting one or both eyes. If these conditions are not corrected early, there is failure of development of normal vision, and the visual acuity will continue to be reduced in the affected eye, even if the underlying problem is corrected at a later stage. This is why it is crucially important that eye defects are identified and corrected as early as possible in children (see Ch. 3).

Another common situation in which amblyopia may develop is squint. In this condition there is usually an adaptive suppression of the image produced by the deviating eye in order to avoid diplopia. This suppression or 'disuse' deprives the visual pathways in that eye of the necessary stimulation to develop normal vision.

Diagnosis

Amblyopia is usually asymptomatic and picked up only by screening. Although screening is easier in older children, amblyopia is more responsive to treatment if diagnosed early.

The diagnosis of amblyopia is reached when there is reduced visual acuity in the absence, or after correction of any organic pathology or refraction error. Other possible aetiologies which meet these criteria include neurological and psychological conditions (occipital cortical lesions and conversion reactions, respectively).

Treatment

The treatment of amblyopia involves providing a clear retinal image by correction of squint, any errors of refraction or removal of cataract, etc., and also by occlusion therapy in which the good eye is covered to force the use of the other eye. This is usually required throughout the waking hours and for a variable length of time. However, it is important that the situation is closely monitored so that the deprivation of stimulation in the occluded eye does not result in amblyopia in that eye. Reassurance and support of the family are important.

✳ KEY DIAGNOSIS

Squint (strabismus)

Aetiology and pathogenesis

The mechanisms underlying the development of binocular vision are not completely understood. Alignment of both eyes is achieved through the function of the 'visual reflexes', which are established in the first few years of life. Thus,

movement of one eye to fixate an object is accompanied by a deviation of the second eye which is proportionate in amount and direction. In the ideal situation there is complete alignment of both eyes allowing the fixation on a particular object (by both eyes) with production of one fused clear image.

Squint denotes misalignment of the two eyes, and can arise from:

1. A sensory pathology that interferes with the production of a clear image. Thus, cataracts, corneal scarring or patching the eye after trauma or surgery, in a child, may lead to habitual disuse of the eye and failure of development of normal vision.
2. Refraction errors, particularly hypermetropia (via the link between accommodation and convergence).
3. Impedance to the eyeball movements: extraocular muscle paralysis/weakness or structural pathology of the orbit.
4. Imbalance of the action of the extraocular muscles.
5. Failure to develop the reflexes necessary for normal binocular vision because of delay in the treatment of any of the conditions listed earlier.

Amblyopia frequently coexists with squints. It may develop as a result of the sensory deprivation imposed by a significant refraction error or other sensory pathology that leads to failure in establishing binocular vision. As mentioned earlier, amblyopia can also develop in a squinting eye with normal sensory function, as in the case of a squint arising from motor pathology. In this situation there is an active suppression of the image produced by that eye to avoid diplopia.

Clinical features

Distinction should be made between latent and manifest squint. In manifest squint, the misalignment is evident almost all the time. In latent squint, the normal alignment is maintained most of the time but misalignment appears when the child is tired.

Diplopia may be present in cases of squint of recent onset (before active suppression and amblyopia develop). Some infants and children may tilt their heads to a particular position in an attempt to align both eyes and avoid diplopia; the presenting feature in such cases may be torticollis.

In paralytic squint, the gaze in the direction of the paralysed muscle will be defective and the misalignment appears or becomes more evident when the eyes look in that direction. The appearance of a paralytic squint indicates the involvement of the motor pathways (the extraocular muscles, cranial nerves III, IV and VI or their central motor pathways).

In hypermetropia, the image produced in the retina is blurred and, in an attempt to achieve a clear image, more accommodation is used. Accommodation and convergence (in-turning) are closely linked, and for each degree of accommodation there is an accompanying degree of convergence. When the child attempts to look at a near object and uses more accommodation in that eye, it deviates inwards.

Congenital esotropia (in-turning) can also occur, and is defined as in-turning of one or both eyes documented in the first 6 months of life. Hypermetropia may be present.

Diagnosis

Mild degrees of squinting and misalignment of both eyes are normally expected to be present in babies in the first few weeks of life. However, if the degree is severe or if it is persistent, further evaluation is necessary.

Squint should be differentiated from pseudosquint, which is a common condition in which the eyes appear to be squinting although the alignment is normal. The impression of misalignment arises because of the presence of a flat broad nasal bridge or epicanthic folds (Fig. 13.1). Normal alignment of the eyes can be confirmed by the pupillary light reflexes and the cover/uncover tests.

In the pupillary light reflex test, the placement in the cornea of each eye of the light reflex from a distant source is compared. If the eyes are aligned, the light reflex appears to occupy the same position in relation to the pupillary circle. Asymmetry denotes manifest squint. In the cover test (Fig. 13.2), the child's attention and cooperation are required. As the child looks at an object, the examiner covers one eye. Movement of the uncovered eye indicates the presence of a manifest squint in that eye. Movement of the covered eye on removal of the cover indicates the presence of a latent squint in that eye.

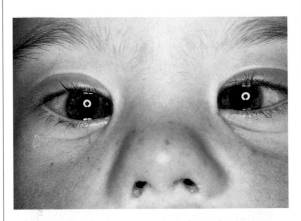

Figure 13.1 A child with marked epicanthic folds giving rise to a pseudo squint. (Reproduced by courtesy of the Wellcome Trust Photographic Library)

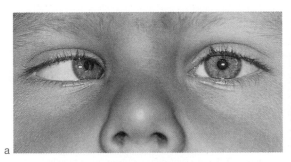
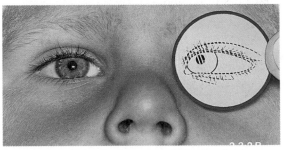

a   b

Figure 13.2 The cover test. **a**: manifest non-paralytic squint in the right eye, the child is using the left eye to fixate objects. **b**: covering the left eye, the right eye is now used to fixate objects. The covered left eye deviates indicating latent squint. (Reproduced by courtesy of the Wellcome Trust Photographic Library)

Management

Suspicion of squint in a child calls for prompt evaluation. In cases of paralytic squint of recent onset, neurological and radiological assessment to exclude intracranial pathology (e.g. tumours, bleeding) is indicated. Equally, some cases of squint of the non-paralytic variety may arise secondary to a serious intracranial pathology (e.g. optic neuritis or papilloedema affecting vision in the squinting eye). Regardless of the implications of the possible aetiology, squint in a child should be promptly evaluated and treated because of the potentially damaging effect on the development of binocular vision.

Treatment of squint involves correction of any sensory or refraction defect, eye patching to deal with any existing amblyopia and, if still necessary, surgical intervention. Pilocarpine or other parasympathomimetic drops are used to treat accommodative squint. The use of botulinum toxin injections to paralyse therapeutically certain extraocular muscles and 'balance out' the eye movements is still at the early stages of evaluation.

Cataract

Cataract denotes opacity of the lens (Fig. 13.3). The significance of cataract relates to its effect on visual function, as well as to the fact that it can be a manifestation of systemic or ocular disease.

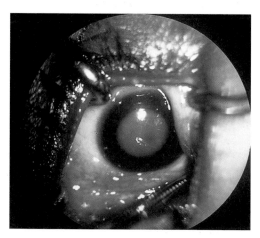

Figure 13.3 Opacification in the lens due to congenital cataracts. (Reproduced by courtesy of the Wellcome Trust Photographic Library)

Congenital cataracts are usually picked up on ophthalmoscopic examination. This should be a routine part of all newborn examination. The presence of cataract is suspected by the absence of bilateral red reflex (see Routine examination of the newborn, Ch. 4). Missing a diagnosis of cataract at this age may lead to amblyopia (see the previous section). Cataract can be acquired as a result of various injuries of the eye such as those due to trauma and infective and inflammatory disorders. The development of cataract is one of the potential ophthalmic complications of long-term steroid therapy – 'steroid ophthalmopathy'.

RED EYE

Infections of the eyelids and conjunctivae

Conjunctivitis is a common condition in childhood (Fig. 13.4). It can arise from infectious (viral and bacterial) or non-infectious causes, including

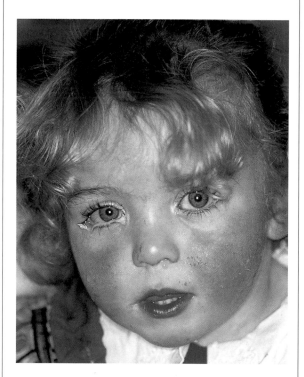

Figure 13.4 A child with severe conjunctivitis. (Reproduced by courtesy of the Wellcome Trust Photographic Library)

allergy or chemical irritation, or can be a manifestation of eye involvement in systemic disease (e.g. connective tissue and vascular disorders; see Kawasaki's disease, Ch. 14).

A *stye* is the infection of the eyelash follicle. This is usually accompanied by tenderness and focal red swelling of the involved eyelid. *Staphylococcus aureus* is the usual causative organism. The treatment involves local antibacterial preparations and frequent warm compresses. Surgical drainage may be required in some cases.

✳ KEY DIAGNOSIS

Conjunctivitis

Bacterial conjunctivitis presents with generalized redness and swelling of the conjunctivae with mucopurulent discharge. *Gram-positive cocci* and *Haemophillus influenzae* are the usual responsible pathogens. The treatment involves bathing the eye frequently to remove the discharge. Frequent instillation of antibacterial eye drops may be required in severe cases.

Both eyelid and conjunctival bacterial infections, if untreated, may progress to more serious infections of the eye and the surrounding tissue, such as orbital and periorbital cellulitis (Fig. 13.5), which require systemic antibiotic treatment and may be associated with intracranial infections. Immunodeficiency states may be associated with recurrent eyelid and conjunctival infections.

Ophthalmia neonatorum is an acute purulent conjunctivitis in the newborn. Historically, gonococcal infection was an important cause, and this form of infection is severe, may result in scarring and blindness, and warrants intensive treatment with systemic antibiotics and local measures. At one stage, prophylactic silver nitrate eye drops were given routinely at birth to all babies, but this resulted in irritant-type conjunctivitis in many. With the diminished likelihood of gonococcal conjunctivitis in neonates in the UK nowadays, routine silver nitrate eye drop prophylaxis is no longer practised.

Chlamydia trachomatis, *Staph. aureus* and *Pseudomonas aeruginosa* are some of the common

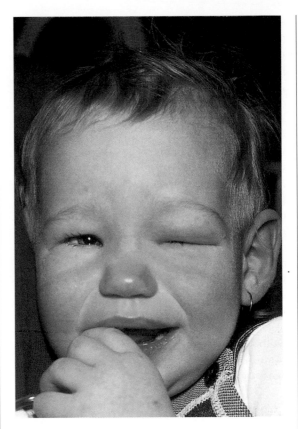

Figure 13.5 Orbital cellulitis in the right eye

pathogens isolated from the eye discharge in neonatal bacterial conjunctivitis. Treatment should include systemic and local administration of the appropriate antibacterial therapy.

Retinoblastoma (see Ch. 11)

CORE PROBLEMS (THE EAR, NOSE AND THROAT)

RUNNY NOSE

✳ KEY DIAGNOSIS

Allergic rhinitis

As with other allergic conditions, there has been a recent dramatic increase in the incidence of nasal allergy in children and adults. Frequently, different forms of allergy coexist in the same individual and run in families (atopy). Some reports estimate that 80% of children with asthma also have some form of nasal allergy.

Aetiology

The offending antigens in nasal allergy are usually inhaled, although a small number of children with a similar presentation may be allergic to ingested allergens. Sometimes ingested antigens may result in symptoms only if combined with exposure to particular inhaled antigens. If the antigens responsible for allergic rhinitis occur only in certain seasons, such as the season of tree or grass pollen, the term 'hay fever' is used. Since the symptoms are seasonal, seasonal allergic rhinitis is another term used. However, other types of allergens, particularly so-called indoor allergens such as house dust mites, animal dander or mould spores, provide continuous exposure resulting in symptoms all year round, so-called perennial allergic rhinitis.

Clinical features

The clinical features include sneezing, which is frequently paroxysmal, rhinorrhoea with a watery, profuse nasal discharge and itching in the nose. Itching, redness and watering of the eyes are also frequently present. Nasal obstruction may be the prominent symptom, sometimes with little discharge. Recurrent ear infections and chronic serous otitis media are possible complications. Recurrent headaches may also be present.

The presence of eosinophils in the nasal discharge points to the diagnosis of allergic rhinitis. In the older child, if the history suggests a particular antigen may be involved, a skin test or Radioallergosorbent test (RAST) may confirm the presence of allergy to that antigen.

Treatment

Avoidance, drugs and immunotherapy are all facets of treatment. Although avoidance is not always achievable, measures aimed at controlling certain exposures are possible. Particular attention should be paid to the child's bedroom, and

measures to minimize house dust mite exposure should be made. If allergy to pets is suggested by the history, particularly if supported by skin and blood testing, avoidance of such exposure should be advised.

Drug therapy includes antihistamines, particularly of the second generation to avoid drowsiness, but care should be taken as some of these have the potential to cause cardiac arrhythmia. Decongestants should not be used topically since, due to the chronic nature of this illness, there is a potential for chronic use and damage to the nasal mucosa. Corticosteroids by nasal spray or drops are very effective, and can be used for those in whom antihistamines failed to control symptoms.

Immunotherapy (a course of injections with minute amounts of the offending antigen to create a state of tolerance) may be considered in selected cases with incapacitating symptoms, but only under the supervision of a specialist and in centres with the necessary expertise. The efficacy of this mode of treatment cannot be guaranteed, particularly if full compliance with the rather lengthy course of repeated injections is not achievable. There is also a risk of generalized anaphylaxis.

PAINFUL EAR

✱ KEY DIAGNOSIS

Acute otitis media

Otitis media (inflammation of the middle ear) is one of the most common diseases in children. Some studies suggest up to two-thirds of all children will have suffered at least one episode of acute otitis media by the time they reach 3 years of age. Many of these children will go on to have at least one recurrent episode of acute otitis media. A degree of middle ear involvement almost universally occurs in the course of colds/rhinitis and other upper respiratory tract infections (see Ch. 6).

The high frequency of this illness in childhood is mainly related to the prevalence of functional and mechanical eustachian tube obstruction, and the consequent loss of protection against contamination of the middle ear by microorganisms present in the nasopharynx. The following features contribute to the malfunction of the eustachian tube in children:

- It is shorter, relatively wider and more horizontal than in adults
- The cartilage in its walls is softer in children than in adults
- Children have relatively large adenoids which are located close to the opening of the eustachian tubes.

Infection of the nasopharynx, allergy, large adenoids or other tumours (polyps, etc.) may all contribute to intrinsic or extrinsic obstruction of the eustachian tube. The presence of congenital abnormalities such as cleft palate or other craniofacial syndromes may be associated with the malfunction of the eustachian tubes and the development of ear infections.

Eustachian tube obstruction leads to negative pressure in the middle ear, and this in turn leads to accumulation of a serous effusion in the middle ear cavity. Contamination of this effusion by organisms refluxed from the nasopharyngeal secretions leads to infection. The commonest bacterial pathogens involved are *Streptococcus pneumoniae* and *H. influenzae*.

Clinical features

Severe ear pain is the most distressing symptom of acute otitis media in children. Typically, the child has a history of a runny nose and other coryzal symptoms over the preceding 2 or 3 days, before sudden onset of ear pain ensues. Frequently, this is accompanied by fever, vomiting and hearing loss. In small infants, this condition often presents with persistent distressing crying which tends to be of rather a continuous pattern as opposed to the intermittent character seen in abdominal colic at this age. Pulling at the ear in a crying infant is another clue to the presence of earache.

Otoscopic examination reveals redness, opacity and bulging of the tympanic membrane with poor mobility.

In spite of treatment, many cases of otitis media progress to perforation of the ear drum. When this occurs, the pain is eased and there is a purulent discharge from the ear canal. Children seen at this stage may be mistaken for having otitis externa, whereas frequently the latter develops as a complication, secondary to irritation of the external ear canal skin by the discharge coming from the middle ear.

Treatment

Treatment includes analgesics/antipyretics. Antibiotics, usually amoxycillin, are often prescribed, but there is little evidence that they have a significant effect on outcome. The benefit of the use of antihistamines and/or decongestants is also debatable. In the majority of cases, a perforation of the ear drum will heal provided the obstruction of the eustachian tube does not persist. Usually the middle ear effusion following acute otitis media is transient. The absence of redness and the lack of fever and acute pain (although discomfort and 'heaviness' may be present) help make the distinction from the acute stage.

Chronic serous otitis media

Aetiology and pathogenesis

Middle ear effusion persisting beyond 3 months following an acute episode of otitis media is termed chronic serous otitis media or chronic secretory otitis media: 'glue ear'. A chronic serous middle ear effusion can sometimes present without a definitive history of acute otitis media.

The precise reason why some children go on to develop this condition continues to be controversial, but blockage of the eustachian tube, thus preventing drainage of middle ear secretions, appears to be a consistent factor. It is likely that there is an interplay of multiple factors, with this relative significance varying from one child to another. Adenoidal hypertrophy is thought by some to be contributory, and thus adenoidectomy is undertaken as a form of treatment. Nasal allergy has been implicated but proof is lacking. There is some evidence that the home environment, passive smoking in particular, is significant. The presence of structural abnormalities, such as cleft palate and other syndromes associated with craniofacial bony abnormalities, may be causative in some children. The possibility of chronic infection has been extensively investigated, but no evidence of this has been found.

Clinical features

The condition is common, with a peak incidence between 4 and 6 years of age. It is commoner in boys and in those with various congenital abnormalities.

The principal manifestation of the condition is bilateral mild to moderate hearing loss of the conductive type. Delayed speech, behavioural abnormalities and even suspicion of mental handicap and social maladjustment may be presenting features that subsequently lead to the diagnosis. There may be sometimes a feeling of fullness, tinnitus and vertigo.

Otoscopic examination reveals a dull tympanic membrane with, on occasion, a fluid level or air bubbles visible behind the membrane. The mobility of the tympanic membrane on tympanometry is impaired. The membrane may be bulging, or retracted because of associated negative middle ear pressure. Age-appropriate screening such as use of the distraction test in infants (Fig. 13.6) may detect hearing loss, but pure tone audiometry is the investigation of choice to quantify the degree of hearing loss (typically in the range of <40 dB in glue ear; see Fig. 3.5).

Management

The treatment of 'glue ears' continues to be controversial. Attempts at medical treatment may be undertaken although convincing proof of the efficacy of this modality of treatment is lacking. Systemic decongestants and antihistamines are frequently used although never shown to be effective in children. Topical and systemic corticosteroids therapy is also of unproven benefit, and systemic use of corticosteroids is not advisable because of the side-effects. Nevertheless, measures to control nasal allergy are reasonable, particularly if the history suggests the presence of a specific allergy.

Further evaluation for the presence of adenoidal tissue obstructing the nasopharynx or an underlying immunological disorder should be

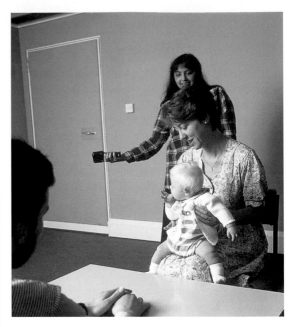

Figure 13.6 The distraction test. (Reproduced by courtesy of the Wellcome Trust Photographic Library)

carried out, particularly if infections elsewhere are present. The presence of structural abnormalities, such as cleft palate or tumours, should be explored and appropriate treatment given. In the absence of any of the above factors, an empirical approach is a trial of antibiotic therapy plus the control of environmental risk factors.

If medical measures fail, and particularly in the presence of significant hearing loss (especially if bilateral), myringostomy and insertion of tympanostomy tubes ('grommets') (Fig. 13.7) may be undertaken. The aim is to improve middle ear ventilation, drain the fluid and improve hearing. As for medical management, firm evidence of the efficacy of this form of surgical intervention is lacking.

Removal of the adenoids may benefit some children but not all. If the underlying cause for adenoidal hypertrophy is allergy, then improvement after adenoidectomy is usually transient and frequently there is regrowth of the lymphoid tissue. Adenoidectomy has been advocated even in the absence of enlargement of the adenoids in children in whom repeated grommet insertion has been ineffective.

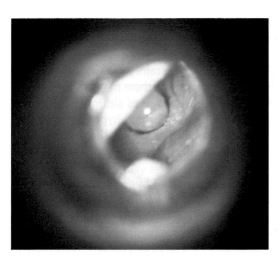

Figure 13.7 Examination of the tympanic membrane showing the presence of grommets. (Reproduced by courtesy of the Wellcome Trust Photographic Library)

RECURRENT SORE THROAT

The tonsils and adenoids are part of the lymphoid tissue that surrounds the pharynx (Waldeyer ring). This tissue provides defence against infection, and there is some evidence that the tonsils are important for the development of the immune system in young children. The tonsils are located in the fauces of the pharynx (pharyngeal tonsils) and are accessible to inspection on throat examination. The adenoids are located in the posterior part the nasopharynx and cannot usually be seen on simple inspection without the use of a pharyngeal mirror.

Both structures are prone to infection and hypertrophy. Acute infections of the tonsils (Fig. 13.8) and adenoids are usually part of the 'sore throat' and upper respiratory tract infection complex, and are discussed in Chapter 6. Chronic infection and/or hypertrophy may affect either the tonsils or adenoids sep   .ely, although frequently both structures are involved.

✱ KEY DIAGNOSIS

Chronic tonsillitis

The main feature of chronic tonsillitis is recurrent or persistent sore throat. There may be a feeling of chronic irritation and dryness. Chronic redness of the anterior pharyngeal pillars and cervical lymphadenopathy are important signs. Contrary to common belief, constitutional symptoms, including poor appetite and slow

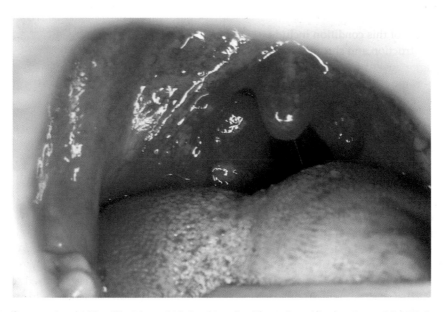

Figure 13.8 Severe pharyngitis with enlarged bilateral tonsils. (Reproduced by courtesy of the Wellcome Trust Photographic Library)

weeping, crusting, bullous formation and worsening of the eczema. Swabbing and culture are helpful in diagnosing skin infection due to other organisms (*Streptococcus*) and also to verify the antibiotic sensitivity of these organisms. Children with eczema also manifest a severe reaction to infection with herpes simplex (eczema herpeticum), and should not be exposed to adults with cold sores.

Treatment

Despite the high prevalence of atopic eczema in children, the treatment of this condition continues to be a major area of controversy. Many of the therapeutic practices, although time honoured, lack scientific evidence. The chronicity of this condition and lack of a specific treatment that can bring about cure encourage many families to seek alternative methods of treatment. Although some forms of alternative medical treatment seem to be promising and work in certain cases, in others they may cause harm.

The fact that steroids are a major part of eczema treatment frequently causes unnecessary and unjustifiable degree of concern among parents. This further fuels the eagerness to seek unorthodox means of treatment.

What follows is a discussion of the principles of treatment. Frequently the appropriate treatment regimen for a particular child is tailored to the individual needs of that child, sometimes based on clues from the history and physical examination, but in others simply by trial and error.

The following are the main lines of treatment of atopic eczema in children:

1. The use of moisturizers. There are no suitably conducted studies showing conclusively the benefits of moisturizer treatment. However, there is a large amount of anecdotal data, as well as a theoretical basis for such treatment. There are a variety of ointments and creams and combinations of these in use: e.g. paraffin (50:50 wax and liquid mix), Vaseline, Diprobase and E45. Various soap substitutes and bath oils are also recommended. Lotions are suitable for moist and weeping lesions, whereas ointments are more appropriate for dry scaly skin.

2. The use of steroids to treat inflammatory lesions. The rule here is to use the minimal potency of steroid creams and ointments, in the minimal dose for the shortest time possible in order to control symptoms. Care should be taken when using these prescriptions on the face where it is not generally recommended to use anything stronger than 0.5% hydrocortisone. The use of steroids over large areas of inflamed skin may result in significant absorption from the skin with possible systemic effects; care should be taken in monitoring these children. It should be understood, however, that withholding steroids when they are necessary may be harmful equally, and may result in unnecessary distress for the child. Steroids containing topical preparations come in different levels of potency; hydrocortisone 0.5–1% products are least potent while betamethasone 0.1% plus clobetasole 0.05% possess the highest potency. The aim should be to use the least potent preparation that is effective in each case. Only preparations of least potency (hydrocortisone 0.5–1%) should be used on the face.

3. Measures aimed at controlling itch should be implemented, since scratching is a major factor in perpetuating eczema. The use of the older family of antihistamines (sedating antihistamines) is recommended, and the sedating effect is probably their major advantage. Paracetamol may also have some anti-itching effect, and a cool environment also reduces itch. Mittens may be used in infants to prevent scratching.

4. The use of systemic antibiotics or antiviral agents. This may be necessary if evidence of secondary bacterial or herpes simplex infection is present. Positive skin swabs for *Staph. aureus* should not be relied upon as evidence of infection, since this organism is almost universally present on the skin of children with eczema.

5. Avoidance. This is a major part of the treatment. Children with eczema are likely to develop reactions to large number of topical agents, including soap, shampoo, creams and

ointments. Sometimes children may react to substances used in the various moisturizing (e.g. lanolin) and steroid creams used to treat eczema, and this possibility should be considered whenever there is no improvement or the inflammation worsens after treatment. Topical antibacterial treatment best be avoided. There is much controversy regarding the role of ingested allergens in perpetuating eczema. The general recommendation is that unless there is definite evidence in the history to suggest this, there is no point in implementing dietary restrictions. Skin testing and the RAST are usually not helpful in this condition.

6 Educating the family. This is a major part of management, and should include a description of the illness and the possible complications, the possible causes and prognosis. It is important to make it clear that no magic cure can be expected, but control of the symptoms is the major goal of treatment. Pre-emptively addressing concerns about the use of steroids, and explaining the fact that much of the publicity is related to ingested steroids, rather than the use of small amounts of topical steroids for short periods.

SKIN INFECTION

✳ KEY DIAGNOSIS

Impetigo

This is the commonest form of skin infection in children. The causative microorganisms are *Staph. aureus* and β-haemolytic *Streptococcus pyogenes*. The infection usually arises at the site of minor skin trauma such as abrasions and insect bites. The early lesion is a small vesicle which ruptures, forming the characteristic honey-coloured crust (Fig. 13.13). Multiple lesions may be grouped together, and the infection may spread on the hands or clothing to other sites of the body.

Characteristically the lesions are painless but pruritic. There is no erythema of the surrounding skin. Systemic upset is absent. There is usually regional lymphadenopathy, and a raised white cell count may be present.

Bullous impetigo is a variant seen principally in infants and young children, and is always caused by *Staph. aureus*. It is characterized by the formation of flaccid bullae which easily rupture, leaving shallow moist erosions.

The diagnosis is made on the basis of the clinical picture and positive culture results of swabs obtained from the lesions. The differential diagnosis includes skin lesions due to herpes simplex, burns or contact dermatitis. Vesicobullous skin disorders such as epidermolysis bullosa, pemphigus or erythema multiforme may have to be considered in the differential diagnosis of bullous impetigo.

Complications include spread of infection to cause more serious conditions such as cellulitis, osteomyelitis or septicaemia, and these should be considered in children with impetigo who manifest constitutional symptoms. Scarlet fever can develop if the strain of β-haemolytic *Strep. pyogenes* causing the impetigo produces the erythrogenic toxin. Non-infectious complications of streptococcal impetigo include post-streptococcal nephritis, but not rheumatic fever.

Treatment includes measures to reduce spread of this highly contagious illness. Local application of mupirocin is usually effective in early localized disease, but systemic antibiotics are usually required. Erythromycin or semisynthetic penicillins given for 7 days is the recommended treatment.

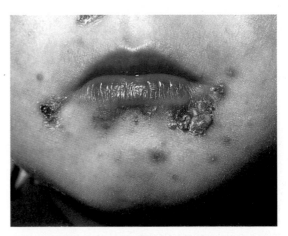

Figure 13.13 Impetigo. (Reproduced by courtesy of the Wellcome Trust Photographic Library)

Scalded skin syndrome

This is a systemic and generalized disease of infants and young children. Constitutional features such as fever and malaise are prominent, and there is excessive tenderness of the skin. There is a generalized erythema and flaccid bullae formation followed by wrinkling and peeling of the skin in large sheets, leaving denuded skin. The epidermis can characteristically be split by gentle force (Nikolski sign). Histologically, cleavage of the blister occurs in the subcorneal plane.

The manifestations of the disease are due to the epidermolytic toxins produced by certain strains of *Staph. aureus* (usually phage group 2, type 71). These toxins cause superficial splitting of the skin. Foci of colonization or infection may be in the nasopharynx, umbilicus or skin abrasions and local manifestations may be minimal or absent. The organisms are rarely recovered from the blood. However, the toxin produced in the absence of specific antitoxin antibodies, spreads haematogenously, leading to the generalized cutaneous manifestations.

Management includes culturing of potential infected or colonized sites and blood cultures. Skin biopsies show the characteristic plane of epidermal splitting. Oral or parenteral administration of anti-staphylococcal antibiotics with local skin care are indicated.

Scabies

This condition is caused by the mite *Sarcoptes scabei*, and infection occurs almost exclusively by direct physical contact with the infected person. This is a common skin infestation worldwide. The manifestations of the illness are due to mechanical burrowing of the mite in the skin and the release of toxic or antigenic substances.

The typical lesions are the burrows, but these are not always seen in young children. Various combinations of red-brown blisters, vesicles, papules and nodules are usually present. Urticarial-type lesions may also be present. Whatever mixture of primary lesions an individual child displays, there are always marks of severe scratching, and frequently some of the initial lesions become eczematized or impetiginized.

The distribution of the lesions is diagnostically helpful; in older children, as in adults, areas of predilection are the interdigital spaces (Fig. 13.14), axilla, buttocks and belt line. In younger children, the face and scalp are also involved as well as the palms and soles.

Intense pruritus, particularly at night, the characteristic lesions and distribution as well as a high index of suspicion of this common skin infestation usually allow a provisional diagnosis to be made. Confirmation of the diagnosis is obtained by microscopic identification of the mite or ova in the material obtained from scrapings of the burrows and from fresh lesions.

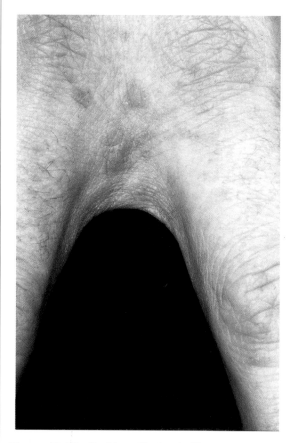

Figure 13.14 Scabies with classical burrows between the fingers. (Reproduced by courtesy of the Wellcome Trust Photographic Library)

The child and all close contacts should be treated simultaneously. Permethrin cream 5% is the treatment of choice, and should be applied from the neck down to all the body surfaces and left overnight. The application is repeated in 1 week. Clothes and bedding should be washed in the normal way, and no disinfectants are necessary.

Headlice

This is a very common infection, particularly among school children. It is caused by a certain species of louse (*Pediculus humanis* var. *capitis*), which spreads via head to head contact or the shared use of combs and towels. This louse does not act as a vector for typhus. The parasite feeds on human blood, but the manifestations of the infection are due to the allergic response to the parasite's salivary juices and faecal material.

Intense pruritus is the hallmark of the condition. The lice are usually invisible, but the nits (sacks in which the ova are contained) are seen on the hair shafts, particularly in the occipital areas and above the ears (Fig. 13.15). Unlike dandruff or other types of scalp scales, nits are difficult to split off the hairs.

Treatment is by the application of permethrin shampoo. Permethrin is not as effective in killing the ova, and repeat application after several days is advisable. Nits can be removed using a fine-toothed comb after wrapping the hair in a towel soaked in vinegar. Vinegar dissolves the chitin which binds the nit to the hair shaft. Other family members should be treated simultaneously.

FURTHER READING

Behrman R E, Kliegman R M, Arvin A M 1996 Nelson textbook of pediatrics, 15th edn. Saunders, London
David T J 1993 Recent advances in paediatrics – 12. Churchill Livingstone, Edinburgh

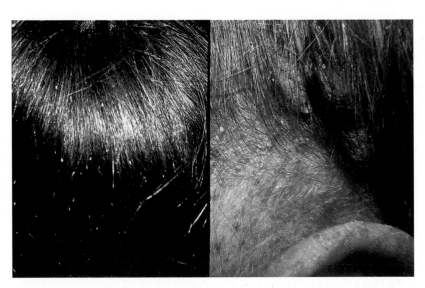

Figure 13.15 Infestation with head lice showing the presence of nits. (Reproduced by courtesy of TALC)

CHAPTER 14

Infection, immunodeficiency and allergy

D. F. Haddad

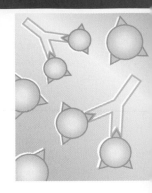

CORE PROBLEMS IN INFECTION, IMMUNODEFICIENCY AND ALLERGY

CORE PROBLEM	KEY DIAGNOSIS	RELATED TOPICS
• Fever with no apparent cause	Meningitis	
• Rash	Exanthemata	Meningococcaemia Henoch–Schönlein purpura[12] Allergic rashes Kawasaki's disease
• Septicaemia and septic shock	Meningococcaemia	
• Congenital HIV infection	AIDS	Congenital infections Immunodeficiency states
• Allergic reaction	Food allergy	Drug reaction Allergic rhinitis[6] Asthma[6]

Where the primary location of a topic is in another chapter, this is indicated by a superscript

ESSENTIAL BACKGROUND

INTRODUCTION

Infections are the most common diagnoses made in children attending clinics and hospitals for emergency consultations. Worldwide, they are the commonest cause of death in childhood.

An infectious illness represents one of several possible outcomes of the interaction between the human body and pathogenic microorganisms. Such interaction involves the body defence mechanisms, and it is largely the balance of forces between the pathogenic microorganism and body defences that determines whether disease will result or not.

The immune system is central to body defences against infections. A knowledge of the functioning of the immune system is essential for the understanding of the pathogenesis of infectious disorders. Immunodeficiency states and allergic disorders are pathological conditions in which disturbances in the function of the immune system are the main pathophysiological feature.

In this chapter, a general outline of the pathogenesis of infections in children, their clinical presentation and principles of treatment is given. Infections of organs/systems are dealt with in their respective chapters. A brief description of immunodeficiency states and allergic disorders is also provided here.

ANATOMY AND PHYSIOLOGY

The environment in utero is normally sterile, but from the moment the membranes are ruptured, the baby begins a lifelong exposure to thousands of different types of microorganisms, which constitute an integral part of the world we live in. Such exposure may or may not result in disease.

Some of the encounters with microorganisms result in a useful coexistence; a well-known example of this is the synthesis of vitamins by bacteria colonizing the gastrointestinal tract. Other encounters may be contained by the body defence mechanisms, and the microorganisms rapidly eliminated in one way or another before they have a chance to cause any harm.

Occasionally, however, a potentially harmful microorganism succeeds in establishing a presence within the host. The body defence systems continually strive to contain the growth of the microorganism and, depending on the balance between the effectiveness of the body defences, the microorganism virulence and its acquired numbers, the outcome of this interaction can be:

1. A carrier state
2. Mild illness (which may or may not confer long-lasting immunity)
3. Severe illness.

Diseases arising from the direct effects of the infectious agents or their products and the immediate body reactions to these effects are called infectious diseases. The terms 'infection/infectious disease' are used interchangeably in this chapter. Note that in some texts the word 'infection' refers to acquisition of the microorganism per se, i.e. regardless whether such acquisition results in disease or the carrier state.

The immune system

Maternal antibodies of the IgG class can cross the placenta and reach the fetal circulation. At term, the concentration of IgG in the fetal blood is higher than that of the mother. This supply of ready made maternal IgG antibody is of great value as it provides passive immunity for the newborn baby. However, the half-life of IgG is only several weeks, and by the age of 4–6 months most of these antibodies will have disappeared.

In the process of evolution, the human body has adopted several strategies to combat infection. These strategies can generally be divided into two main groups, non-specific and specific.

The first (*non-specific*) line of defence includes physical barriers (intact epithelia, skin), physical factors (motile cilia), unfavourable chemical microenvironment (gastric acidity), mucus and mucosal antimicrobial agents, as well as the competition among the different microbial colonies. These are 'non-specific' defence systems, i.e. they provide protection against various types of injuries and infections.

The second (*specific*) line of defence consists of a system of cells and protein molecules which act in an orchestrated manner to contain invasions by microorganisms that have breached the barriers of the first line of defence and succeeded in gaining access to the body's internal environment (bloodstream, deep layers of tissues). These cells, proteins and mediators constitute the specific defence systems which make up the immune system.

One of the main properties of the immune system is that its ability to provide protection against infection by a particular microorganism is greatly enhanced by repeated exposures to that microorganism, i.e. an 'immune experience' is required for the full effectiveness of the immune system to be expressed.

Although the functional capacity of their immune systems is probably comparable to that of adults, infants and young children are at a disadvantage in terms of protection against infections because of lack of immune experience and underdeveloped physical barriers (low gastric acidity, inadequate coughing, etc.).

In neonates, the umbilical stump represents a natural breach of the skin, and this site frequently acts as a port of entry for infection. The situation with premature babies is further compromised by low levels of maternal antibody, thin skin and immaturity of the immune system.

A brief outline of the components of the immune system is provided next. For an overview of the function and interaction of the different components of the immune system, refer to Beyond core: a review of the immune system.

The immune system consists of three components: phagocytes, the complement system and lymphocytes.

The *phagocytic cells* (neutrophils, monocytes and macrophages) constitute an essential part of the inflammatory response, and are abundant both in the circulation and tissues. When needed, more cells can be mobilized into action from various stores and compartments. Phagocytic cells are then diverted to the areas of action by chemotaxis. Phagocytic cells internalize and digest invading microorganisms, and they possess powerful mechanisms for microbial killing. Phagocytic cells do not display functional specificity. They can be deployed rapidly, and are an effective mechanism for containing and limiting damage caused by a wide range of injuries including those produced by infections.

The *complement system* consists of several components which are activated in a cascade fashion and produce a complex that is capable of attacking the invading microorganism. In addition, other products of this activation include chemotactic factors and substances that aid phagocytosis and contribute to the inflammatory response.

There are more than 30 glycoprotein molecules which constitute the various components of the complement system (C1 to C9) together with the related regulators, accessory factors and receptors. These molecules are largely present in plasma but also on the surfaces of certain cells. In addition to its role in the immune response and inflammation, the complement system interacts with other plasma cascade systems, namely the coagulation, kinin and fibrinolytic systems (details of which are found in standard textbooks of physiology).

A REVIEW OF THE IMMUNE SYSTEM – 1

When they encounter the antigenic structure that they are programmed to react to, both B and T cells undergo a process of transformation, at the end of which two types of cells are produced: effector cells and memory cells.

The effector cells, in the case of B lymphocytes, are plasma cells that manufacture antibodies directed to the specific antigenic structure. In the case of T cells, effector cells may be helper, cytotoxic or suppresser cells or a combination of these.

The antibodies may themselves neutralize toxins or effect killing of the microorganisms, and may bind with their antigens to initiate the classical complement pathway, thus enlisting this important defence mechanism. Moreover, with or without complement, a microorganism that has succeeded in evading the phagocytic cells can be readily made available for phagocytosis by antibody coating. The half-life of most antibodies does not exceed several months. However, the repeated exposure to the common antigens, including those borne by the common environmental microbes, serves as a continuous trigger for manufacturing specific antibodies. Therefore, a significant titre of ready made antibodies against common microorganisms is usually achieved by children as they progress in age and maturity.

The cytotoxic T lymphocytes are capable of directly reacting with the specific antigen that triggered their production and, in the case of a living organism bearing that antigen (i.e. a bacterium), are capable of killing it. Helper and suppresser cells participate in the regulation of the overall immune response to the specific antigen, including that of B cells. They also influence the function of the phagocytes and the inflammatory response.

On subsequent encounters with the same antigen that has previously triggered an immune response, the pool of cells capable of reacting with it will now include the memory cells produced during the previous (primary) immune response. The participation of memory T and B cells will effect a swift and augmented response which, in the case of microorganisms, exceeds their ability to multiply, and thus the balance is decisively tilted in favour of the body defences. Memory cells are among the longest living human body cells (some have been documented to survive for more than 30 years). These properties of memory cells are the basis of immune experience and active immunity.

A REVIEW OF THE IMMUNE SYSTEM – 2

Although each of the components of the immune system is capable of inflicting damage on microorganisms on its own, their effectiveness is greatly enhanced when their activities are coordinated.

The phagocytic cells, inflammatory reaction, and alternative and MBL complement pathways can be viewed as rapid-response defence forces, which can be deployed at any time against unfamiliar invaders. They do not require the sophisticated system of recognition of the exact identity of the antigen. Together with ready made antibodies, they are available for immediate action.

The response mounted by lymphocytes, on the other hand, is characterized by specificity. It is directed against a well-defined specific trigger, and requires familiarity with the target to be fully effective. Lymphocytes and the products of their activation perform the following functions:

- Effect microbial killing and neutralization of viruses and toxins
- Boost the activity of the complement system by activation of the classical pathway
- Aid phagocytic activity by rendering certain microorganisms more susceptible to phagocytosis
- Contribute to the inflammatory reaction by the production of cytokines and other mediators
- Control the overall response by either up-regulating or down-regulating the activity of the other participants.

The complement system can be activated via two routes: the classical pathway, which is initiated by the antibody–antigen complex (as well as by a special protein called mannan-binding lectin (MBL)), and the alternative pathway, which is usually triggered directly by microbial products (the lipopolysaccharide of Gram-negative bacteria or the techoic acid of Gram-positive bacteria).

Three types of *lymphocyte* are recognized: B cells, T cells and NK (natural killer) cells. As their name suggests, the last possess natural non-specific ability to kill other cells. B and T cells are equipped with a sophisticated system for antigen recognition.

Temperature control

Alteration in body temperature is a cardinal feature of disease due to infection; a brief discussion of the mechanisms, implications and diagnostic significance of fever and hypothermia is provided in this section.

Young children are at a disadvantage in terms of heat preservation, with a large body surface area relative to body mass and thin skin with little subcutaneous fat favouring heat loss. Hypothermia frequently complicates the course of serious illnesses in children, including those due to infections. This is particularly true of neonates and sick children during transportation. Monitoring of body temperature should be part of the routine observation of sick children, and measures directed at preservation of body heat (optimal room temperature and humidity, wrapping, radiant heat source, etc.) implemented as required.

Hypothermia

If severe and prolonged, hypothermia may trigger a series of pathological reactions that lead to severe metabolic and haemodynamic disturbances including hypoglycaemia, acidosis, disseminated intravascular coagulation and shock. The ability of the body immune systems to fight infection is also impaired at lower body temperatures.

Hypothermia, rather than fever, is likely to be present in young children and neonates with severe illness due to infection. Sometimes such children may have minor or no alteration in body temperature. Failure to document fever in a sick child should never be relied upon as a criterion to rule out the possibility of infection as an underlying cause of illness. Indeed, absence of fever at presentation is one of the reasons for missing the diagnosis of meningitis in young children.

Fever

Fever is one of the more consistent features of disease due to infection in older infants and children, and frequently it is the main reason for seeking medical advice. Although infections are by far the most common underlying cause of fever in children, non-infectious causes may also result in fever. Dehydration, inflammatory disorders (e.g. inflammatory bowel disease, connective tissue and vasculitic disorders), malignancy and endocrine disorders (e.g. hyperthyroidism) may all result in elevation of body temperature; these conditions should be considered in febrile children if, after careful evaluation and investigation, no other indication of an infective process is found.

Fever is present when the core body temperature rises above 38°C. This corresponds to an axillary temperature of 37°C. The magnitude of the rise in temperature does not necessarily correlate with the severity of the underlying infection or with the type of the infection – viral or bacterial.

Fever brings about several adaptive physiological changes: the heart rate rises by probably 10–20 beats/min for each 1°C elevation in temperature, the pulse is bounding, and the overall picture is that of a hyperdynamic circulation. The respiratory rate also increases, on average by five breaths for each 1°C, and there may be muscular retractions and grunting. Mottling of the skin may be present, particularly if tepid sponging has been attempted to lower the temperature. These clinical signs may erroneously suggest an underlying cardiac or respiratory disorder. Frequently, reassessment at a later stage when the temperature has been brought down is necessary in order to confirm or exclude the presence of such disorders. The response to fever in young children includes the possibility of febrile seizures (see Ch. 10).

Fever is usually accompanied by unpleasant subjective feelings including headache, tiredness and lack of energy. There is a debate as to whether there are physiological benefits of fever, particularly since some of the immune functions seem to be more active at higher body temperatures. There is, however, no convincing evidence that the outcome is any better in subjects whose fever is not treated. Until such evidence is produced, it is advocated that steps are taken to treat fever. Of course, in children with a history of febrile fits, the case for treating fever is clear cut.

Treatment

Antipyretic drugs used in children are paracetamol and ibuprufen. Both seem to be of comparable efficacy and both have an excellent record of safety. Paracetamol is given at dose of 60 mg/kg/day, divided in 4–6 doses. This drug has no significant side-effects if the recommended dose is not exceeded. Allergic reactions are extremely rare. Overdose may lead to fatal liver damage (see Ch. 15). The use of ibuprufen as an antipyretic has only recently been adopted on a wide scale in children. Although this drug too has had a good record of safety so far, there are some concerns about its anti-inflammatory properties with the potential to mask the clinical features of, and to interfere with, the host's immune response to certain infections (e.g. invasive streptococcal disease). Encouraging fluid intake and ensuring cool surroundings are other measures for controlling high temperature (see also Beyond core: heat control).

THE MICROBIOLOGY OF CHILDHOOD INFECTIONS

Bacterial infections

In the neonatal period, Gram-negative coliform bacteria and group B streptococci are the most common organisms responsible for systemic infections. This largely reflects the fact that there is a relatively high percentage of carriage of these organisms in the female genital tract.

BEYOND CORE

HEAT CONTROL

Normal body temperature is regulated by the hypothalamus, which maintains an equilibrium between heat production and heat loss. Such equilibrium is normally set in a narrow range (36–38°C core body temperature). Alteration in body temperature can occur if the balance between heat production and heat loss cannot be achieved or maintained, such as in prolonged exposure to heat or cold, abnormal basal metabolic rate (hypo- or hyperthyroidism) or impairment of sweat production (atropine poisoning or congenital absence of sweat glands). However, far more commonly the cause of the fever is a disturbance in the temperature control centre in the hypothalamus. Under the influence of exogenous and/or endogenous pyrogens (such as those produced during infection), and through a sequence of reactions in which prostaglandins and other substances are involved, the hypothalamic centre is reset at a higher temperature. Heat production and loss mechanisms are then modulated to achieve a new state of equilibrium.

Based on this concept it is possible to understand the subjective and objective phenomena that frequently accompany fever. In the initial stage, immediately after the hypothalamic 'thermostat' is reset at the higher temperature, receptors in the skin and elsewhere in the body sense skin and body temperature to be lower than the newly desired level, leading to a feeling of cold or chills that frequently accompany the fever. In order to raise the body temperature, heat conservation mechanisms are employed, including skin vascular constriction, leading to pallor frequently seen in febrile subjects. Heat production mechanisms are also mobilized, and additional heat generated through repetitive muscular contraction (rigors).

Both the rigors and feeling of chills usually disappear when the body temperature is raised to the newly set level. When the fever is resolved, either by the illness following its natural course or by antipyretics such as paracetamol, the thermostat is reset at the lower (normal) temperature, and the reverse happens, with flushing and sweating helping to get rid of the excess heat. The febrile patient feels hot during this phase.

In immunocompetent children, beyond the neonatal period, the relative significance of the various organisms as causes of infection varies with age. However, three organisms account for most cases of septicaemia and meningitis:

1. *Neisseria meningitidis* (meningococcus) is the commonest cause of bacterial meningitis and primary septicaemia in children beyond the neonatal period.
2. *Streptococcus pneumoniae* (pneumococcus) is the commonest cause of bacterial otitis media and lobar pneumonia in all ages beyond the neonatal period. It is the second most common cause of meningitis. This organism is also responsible for most cases of primary occult bacteraemia and primary peritonitis.
3. *Haemophilus influenzae* type b (Hib, the capsulated type) is responsible for most cases of epiglottitis. This organism used to account for most cases of meningitis, septicaemia and septic arthritis in children between 6 months and 5 years of age, and was the second most common cause of otitis media and pneumonia in this age group. However, since the introduction of the Hib vaccine (1992 in the UK), the incidence of serious infections caused by this pathogen, including that of epiglottitis, has fallen dramatically. Above 7–8 years of age, infections with *H. influenzae* type b were rare in the prevaccination era. By this age, children attain a protective level of immunity against this organism, which is both ubiquitous and has little antigenic variation (unlike the pneumococcus).

However, as the pattern of carriage and circulation of this organism is altered by Hib vaccination (which does not confer lifelong immunity), the pattern of susceptibility to disease caused by this organism may also change.

All of these three organisms share the feature of a polysaccharide capsule. This may explain their relative success in causing invasive infections in children; the polysaccharide capsule is hydrophilic and the phagocytes are not able to achieve the level of proximity to the antigens on the capsule that is required for phagocytosis. The organisms must first be primed by antibody (opsonization) for successful phagocytosis. Children, with their limited 'immune experience', possess low levels of these antibodies.

Two other pathogens are implicated in a considerable number of childhood illnesses caused by infection: *Staphylococcus aureus* and *Escherichia coli*.

Staph. aureus is responsible for the majority of cases of osteomyelitis and septic arthritis in children (see Ch. 12). As is the case with adults, this organism accounts for most cases of skin and soft tissue infections. *Staph. aureus* is capable of producing a number of toxins which are responsible for some serious syndromes, such as the toxic shock syndrome and food poisoning.

E. coli is the commonest infectious agent involved in urinary tract infections in children. It also accounts for a significant number of cases of food poisoning and colitis. This organism, as well as other enteric bacteria, is responsible for the majority of cases of sepsis associated with abdominal surgical conditions. Both *Staph. aureus* and *E. coli* may be implicated in septicaemia and/or meningitis. This usually occurs as an extension of the primary condition and 'spilling over' of the infection in the bloodstream, but only rarely as a primary infection.

Streptococcus pyogenes is the principal bacterial organism responsible for bacterial tonsillitis/ nasopharyngitis. It also accounts for some cases of skin infections and pneumonia. This organism produces a number of toxins, one of which is responsible for the cutaneous manifestation of scarlet fever. Other toxins produced by this organism are implicated in some cases of vasculitic disorders and the toxic shock syndrome. Recently, a cluster of cases of soft tissue infection – 'necrotizing fasciitis' – caused by a particularly virulent strain of *Strep. pyogenes* has renewed interest in this common pathogen, ('the flesh eating bug'). Non-infective complications of streptococcal infections include rheumatic fever and glomerulonephritis. There is currently a resurgence of rheumatic fever in USA.

Chlamydia and *Mycoplasma* species are implicated in a significant number of infections in children, including chest infections, the so-called atypical pneumonias.

It should be stressed that this specificity or predilection for a certain microorganism to cause a particular disease or result in infection in a specific site is only relative, and there frequently is a great deal of overlap. For example, whooping cough is usually caused by *Bordetella pertussis*, but a very similar illness can be caused by other bacteria (*Bordetella parapertussis*) or viruses (adenoviruses).

Viral infections

Most 'infectious episodes' in children, as in adults, are due to viruses, which cause the vast majority of cases of upper respiratory tract infection (URTI) and gastroenteritis in the temperate regions of the world. In this section, a brief outline of the common childhood viral infections is provided.

The term *congenital infection* refers to the acquisition of infective agents by the fetus, in utero, through transplacental spread of maternal infection. Varying degrees of injury and deformity may result, and some of these infections may persist postnatally. Prominent among these are the viral infections: rubella, cytomegalovirus, infection, human immuodeficiency virus (HIV) infection, parvovirus infection and chickenpox. Non-viral congenital infections include toxoplasmosis and syphilis.

In the *neonatal period*, infections with herpes simplex virus can have devastating consequences. Herpes simplex encephalitis is a particularly severe form of encephalitis, and is associated with poor prognosis. It is usually caused by HSV type 2 acquired from carrier mothers, but cases due to HSV type 1 acquired from adults and older children do occur. If the first exposure to HSV occurs later in infancy, it may lead to extensive oral mucosal ulceration with systemic upset (herpetic stomatitis). Further encounters/ reactivation in an immune subject result in localized mucocutaneous ulceration, the cold sore.

In the *first few months of life*, infants benefit from the passive immunity conferred by the IgG of maternal origin and thus the incidence of colds, flu, etc., is less than that in older infants and children. Nevertheless, some viruses start to pose a threat from early on. An important example is the enterovirus group, which is responsible for a wide range of disorders from mild gastrointestinal upsets, skin rashes, mild URTI to severe cases of encephalitis and carditis.

Infections caused by viruses which are naturally widespread, have little antigenic variation, and which confer long-lasting immunity tend chiefly to cause disease early in life. Prior to the introduction of effective vaccines against them, poliomyelitis, measles, German measles and mumps (Fig. 14.1) used to belong to this group of 'childhood-specific' diseases.

Two viruses continue to be predominantly associated with significant disease in *young children*. These are the respiratory syncytial virus (RSV) and rotavirus. In young children they are the commonest causes of chest infections (bronchiolitis and bronchopneumonia) and gastroenteritis, respectively. In children older than 4 years and in adults, RSV and rotavirus are generally associated with little or no symptomatic disease.

The specific disease entities caused by infection, viral and bacterial, are discussed in the chapters on the relevant systems.

INFECTIONS AND IMMUNODEFICIENCY STATES: AN OVERVIEW

Infectious disorders

Although the pathogenesis of infectious disorders can follow different patterns, in essence there are two routes for the development of disease from the stage of acquisition of the microorganism: local spread and haematogenous dissemination. In either case, the production of toxins by the microorganism and/or the host's reaction to the infection may give rise to pathological features that dominate the clinical picture. Figure 14.2 is a schematic representation of this concept applied to bacterial infections. In viral infections, the pathogenesis of disease may be further complicated by cycles or loops of initial invasions of certain target tissues before the major wave of haematogenous spread occurs.

Immunodeficiency states

Immunodeficiency states can be congenital or acquired, and they can involve any of the components of the immune system. The study of immunodeficiency has received increasing attention in recent years. The improved survival of children with malignancy, the acquired immune deficiency syndrome (AIDS) and recipients of organ transplants has increased the number of children with immunodeficiency states requiring skillful management and understanding of the nature of their disease (for a general framework for the categorization of immunodeficiencies in children, see Beyond core: classification of immunodeficiency states).

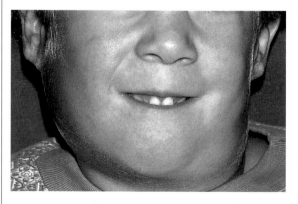

Figure 14.1 Facial swelling secondary to salivary gland enlargement classical of mumps. (Reproduced by courtesy of the Wellcome Trust Photographic Library)

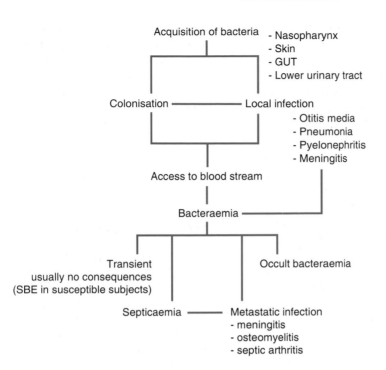

Figure 14.2 The pathogenesis of bacterial infections

Immunodeficiency should be suspected in children who present with frequent infections, especially if these are of invasive nature (pneumonia, meningitis). Children who suffer particularly severe forms of common childhood infections, or who display susceptibility to infections by microorganisms of low virulence, should also be evaluated for possible immunodeficiency.

Recurrent URTIs and gastroenteritis are a 'normal' feature in children, particularly when they start attending nursery or school. This probably reflects increased exposure coupled with lack of immune experience. An unacceptably frequent number of these infections is usually due to causes other than immunodeficiency; such causes include allergy, adenoidal hypertrophy, the presence of asymptomatic carriers within the household or poor hygiene. Nevertheless, IgA deficiency, the commonest form of immunodeficiency in children, is also associated with increased frequency of URTIs, gastroenteritis and urinary tract infections (IgA plays an important role in the protection of mucosal surfaces), and should also be included in the differential diagnosis. It is difficult to define what is the 'acceptable' frequency of URTIs in normal children. Generally, it is thought that for a normal toddler 6–8 such infections per year can be expected. An associated failure to thrive should always raise concern.

In addition to increased susceptibility to infections, immunodeficiency states are associated with a higher incidence of malignancy and autoimmune disorders. A listing of some of the important presenting features suggestive of the various categories of immunodeficiency states is given in Table 14.1.

Because the components of the immune system function in an interdependent manner, severe defects of any of them may lead to increased vulnerability to infection caused by a wide range of microorganisms. Chronic diarrhoea, severe eczema and failure to thrive are other features generally associated with immunodeficiency states. Lymphopenia,

CLASSIFICATION OF IMMUNODEFICIENCY STATES

Congenital immunodeficiencies

The phagocytic cells	The complement system	The lymphocytes
Neutropenia Chronic granulomatous disease[a] Leucocyte adhesion deficiency[b]	Deficiency of the early components Deficiency of the late components Properdin deficiency[c]	T cell: DiGeorge's syndrome B cell: agammaglobulinaemia, IgA deficiency Combined T and B cell deficiencies

Acquired immunodeficiency states

Infections	Drugs[d]	Others
Postviral HIV infection	Steroids Cytotoxic therapy Irradiation	Malnutrition Burns Stress

[a] In this X-linked disease the number of neutrophils is normal but their ability to kill some microorganisms is defective

[b] Leucocyte mobility and recruitment at the site of infection are impaired

[c] Properdin is one of the protein molecules which participate in the alternative pathway of complement activation

[d] Although antibiotics do not directly act on the immune system, they can alter the 'ecological' balance of the body by indiscriminate killing of non-pathogenic bacteria. The increased susceptibility to fungal infections among children treated with broad-spectrum antibiotics is a common and well-known example

Table 14.1	Immunodeficiency states
System	Clinical features
Phagocytic cells	Recurrent skin and bone infections Recurrent lymphadenitis (chronic granulomatous disease)
Complement system	Early components: systemic lupus erythematous and glomerulonephritis Late components: meningococcal disease Alternative pathway: meningococcal disease
T lymphocytes:	Severe illness caused by live virus vaccines or BCG. Reactivation of tuberculosis Unusually severe illness caused by common 'ordinary' viruses of childhood Severe and chronic forms of *Candida* infection *Pneumocystis carinii* pneumonia Some types of malignancy, e.g. Kaposi's sarcoma
B cells	Recurrent bacterial invasive disease (meningitis, pneumonia)

neutropenia and/or morphological abnormalities of the white blood cells are to be found in some of the immunodeficiency states. The diagnosis of immunodeficiency, however, frequently relies on the services of specialized laboratories.

Later in this chapter a discussion of the main characteristics of AIDS in children is provided.

Nevertheless, the study of the numerous immunodeficiency states and syndromes is beyond the scope of this book, and the reader is directed to the further reading list provided at the end of the chapter.

CORE PROBLEMS

The clinical features produced by infection can be so protean and diverse that infections may be included in the differential diagnosis of almost any clinical presentation. Infections generally produce local and systemic manifestations; both of these categories can be specific or non-specific for a particular infective agent. For example, pain on swallowing and redness of the pharyngeal wall are non-specific local features of pharyngotonsillitis. However, the presence of tonsillar follicular exudate, petichiae on the soft palate and painful anterior cervical lymphadenopathy are more specific features associated with streptococcal pharyngeal infection. Fever and malaise are systemic features which can be produced by pharyngeal infection caused by almost any microorganism, while the presence of an erythematous fine papular rash is a more specific feature strongly suggestive of scarlet fever – an infection caused by a particular strain of *Strep. pyogenes* (a strain that has acquired the ability to produce an erythrogenic toxin as a result of being infected by a phage virus).

Fever and rash, which are two of the more consistent systemic features of infectious disorders, and septicaemia and meningitis, which represent the more severe forms of disease caused by infection, are discussed further in this section. The clinical presentations produced by infection of specific anatomical structures are addressed in the chapters on the relevant organ systems.

FEVER WITH NO APPARENT CAUSE

In the vast majority of children with fever, the underlying cause is related to infection. Frequently this is a mild, self-limited and localized infection, which is most commonly caused by a virus. Usually, no specific treatment is indicated, and encouraging fluid intake and the use of analgesics/antipyretics are all that is required.

Less commonly, infection may be caused by bacteria. However, the clinical picture produced is often identical to that caused by viral illnesses, and making the distinction between these two, on clinical grounds, is frequently impossible. In bacterial infections, antibiotic treatment may shorten the duration of illness and reduce the chances of complications. Table 14.2 lists some of the general clinical characteristics of bacterial and viral infections in children.

Some children with fever due to infection may present with no obvious focus of infection, and careful examination fails to reveal the underlying illness. If the child is relatively well and there is no reason to consider him or her at risk of a serious infection, the likelihood is that the child is suffering from a non-specific viral illness. However, it must be emphasized that such a picture may be produced by the atypical presentation of some common and even serious childhood infections. The following list should be considered in every such child:

- Meningitis
- Otitis media
- Urinary tract infection
- Pneumonia
- Primary bacteraemia
- Viral infections with little in the way of prodromal symptoms and signs (e.g. roseola infantum).

It is important to note that in the early stages of a serious infection such as meningitis, there are few specific features, and the child may not look very sick. Unless it is appreciated that fever with no obvious cause is significant, and warrants a careful search for the cause, it is possible to miss the diagnosis and thus lose the opportunity for early effective treatment. Likewise, urinary tract infections, pneumonia and ear infections are not always straightforward to diagnose, particularly in young infants. A specific effort should be made to exclude these infections.

Table 14.2 Features suggestive of bacterial and viral infections	
Bacterial infection	*Viral infection*
History of exposure to a subject known to have had bacterial infection	History of exposure to a subject known to have had viral infection
Features localized to one area or system Secretions are usually purulent. Toxic appearance in serious infections	Multisystem features, including runny nose, skin rashes and diarrhoea. Secretions are non-purulent. Toxic appearance is rare
Neutrophilia, raised C-reactive protein (CRP) level and positive cultures	Neutrophilia infrequently present, CRP level usually not significantly raised
Response to antibiotics	No response to antibiotics[a]

[a] In addition to viral infections, other possible causes for failure of a presumed bacterial infection to respond to the 'appropriate' antibacterial treatment include resistance, infection by atypical agents (e.g. *Mycoplasma*) or the presence of a non-infective cause

Frequently, this will involve observation and reassessment and sometimes ordering investigations such as urine analysis, microscopy and culture, chest radiography, and/or lumbar puncture (in the last case, only if it is considered safe; refer to Ch. 10), as necessary.

Primary bacteraemias are said to occur with significant frequency in children with temperatures above 39°C with no obvious cause. A white blood cell count above 15 000 makes the possibility more likely. Blood cultures should be obtained from all such children.

Febrile children who present with no obvious focus of infection but who look sick should be managed as cases of septicaemia until proven otherwise. This means that some children with viral infection will receive antibiotics unnecessarily, but this is a worthwhile price to pay in order to avoid delays in the treatment of a potentially fatal infection. Non-infectious causes of fever include drug reactions and connective tissue disorders (e.g. juvenile chronic arthritis (see Ch. 12) and Kawasaki's disease (see Beyond core: Kawasaki's disease)).

✱ KEY DIAGNOSIS

Meningitis

Meningitis is one of the most serious infections of childhood and, unless identified and treated at an early stage, may result in death or chronic sequelae. Meningitis can be caused by a wide range of viruses, bacteria and other microorganisms. Viral (aseptic) meningitis is the commonest form of this infection. However, its course and prognosis is usually much more benign than bacterial meningitis. Viral meningitis is usually part of a generalized viral infection and frequently may not declare itself by more than a coryzal or flu-like illness which is slightly more severe than usual and in which headache, vomiting, photophobia and/or irritability may be prominent.

Meningitis and encephalitis are two forms of generalized central nervous system infection, and can be viewed as two points on a continuum of involvement of the brain and its covering membranes. Usually both are involved to a varying degree, and the term 'meningoencephalitis' is frequently used (see Ch. 10).

Beyond the neonatal period, *N. meningitidis*, followed by *Strep. pneumoniae* and *H. influenza* type b are the most common bacteria implicated. The pathogenesis of meningitis is similar to that of septicaemia (see later). In meningitis, the bacteraemic phase leads to the spread of bacteria to the meninges, where they initiate a local infection and trigger an inflammatory response. Rarely, meningitis results from extension of infection of an adjacent focus (e.g. otitis media, orbital cellulitis).

Gram-negative bacteria and group B streptococci are the most commonly implicated organisms in neonatal meningitis (see Ch. 4).

Clinical features

In typical cases, there usually is a preceding upper respiratory tract or gastrointestinal illness of a few days duration. This is followed by features of systemic infection as well as symptoms and signs of meningeal irritation.

Features of systemic infection are those of a septicaemic illness (see Septicaemia (p. 285) and Septic shock (p. 285)) with elevation of temperature, poor feeding, pallor, muscle and joint pain as well as a range of cutaneous lesions which may include petechial rash, ecchymoses and maculopapular eruptions. In advanced untreated cases the condition progresses to septic shock with hypotension and features of multiple-organ dysfunction.

The symptoms of meningeal irritation include headaches, photophobia, and neck and back pain. Irritability, drowsiness, vomiting and unwillingness to be handled are other features pointing to central nervous system involvement. The presence of any of these symptoms in a child with fever should always raise the possibility of meningeal irritation and central nervous system infection.

Signs of meningeal irritation

- Neck and back stiffness: these can be demonstrated by active or passive movements. The child is asked to press the chin against the chest or, in the sitting position with the hips and knees flexed, to kiss his or her knees; in the presence of meningitis this proves impossible because of pain in the neck and back. Attempts at passive flexion of the head are made by placing the palm of one hand underneath the occiput while the other gently presses over the chest (another way of eliciting the same sign is to hold the head of the child with both hands and gently flex the head). In an infant, often the best technique is to observe the child's ability to follow a brightly coloured toy.
- Kernig sign: in the supine position, with the hip and knees flexed, extension of the knee is limited by pain in the back.
- Brudzinski sign: in the supine position, flexion of the neck results in an involuntary flexion of the hips and knees.

Features of increased intracranial pressure are frequently present. However, papilloedema is unlikely in uncomplicated cases of meningitis, and its presence points to a more chronic process such as abscess or empyema. In young children with an open anterior fontanelle, bulging of the fontanelle (see Fig. 14.3) is a useful sign of increased intracranial pressure (see Ch. 10). Seizures can occur due to the central nervous system infection or electrolyte imbalance. If they persist beyond the fourth day of the illness they are usually difficult to control and are associated with poor prognosis.

Meningitis of a sudden onset and following a fulminant course is seen particularly in cases of meningococcal meningitis. In these cases the manifestations are mainly those of the septicaemic state and death may occur within 24 h. Rarely, meningitis due to pneumococci and *H. influenzae* may follow a rapid course. Atypical presentations of meningitis can occur, and unawareness of this fact may result in the diagnosis being missed, with disastrous consequences.

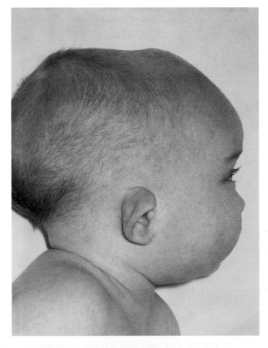

Figure 14.3 A child with meningitis showing a bulging fontanelle. (Reproduced by courtesy of the Wellcome Trust Photographic Library)

Atypical presentations

- In a young infant, the course may resemble that of neonatal meningitis in which the manifestations are mainly non-specific. These infants present with poor feeding, and sometimes vomiting, jaundice and sleepiness. Frequently the main presenting complaint is a non-specific observation, usually made by the mother, that the child is not looking right or is not his or her usual self. Temperature instability and hypothermia are more frequently seen than fever. Fitting may also be difficult to recognize in these infants. Fullness of the anterior fontanelle may be present, but the tense, bulging anterior fontanelle seen in older infants is a late sign.

- Children who have received antibiotics in the preceding days (for the prodomal symptoms or a concomitant infection) may have a modified course and not display all the typical features. The presence of another focus of infection such as an ear infection, tonsillitis or pneumonia may distract the attention of the physician from the presence of meningitis. It is always important to make sure that the degree of systemic upset is proportionate to the working diagnosis. Failure to improve, in spite of adequate antibacterial treatment for a diagnosed infection and particularly if progressive deterioration occurs, should alert the physician to the possibility of a second focus of infection, such as meningitis.

- Meningitis is one of the differential diagnoses of fever with no obvious focus: (see earlier).

Investigations

Leucocytosis and neutrophilia with a shift to the left (towards more immature forms) are frequently present. Elevated C-reactive protein (CRP) levels and an erythrocyte sedimentation rate (ESR) are present and help to differentiate bacterial from viral meningitis. However, both the ESR and CRP level may be normal in the early stages of bacterial meningitis. Thrombocytopenia and evidence of disseminated intravascular coagulation (DIC) may be present, particularly in the rapidly progressive pattern of presentation. The blood culture is usually positive, revealing the responsible bacteria in 90% of cases of childhood meningitis.

The 'gold standard' for the diagnosis of meningitis is positive findings on analysis of cerebrospinal fluid (CSF) obtained by lumbar puncture. Lumbar puncture should be performed whenever bacterial meningitis is suspected except in the presence of contraindications, particularly where raised intracranial pressure is suspected (see Ch. 10). If the lumbar puncture is delayed because of the presence of any of the contraindications, immediate empirical treatment with antibiotics should be started. Lumbar puncture may be performed later when the contraindication is no longer relevant (e.g. after treatment of increased intracranial pressure or on obtaining a negative computerized tomography scan for a suspected focal lesion such as a brain abscess).

When performing a lumbar puncture, the CSF pressure should be first noted. Samples should then be taken and sent for microscopy, cell count and differential, biochemical analysis for glucose and protein, and microbiological processing for Gram staining, culture and viral studies. In certain cases, further testing for the presence of antigens may be required (see below).

> **CSF analysis in bacterial meningitis**
> - High CSF opening pressure (the child should be in an extended posture and not crying)
> - Increased cell count with dominance of neutrophils
> - High protein and low sugar levels
> - Presence of microorganisms on Gram staining
> - Positive culture

> For the CSF normal values, refer to Ch. 10

In the early stages of meningitis, the only finding may be a positive culture, and thus an initial normal CSF analysis should not delay treatment if there are sufficient clinical grounds.

In partially treated meningitis, Gram staining and culture are less likely to be positive. However, the biochemical and microscopic abnormalities persist, although the CSF neutrophilia may be less striking. Detection of bacterial antigens by various techniques (enzyme-linked immunosorbent assay (ELISA), polymerase chain reaction (PCR), etc.) may also be helpful. After a traumatic lumbar puncture (puncturing of a blood vessel resulting in blood contamination of the CSF sample), it may be difficult to interpret the CSF cell count and protein concentration. However, the Gram stain and culture are usually not affected. In aseptic (viral) meningitis, the CSF shows a lesser degree of pleocytosis, and lymphocytes predominate; the CSF sugar level is usually normal (in mumps aseptic meningitis, however, the CSF sugar level may be low), and the protein elevation is less marked.

Treatment

A third-generation cephalosporin such as ceftriaxone or cefotaxime should be used to cover the three main organisms implicated in childhood meningitis (i.e. *N. meningitidis, Strep. pneumoniae* and, less commonly, *H. influenzae*). The third-generation cephalosporins are also active against Gram-negative coliform bacteria and group B streptococci, which are the usual pathogens isolated from neonates with meningitis. However, in the neonatal period, because meningitis can also be caused by *Listeria monocytogenes*, amoxycillin is added to the regimen. In a few cases where there are grounds to suspect staphylococcal infection (e.g. presence of VP shunt), antistaphylococcal treatment should be added. The initial antibacterial therapy should be modified according to the sensitivity profile of the organism cultured from the blood and CSF.

Antibiotic doses for meningitis are higher than the average recommended dose for most other types of infection so as to ensure an effective concentration of antibacterial drug in the CSF. The spectrum of antibacterial activity, safety at high concentrations as well as the ability to penetrate the inflamed blood–brain barrier are the three important considerations that govern the choice of antibiotic treatment for this condition. Third-generation cephalosporins seem to perform very well on each of these counts. The doses used for cefotaxime are 200 mg/kg per day divided in four doses. The duration of treatment is on average about 7 days for meningococcal meningitis and

10–14 days for *H. influenzae* and pneumococcal meningitis, provided the response to treatment is favourable and there are no complications.

There is some controversy about the role of steroids in the treatment of meningitis. One view is to give dexamethasone at the outset with antibacterial treatment and to continue for the first 2 days (the rationale behind this recommendation is discussed in Highlights and Hypotheses: the use of steroids in infection).

Appropriate therapeutic steps should be taken in the presence of increased intracranial pressure (see Ch. 10).

Fluid balance disorders are common, and children with meningitis are at risk of developing the syndrome of inappropriate antidiuretic hormone (ADH) secretion. This may aggravate cerebral oedema and contribute to seizure activity in this condition (see Ch. 10). Parameters of hydration including fluid intake and output, body weight, physical signs of over- or underhydration as well as urine osmolality, and serum sodium levels should be monitored. If these indicate the presence of inappropriate ADH secretion (hyponatraemia in a child with normal renal and adrenal function with urine which is not maximally dilute despite a low plasma osmolarity), the fluid intake should be reduced to between two-thirds to one-half maintenance. However, it is important to maintain adequate perfusion.

Anticonvulsants should be administered to control seizures as required. Phenytoin is the preferred agent, since it is the least likely to result in depression of consciousness (level of consciousness is a valuable sign for monitoring in this condition). Other possible triggers of seizure activity should be considered, including hyponatraemia, other electrolyte imbalances and hypoglycaemia.

Supportive treatment includes adequate ventilation and circulation, the use of antipyretics and analgesia, and maintenance of good hydration and adequate blood sugar levels. Monitoring of these physiological parameters and correction when required are crucial. Daily assessment of the neurological status, head circumference, and presence of complications or

HIGHLIGHTS AND HYPOTHESES

THE USE OF STEROIDS IN INFECTION

The controversy over the use of corticosteroids in the treatment of infections has continued for many years.

Decades ago it was noted that the use of effective antibiotics in the treatment of certain types of infection was, paradoxically, associated with initial worsening and sometimes with a shock-like reaction. This phenomenon was noted to occur in particular subacute infections, where lack of specific symptoms delays diagnosis and allows the bacterial load to increase (syphilis, relapsing fever). The initiation of treatment with an antibiotic for which the responsible organism is highly sensitive (e.g. penicillin in syphilis) was thought to be associated with large-scale killing of bacteria and release of bacterial products, and hence the untoward reaction (Jarisch–Herxheimer reaction). The use of steroids was thought to block this reaction, and was advocated as an adjunct treatment.

In severe meningococcal disease, adrenal haemorrhages have been shown to be responsible for some cases of shock and refractory hypotension (Waterhouse–Friderichsen syndrome). The use of steroids is known to be beneficial in these cases. Furthermore, in meningitis, brain oedema is a major pathophysiological factor, and the use of steroids, dexamethasone in particular, has been shown to be of value.

More recent work has provided further support to the use of steroids in meningitis:

- Some studies have shown a reduction in the incidence of complications such as deafness associated with certain types of meningitis in children treated with corticosteroids.
- In many cases, where a second CSF examination is performed 12–24 h after the initiation of antibacterial therapy, there is an increase in the number of inflammatory cells in the CSF. Although this may simply reflect the time-scale according to which body responses develop, at least partly it is explained on the basis that killing of the infecting organisms and release of bacterial products stimulates the immune mechanisms with release of inflammatory mediators, thus aggravating the inflammation and possibly precipitating further damage.

Arguments against the use of steroids in meningitis have not, however, been in short supply. Their long list of potential side-effects, particularly immunosuppression, have always made clinicians uneasy about the use of corticosteroids in severe infections, and clinical practice has shown that these fears are not unfounded; there have been reports of delayed sterilization of the CSF and case reports of gastrointestinal bleeding associated with the use of steroids in meningitis.

Because of the safety of the third-generation cephalosporins and our ability to give them in high doses combined with their excellent penetration of the inflamed blood–brain barrier, the concentration achieved in the CSF can be several times that of the MIC (minimal inhibitory concentration). This may effect a large-scale killing of the infecting microorganism with massive release of endotoxins and the potential for further inflammatory tissue injury is high. Delayed sterilization of the CSF has not been documented in children with meningitis who were given steroids but who were treated with third-generation cephalosporins.

Hence, it is currently recommended that the first dose of dexamethasone is administered just prior to the first dose of antibacterial therapy (to prevent the release of proinflammatory mediators in response to toxins liberated from killed bacteria). The recommended treatment dose and duration are 0.6 mg of dexamethasone per kilogram per day divided into four doses, and given intravenously over a period of 2 days.

---

other foci of infection should be performed. Neurological deficits may be due to an acute involvement of the relevant area of the brain or increased intracranial pressure, infarction, abscess formation or pressure from a subdural infusion. Early scanning and appropriate treatment are mandatory.

The persistence of fever may be due to lack of response (bacterial resistance, inadequate dosage, faulty administration, etc.) or an adverse reaction to the antibiotic administered. Additional causes include the presence of coexistent infection, and the presence of complications such as subdural effusion or brain abscess. Focal pathology in the brain should be excluded before a second lumbar puncture is performed to assess the response to the prescribed antibacterial treatment.

Prophylaxis

Children with meningococcal meningitis and their contacts may qualify for chemoprophylaxis as described in the section on meningococcaemia (see later). For cases of *H. influenzae* and pneumococcal meningitis, indications for chemoprophylaxis should be decided according to the age, vaccination and immune status of contacts as well as the type of contact.

Complications

Acute complications include shock, respiratory arrest, acute increase in the intracranial pressure (cerebral oedema), cerebral infarction, abscess formation and subdural effusions.

Chronic complications include chronic neurological sequelae such as deafness, blindness and focal neurological deficits. It is important to note that the incidence of these complications decreases with time. Thus, some studies have shown that at discharge up to 40% may show abnormalities on neurological examination, but 2 years later only 10% demonstrate specific neurological deficits. The incidence of hearing loss has been estimated at approximately 30% which, in 12% of cases, interfered with speech. Hydrocephalus and focal neurological deficits are less common.

RASH

Skin eruption is a common feature of disease in children. Frequently, the rash is transient, non-specific and is of little diagnostic value. Sometimes, however, the rash has characteristics that are specific for a particular disease and serves as a useful clue to the diagnosis (e.g. meningococcaemia). In certain cases, the rash is the main feature of the illness (e.g. exanthemata such as measles and chickenpox).

The diagnostic approach to a child with skin rash should follow a systematic and logical scheme. Two groups of features need to be addressed:

BEYOND CORE

KAWASAKI'S DISEASE

The aetiology of Kawasaki's disease (mucocutaneous lymph node syndrome) is unknown but thought to be infection or toxin related. It occurs in prepubertal children characterized by diffuse vasculitis of small and medium-sized vessels. There is no definitive laboratory test, and the diagnosis is made on the basis of five of the six major clinical features, including fever. Coronary artery aneurysm, which occurs in up to 20% of cases, is the most important associated feature (see below), and may result in fatal infarction. Early treatment with aspirin and γ-globulin reduces the risk of aneurysm formation. Thrombocytosis and desquamation, which occur in the second and third weeks of the illness, are particularly helpful in confirming the diagnosis.

Major clinical features

High swinging fever:	abrupt onset, up to 40°C
Non-purulent conjunctivitis:	may be accompanied by a mild uveitis
Oral changes (mucositis):	diffuse inflammation of oropharynx, tongue and lips, which are swollen and cracked
Changes in the extremities:	erythema of palms and soles with non-pitting oedema of hands and feet followed by desquamation
Polymorphous rash:	usually macular sometimes macular papular, but can take almost any form
Cervical lymphadenopathy:	found only in 50% of cases, usually as a single node >1.5 cm in diameter

Associated features: asceptic meningitis, arthritis, cardiovascular (pericarditis, myocarditis, coronary artery aneurysms, peripheral artery aneurysms), gastrointestinal (diarrhoea, hepatitis, hydrops of gall bladder), thrombocytosis.

1. The characteristics of the rash

- The nature of the skin lesions
- The distribution of the rash
- Its course and progression

2. Other features of the illness

The characteristics of the rash

The nature of the skin lesions

A skin rash is made up of multiples of individual skin lesions which may be of one or more type. The following is a brief outline of the more common types of rashes seen in children.

Maculopapular rashes are the most common type of skin eruptions accompanying infectious diseases in children. Non-specific viral illnesses are probably the most common underlying illness, but the rash of measles and rubella is also of this type. Some bacterial infections and non-infectious disorders (e.g. connective tissue disorders) may also be accompanied by a maculopapular rash. The rash of scarlet fever tends to be fine papular (the fine papules are easier felt than seen) on a background of erythema.

The *vesicular and vesiculobullous rash* is typically seen in infections with the herpes group of viruses including chickenpox and herpes simplex. Some skin bacterial infections (e.g. staphylococcal impetigo) are associated with vesiculation and bullous formation (see Fig. 13.12). Several non-infectious primary skin disorders are vesiculobullous in nature.

Petechiae and ecchymoses are seen in severe septicaemic states, particularly those due to meningococcal disease. However, some viral infections may present with similar rashes. Non-infectious causes include states associated with bleeding tendencies (e.g. thrombocytopenia (see Fig. 11.8), leukaemia and coagulation disorders) and vasculitis, the most common of which is Henoch–Schönlein purpura (see Ch. 12) in which the lesions are characteristically palpable (see Fig. 11.9). Non-accidental injury is an important condition to consider in the differential diagnosis.

The distribution of the rash

The rash of measles tends to be dense all over the body (Fig. 14.4), while that of rubella (Fig. 14.5) is

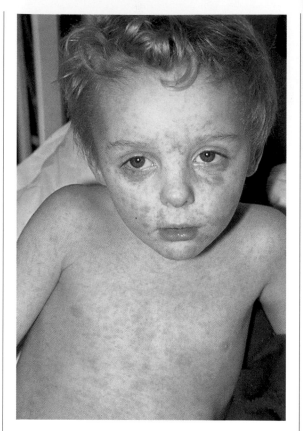

Figure 14.4 A child with a typical rash of measles. (Reproduced by courtesy of the Wellcome Trust Photographic Library)

less striking. The rash of chickenpox is more dense on the trunk than the extremities (centripetal). The distribution of the rash in Henoch–Schönlein purpura can be diagnostic, being typically limited to the lower extremities and buttocks.

Course and progression

This is an important feature of skin rashes; for example, the rash of measles usually starts behind the ear, involves the face, then extends to the trunk before it reaches the extremities, usually on the third day. This contrasts with allergic rashes and drug eruptions in which the rash spreads rapidly (minutes/hours).

The course of the rash may not only involve spread to different parts of the body but also the evolution of the skin lesions themselves. For

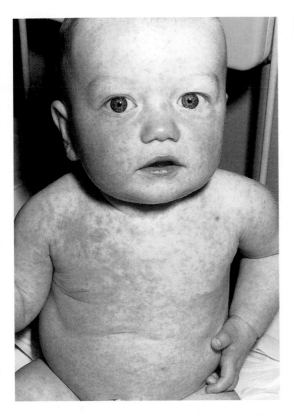

Figure 14.5   An infant with the exanthem of rubella

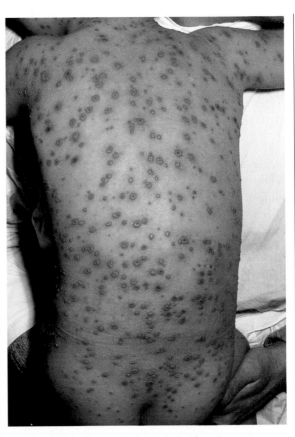

Figure 14.6   A child with a rash typical of chickenpox. (Reproduced by courtesy of the Wellcome Trust Photographic Library)

example, in chickenpox the lesions start as macules that change to papules, evolve into vesicles and occasionally into pustules (if secondary bacterial infection ensues). The vesicles and pustules eventually rupture, and the raw surface dries to form scabs (Fig. 14.6). This course of events is characteristic. A striking feature in chickenpox, however, is that skin lesions at different stages of development can be seen during most of the course of the rash.

Desquamation is a late feature of both scarlet fever and Kawasaki's disease (see Fig. 14.7 and Beyond core: Kawasaki's disease).

Other features of the illness

The diagnosis of an illness accompanied by a skin rash frequently rests not on the characteristics of the rash itself but on the presence of certain other features of the illness that are suggeestive of a particular diagnosis. Children frequently present with 'non-specific' rashes, and looking for such

features is an essential part of the evaluation of these children.

The natural course of most infections runs the following pattern:

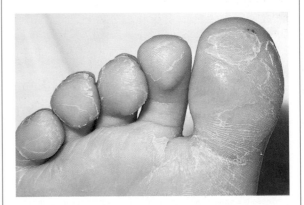

Figure 14.7   Desquamation of the toes seen in Kawasaki's disease

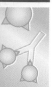

Contact\contraction of the infection → Incubation period →

Prodromal phase → Full clinical picture

Information about each of these phases of the disease should be gathered.

The epidemiological history

Through enquiry about contact with a similar illness, or awareness of the presence of an infectious disease in the community that causes a similar clinical picture, a provisional diagnosis or differential diagnosis can be made. For example, the knowledge of the presence of a few rubella (German measles) cases in the neighbourhood, might prompt the clinician to consider this diagnosis in a 1 year old infant with a cold and a rash, and it may then be prudent to advise the avoidance of contact with pregnant women even before the full clinical picture develops.

Obviously, numerous other considerations come into play here, including the type of contact, the susceptibility of the subject and the infectivity of the illness in question. It is most important, however, to remember that what is gained from the epidemiological data is simply circumstantial evidence. The possibility of other diagnoses should never be neglected.

Incubation period

This is the period from the time of acquisition of the infectious agent of a particular disease to the time of appearance of the first symptoms and signs of that disease. It is thought that during this period the infectious agent multiplies and invades the target organs and tissues. Only when the infecting agent numbers attain a certain level (this varies widely in different diseases, and also depends on the virulence of a particular strain, the immunity of the host, etc.), and tissue involvement reaches a certain stage (again variable), that symptoms and signs develop (Table 14.3).

The prodromal period

This is defined as the period from the time of appearance of the first symptoms and signs (usually non-specific) to the time of appearance of the main specific features of the illness (in exanthemata this is usually the rash).

Characteristics of this period may be of great diagnostic value; in measles, for example, the prodromal period is prominent and characterized

Table 14.3	The incubation periods of some of the infectious diseases commonly seen in children[a]		
Disease	Infective agent	Incubation period[a]	Infectivity period
Meningococcaemia	*N. meningitidis*	Few hours to few days	Until chemoprophylaxis is given
Pertussis	*B. pertussis*	7–14 days	From prodromal stage through 4th week
Measles	RNA virus	11–14 days	From 5th day of incubation through 4th day of rash
German measles	RNA virus	18 days	From 1 week before to 1 week after the rash
Chickenpox	DNA virus	18 days	2 days before the rash until all lesions are scabbed
Mumps	RNA virus	18 days	From 1 week before the swelling until it subsides
Scarlet fever	*Strep. pyogenes*	3 days	Variable. 2 days into treatment
Roseola infantum	DNA virus	? 10 days	?

[a] These are approximate figures; there is always a range for the incubation periods, which for some infectious illnesses may be quite wide

by high fever, cough, symptoms of cold, and conjunctivitis. The temperature reaches its peak on the day the rash appears, and plateaus for a day or two after the appearance of the rash, before steady improvement begins.

The situation in measles sharply contrasts with two other illnesses that may have skin rashes very similar to that of measles. These are German measles and roseola infantum.

In German measles, the prodromal period is characteristically mild; its only significant feature is the presence of posterior–cervical, retroauricular and/or postoccipital lymphadenopathy.

In roseola infantum, the prodromal period is characterized by high fever, but with absence of other symptoms and signs. This usually poses a diagnostic difficulty, and children with this illness are frequently admitted to hospital for observation. The problem is compounded by the fact that the temperature usually rises rapidly in this disease; thus susceptible children are likely to suffer from a febrile fit in the course of the febrile period. The distinctive, almost pathognomonic feature of this illness is rapid resolution of fever as the rash appears.

The absence of a prodromal period before the appearance of a skin rash favours an allergic rather than infectious aetiology of the rash.

Accompanying features
These are the other symptoms and signs, which are present at some stage of the illness and may point towards the underlying disease process. Some of these features may coexist with the rash, appear in the prodromal period or persist after the rash has disappeared.

Diagnostically useful findings
- Koplik spots in measles. These are white small dots surrounded by an area of redness and are to be found on the buccal mucosa, typically opposite the lower posterior maleolars. Koplik spots appear transiently, late in the prodromal period, and are pathognomonic of measles.
- Strawberry tongue in scarlet fever. This results from swelling of the papillae, which project

from the tongue surface. The sign is noted from the early stages of the illness, and persists for several days after the appearance of the rash. Although the 'strawberry tongue' sign can also be found in some other infectious and non-infectious disorders, scarlet fever and other streptococcal infections are the most common underlying diagnoses.
- Cervical lymphadenopathy in rubella. Characteristically retroauricular, postoccipital and posterior cervical lymph nodes are considerably enlarged and tender. This tends to occur shortly prior to the appearance of the rash, and persists for several days.

✳ KEY DIAGNOSIS

Exanthemata

The principal features of the important exanthematous disorders in children have been discussed in the previous section, and are summarized in Table 14.4 together with some of the 'childhood-specific' infectious disorders.

SEPTICAEMIA AND SEPTIC SHOCK

The term 'septicaemia' refers to severe illness, resulting from invasion of the bloodstream by bacteria and/or the release of toxins, together with the effects of the body's reaction to these events. In clinical practice, septicaemia is almost always included in the differential diagnosis of acute severe illness of undetermined aetiology.

Aetiology and pathogenesis
Bacteria gain access to the bloodstream repeatedly but transiently in healthy and normal individuals. Activities such as tooth brushing and straining may be accompanied by 'escape' into the bloodstream of small numbers of bacteria, from where they are normally present in the oral cavity and upper respiratory or lower gastrointestinal tracts. Instrumentation of these areas (dental extraction or endoscopy for example) may also be accompanied by similar spilling over of microorganisms into the bloodstream. However, provided the body defence and immune systems

Table 14.4   The important features of some of the childhood-specific infectious disorders, including exanthemata

Disease[a]	Prodromal period	Rash	Diagnostic features	Comments
Meningococcal septicaemia	Can be abrupt with rapid progression	Petechial	Rash typically occurs in the sick child	Variants with a mild start possible
Pertussis[b]	Cold-like illness for a few days		Paroxysmal cough followed by whoop or vomiting	Apnoea and vomiting more likely in small infants
Measles	Prominent cough, fever and conjunctivitis	Maculopapular, starts on the face and spreads	Koplik spots in prodromal period	Temperature peaks as rash appears and plateaus for 2 days
German measles	Mild cold-like illness	Maculopapular, rapidly spreads and fades	Enlargement of lymph nodes at the back of the neck, ears, occiput	Rash can be scanty and prodromal symptoms mild
Roseola infantum	High fever with little else	Maculopapular	Temperature rapidly drops as rash appears	Febrile fits in susceptible children
Chickenpox	Mild febrile illness	Maculopapular, evolves into vesiculo-pustular	Presence of skin lesions at different stages at the same time	Rash may be scanty, but can be severe in children with eczema
Mumps[b]	Mild febrile illness		Typical swelling of salivary glands	Other glands and testes may be involved
Scarlet fever	Sore throat	Fine papular on a flushed skin	Sore throat, strawberry tongue and the rash	Peeling of the skin may follow

[a] Severe and mild cases, as well as atypical forms, can occur. Modified and atypical cases are likely if disease occurs in an immunized child. Children who present with particularly severe forms of these illnesses should be evaluated for possible immunodeficiency
[b] Pertussis and mumps (see Fig. 14.1) are not members of the exanthemata; rashes are not characteristic clinical features in these illnesses but they are included here as 'childhood-specific' diseases

are intact, these microorganisms are rapidly dealt with and eliminated. In the absence of factors that favour the settling of bacteria in certain areas (defective heart valves, bone infarcts, etc.) these short-lived excursions of bacteria into the bloodstream result in no harm.

Persistence of bacteria in the bloodstream accompanies states of significant focal bacterial infection. Thus, in some cases of bacterial pneumonia, septic arthritis or pyelonephritis, bacteria are present in the bloodstream and persist for a variable period during the illness. In

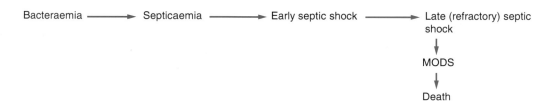

Figure 14.8   Evolution of septicaemia

these situations, the presence of an active focus of infection acts as a source of continuous supply of bacteria entering the bloodstream in large numbers. Body defence and immune systems normally act to contain these incursions and prevent the bacteria from multiplying within the bloodstream or establishing further foci of infection in other areas. If the balance is tilted in favour of the microorganism for any reason (virulence, weakened host defences, local causes), the bacteraemia may result in seeding of the microorganism in other areas, i.e. haematogenous spread of infection. Septicaemia occurs when the presence of multiple foci of infection, the multiplication of the microorganisms and/or massive release of toxins within the bloodstream evoke the host systemic inflammatory response syndrome (SIRS), which may lead to shock and the multiple-organ dysfunction syndrome (MODS) (Fig. 14.8).

Clinical features

The clinical manifestations of early septicaemia are frequently difficult to separate from those of the preceding infection, and the clinical picture of the underlying illness simply merges into that of

---

BEYOND CORE

THE PATHOGENESIS OF SEPTICAEMIA

Septicaemia is no longer thought of as a direct result of microbial invasion or a direct effect of microbial toxins, but rather that it represents a severe generalized reaction of the host to infection. Such a reaction leads to the systemic inflammatory response syndrome (SIRS), which underlies the principal features of septicaemia and can lead to the multiple organ dysfunction syndrome (MODS), characteristic of the advanced stages of the septicaemic state. This explains why some children with viral and other non-bacterial infection may present a clinical picture indistinguishable from that of bacterial sepsis. In fact, some of the non-infective conditions (e.g. connective tissue disorders) may produce a similar clinical picture. Hence, together with infections, they are frequently included in the differential diagnosis of this clinical presentation.

Another important observation which can be explained by this model for septicaemia is the fact that the morbidity and mortality of septicaemia continues to be high despite the discovery and use of new 'super-effective' antibacterial agents. At present, much of the research conducted in this area is focused on the host's response and ways to modify it.

The mode and sequence of activation of the various body mechanisms which culminates in the SIRS are complex and not completely understood. A central role is played by the various bioactive substances, that are collectively known as 'mediators of inflammation'. In laboratory animals, almost all the manifestations of septicaemia can be reproduced by injecting these animals with tumour necrosis factor α (TNFα).

The most crucial effect of the action of the mediators released in response to the SIRS is on the vascular endothelium. Initially this leads to peripheral vasodilatation, and the blood volume proves inadequate for the expanded intravascular space. Tachycardia and increased cardiac output may maintain the blood pressure for a while, but hypotension eventually results (warm septic shock). Later, as the vascular endothelium loses its integrity, leakage into the extravascular space occurs. This, together with depressed myocardial contractility, further impairs the circulation, and compensatory vasoconstriction supervenes (cold septic shock). The local effects of leakage in the lungs lead to the adult respiratory distress syndrome, causing hypoxia and carbon dioxide retention.

Once the sequence of events leading to SIRS is initiated, a relentless progression begins, which is not halted until appropriate intervention takes place. Beyond a certain point, such progression will not respond to any intervention (refractory septic shock).

septicaemia, giving the impression of a gradual deterioration in the overall well-being of the child. Sometimes there is a distinct worsening as the septicaemic state develops on a background of mild infection or bacteraemia and, particularly with virulent organisms and/or massive infecting doses, the onset of the symptoms of septicaemia is abrupt.

In addition to the deterioration in the child's general condition, the onset of septicaemia is marked by alteration in the pattern of fever or by hypothermia. Frequently, rigors, pallor, tachycardia and tachypnoea are also present. A range of cutaneous lesions may appear, and these include petechiae, ecchymoses, diffuse erythema and peripheral gangrene (purpura fulminans). Untreated, the septicaemic state invariably progresses to septic shock. Shock is defined as a state of tissue hypoperfusion, and the clinical features reflect the hypoperfusion of the organs accessible for clinical evaluation (i.e. brain, kidneys and skin):

- *Early (warm) septic shock.* In addition to hypotension and the features of sepsis listed above, there are changes in the mental state such as confusion/drowsiness, and oliguria. The skin, however, feels inappropriately warm because vasodilatation is the pathophysiological mechanism of the early stage of this type of shock. Hypoxaemia reflects the unmet increased tissue demand for oxygen, and cyanosis may be present.
- *Late septic shock.* The compensatory cutaneous vasoconstriction overrides the vasodilatation, and the skin feels cold. Initially this is restricted to the hands and feet, but as the shock state deepens the coolness level creeps up to the thighs and shoulders. The capillary refill time (blushing of the blanched area created by pressing the skin over the sternum) is also prolonged (normally less than 2 s).

In the advanced stages of septic shock, the hypoperfusion leads to multiple-organ dysfunction with disruption of the vital physiological functions of the body. Prominent among these is the development of the adult respiratory distress syndrome or shock lung, myocardial dysfunction, DIC and acute renal failure.

There may also be features relating to focal infection, such as pneumonia or meningitis, which are frequently the source of the septicaemia. However, local infection may develop as a result of the septicaemic state when bacteria settle in the various tissues and organs. Other notable features may include those of an underlying immunodeficiency disorder or the presence of an intravascular device that may act as the port of entry for the microorganisms and, subsequently, a reservoir of infection which may be difficult to eradicate.

Investigations

Abnormalities of the white blood cell count are frequently present; usually there is a leucocytosis with a shift to the left in cases of bacterial infection. However, leucopenia may be present, and is associated with a poor prognosis. Positive blood cultures are frequently obtained, but the organisms take time to grow. Gram staining of the blood or skin lesions may demonstrate the microorganism. There may be thrombocytopenia and evidence of DIC, which includes, in addition to deformed red blood cells on the blood film, prolonged prothrombin and partial thromboplastin time, reduced fibrinogen levels and increased D-dimer levels. Later, the investigations reflect the MODS. Cultures of the urine and CSF may or may not be positive.

Treatment

Children with septic shock should preferably be cared for in an intensive care unit, with the capability for continuous close monitoring and where skilled expertise is at hand. Broad-spectrum antimicrobial agents should be given as soon as the diagnosis of septicaemia is suspected and specimens for culture obtained. The choice of antibiotic is usually made according to age and the circumstances surrounding the development of septicaemia. Thus, antistaphylococcal agents should be added when the septicaemia develops in a hospitalized child, particularly if intravascular devices (long lines, arterial lines) are present. Antifungal agents may also be considered in some cases. In immunocompromised children, the choice of antibiotic will depend on the particular type of immunodeficiency, and the appropriate protocols should be consulted. In abdominal sepsis, metronidazole should be added to provide cover against anaerobes. For septicaemia acquired in the community by previously healthy children, the commonest organisms are *N. meningitidis*, *Strep. pneumoniae* and *H. Influenza* (less common since the introduction of Hib immunization); a third-generation cephalosporin such as cefotaxime or ceftriaxone is a reasonable initial choice. When the culture results are available, the antibacterial therapy should be modified according to the sensitivity profile of the cultured organism.

Intravenous fluid therapy using isotonic solutions, such as normal saline, is usually effective in the early stages of shock. Although concern has been recently expressed regarding the use of albumin in acutely ill adults and children, there is no convincing evidence that its use in septicaemic children is associated with a worse outcome. Inotropic agents, such as dopamine and dobutamine, may also be required. If hypotension persists, catecholamine infusion should be started. These inotropes should always be given under close monitoring in the intensive therapy unit which includes measurement of central venous pressure. Vasodilator agents may be of benefit in the late phase when the peripheral resistance is high.

Supportive treatment includes maintenance of adequate ventilation and circulation, control of DIC and management of renal failure, electrolytes and acid–base disturbances. Close monitoring is crucial.

Treatment aimed at modifying the inflammatory response is being investigated. In certain cases, transfusion of immunoglobulins and the use of corticosteroids seem to be beneficial. In spite of the importance of tumour necrosis factor α (TNFα) and other proinflammatory mediators in the pathogenesis of septic shock, use of anti-TNF antibodies has been disappointing. In immunodeficiency states, the use of granulocyte transfusions and immunoglobulins may be of benefit.

Disseminated intravascular coagulation

DIC is a serious condition that can be triggered by a number of different types of pathology, including septicaemia. It is characterized by disruption of the normal equilibrium between the coagulation and fibrinolytic pathways, with the result that both processes are, to varying degrees, activated and both intravascular thrombosis and bleeding occur concurrently.

These events are due to endothelial injury, most commonly resulting from shock, but also from trauma or other causes. Activation of other cascade systems (complement, kinin) which are interlinked with the coagulation and fibrolytic pathways is also involved. The manifestations vary from case to case depending on whether the coagulation events or bleeding predominate. Thus, there may be excessive bleeding from intravascular sites and surgical wounds and/or tissue infarction and necrosis because of ischaemia.

The haematological picture shows thrombocytopenia, low levels of fibringen and high levels of D-dimers (fibrinogen degradation products) as well as haemolytic anaemia (microangiopathic haemolytic anaemia). The treatment of this condition is still unsatisfactory, and is usually directed at controlling the particular manifestation of the condition in the individual child. Thus, if bleeding phenomena dominate, fresh frozen plasma may be useful, while heparin or fibrinolytic agents may be employed in cases of intravascular thrombosis and tissue necrosis. Treatment of the underlying cause is crucial.

There are some aspects of the clinical manifestations of septicaemia which vary according to the microorganism involved. Septicaemia due to *N. meningitidis* is the most common type of septicaemia in immunocompetent children beyond the neonatal period. Not infrequently, meningococcaemia follows a fulminant course, with rapid progression from what seems to be a mild illness to a state of shock or even death in few hours. Disease due to *N. meningitidis* is endemic in many communities, and has the potential to cause major epidemics. A more detailed discussion of this type of septicaemia is therefore provided.

✳ KEY DIAGNOSIS

Meningococcaemia

Acute meningococcal septicaemia is one of paediatrics true emergencies. There are few other situations in paediatric practice in which early recognition and prompt intervention may truly mean the difference between life and death. Although the meningococcus may cause a range of localized infections, subacute and chronic conditions, any infection caused by this organism in a child should be regarded as a potential source of acute meningococcal sepsis.

Aetiology

The meningococcus is a Gram-negative diplococcus (arranged in pairs, frequently referred to as biscuit shaped). It is a fastidious organism and there are certain requirements which have to be met for it to grow in culture; thus it is an unlikely contaminant.

There are several sero-groups, divided according to the antigen structure of the capsular polysaccharide. Groups A, B and C are the ones usually implicated in disease, with group A responsible for the major epidemics, particularly in the developing countries. Groups B and C are implicated in sporadic cases and small epidemics in the Western world.

Pathogenesis

N. meningitidis is carried in the nasopharynx of 2–30% of the normal population; this percentage may be even higher in closed communities and during epidemics. Acquisition of the organism usually occurs by the respiratory route and, in the majority of cases, this leads to asymptomatic carriage. Dissemination through the bloodstream and invasive disease may then occur.

When meningcocci gain access to the circulation, the polysaccharide capsule provides protection against phagocytosis. However, two host defence factors play a crucial role in containing the invasion and clearing the blood from the meningococci: these are the presence of a normal complement system and the presence of ready made antimeningococcal antibodies. Such antibodies may have been produced as a result of preceding nasopharyngeal carriage of the organism or in response to infection with other bacteria that have antigens similar to those of the meningococcus.

Newborns are protected by antibodies of maternal origin, but these decline so that between the ages of 4 months to 2 years, infants are poorly protected against this organism, and hence the highest incidence of meningococcal disease is in this age group. Immunodeficiency states are associated with severe and sometimes recurrent meningococcal disease.

Clinical features

Dissemination of the meningococci to the bloodstream may result in several clinical syndromes that vary in severity.

In 'occult' bacteraemia, the child presents with fever and non-specific upper respiratory or gastrointestinal symptoms with or without a macular-papular, measles-like rash. Untreated at this stage, the disease may progress to meningococcaemia/meningitis, or recovery may be spontaneous. These cases of meningococcal bacteraemia are difficult to recognize, but a blood culture should be obtained from children with high fever and high white blood cell count. Such a presentation is increased in frequency during epidemics, and a high index of suspicion during these times aids recognition.

Meningococcal septicaemia usually starts with a flu-like illness with fever. At this stage there may or may not be few petechiae or other types of skin rash. This is followed by a rapid progression to the full-blown illness, with the child acutely ill with hypotension and poor perfusion, petechial rash (Fig. 14.9), ecchymoses and gangrenous skin lesions in severe cases. Localized foci of infection may include meningitis, septic arthritis, carditis and pneumonia. In established shock there is severe hypotension and multiorgan failure.

A chronic course for meningococcaemia is rarely seen, and is confined particularly to older children and adults. There may be fever, joint pain and various types of rashes; the course is slow, and the illness may drag on for several weeks. Escalation and acute complications such as meningitis can occur.

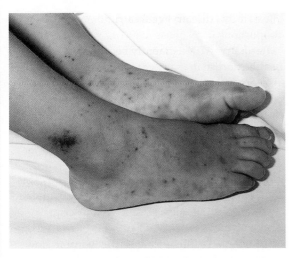

Figure 14.9 Classical purpuric rash seen on the lower extremities in meningococcal septicaemia

Investigations

The definitive diagnosis rests on culturing the meningococcus from the blood, CSF or skin lesions. Gram staining of the skin lesions may offer a rapid diagnosis, and detection of bacterial antigens and nucleic acid sequences by various techniques (ELISA, PCR, etc.) may be helpful in cases with negative cultures. There is usually an increase in the CRP level, leucocytosis or leucopenia, and evidence of DIC. In children diagnosed with meningococcal disease, investigation of the immune system (particularly of the complement pathway) is warranted.

The differential diagnosis includes septicaemia caused by other bacteria, such as *H. influenzae*, as well as certain viral infections, particularly those caused by coxsackie- and echoviruses. Vasculitic diseases, including Henoch–Schönlein purpura, may sometimes be confused with meningococcaemia. Idiopathic thrombocytopenic purpura, erythema multiforme and some hypersensitivity drug reactions can result in similar skin manifestations.

Acute complications are those of severe multiple organ failure and DIC. Skin sloughing and gangrene of extremities can also occur. Late complications may be related to immune complex disease, and are manifested by arthritis, skin rashes and pericardial effusion.

Treatment

Although the majority of the meningococcal strains are sensitive to penicillin, there has been an emergence of resistant strains. Hence, the current recommendation for hospital treatment is to give cefotaxime at a high dose of 200 mg/kg per day (in four divided doses) for 7 days. Ceftriaxone is another third-generation cephalosporin of comparable efficacy with the added advantage of once-daily dosing. Supportive therapy should be given as described for septicaemia and septic shock in the previous section.

If the condition is first suspected outside hospital, the first dose of antibacterial treatment (intravenous cefotaxime 50 mg/kg) should be given in the office and, if intravenous access proves difficult, intramuscular penicillin at a dose of 300 000 IU (600 000 IU in children above 6 years of age) should be given immediately before making arrangements for the child to be taken to hospital.

Mortality continues to be high for meningococcaemia, and is probably somewhere around 10%. Long-term sequelae are related to organ damage (e.g. skin gangrene, renal failure) and the presence of an associated meningitis (see next section). Poor prognostic indicators are rapid spread of the petechial rash, hypotension, hypothermia, a low platelet count and a low white blood cell count. High levels of endotoxin and TNFα are also associated with poor prognosis.

Prevention

Close contacts in the household should be given chemoprophylaxis with rifampicin 10 mg/kg per dose, twice a day for 2 days. All contacts should be monitored, and should be assessed if they develop fever. Chemoprophylaxis should be given as soon as possible because meningococcaemia is known to develop very soon after colonization of the nasopharynx, and sometimes secondary cases present with the index case at the same time (ciprofloxacin is another drug used for chemoprophylaxis in contacts).

Affected children themselves qualify for chemoprophylaxis since the meningococcus may still be harboured in the nasopharynx despite having received a course of treatment with resultant clearing of infection from the blood and

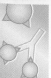

deep tissues. Rifampicin is usually given at the conclusion of treatment, but is unnecessary if ceftriaxone is used for treatment of the acute illness.

Immunization is effective against certain strains of the meningococcus, including A and C. There is, however, no currently available vaccine which is effective against the B strain, and vaccination is generally not very immunogenic in children below 2 years of age. The administration of antimeningococcal vaccine is indicated for children travelling to areas where infections with the type A strain are endemic.

The wide use of *H. influenzae* vaccine in the Western world has dramatically decreased the incidence of serious infection caused by this organism, including septicaemia and meningitis. For *H. influenzae*, chemoprophylaxis of unvaccinated children should be undertaken with rifampicin at a dose of 20 mg/kg per dose, once a day for 4 days.

CONGENITAL HIV INFECTION

Over the relatively short period of the past 20 years, HIV infection and AIDS have become a major worldwide health concern. The absence of symptoms of disease for a relatively long period following the acquisition of the virus, the spread through several routes including homosexual and heterosexual practices, intravenous drug abuse, blood products and vertical transmission, as well as the ease of transfer and travel in the modern world are among several factors which have allowed this disease to attain pandemic proportions.

Paediatric AIDS is rapidly becoming a major health concern in many communities in the Western world. In some developing countries, the problem has reached proportions that stretch their health, social and economic resources to the limits (see Ch. 20).

Aetiology

AIDS is caused by the retrovirus HIV type 1. This is an enveloped RNA virus endowed by a special type of DNA polymerase, reverse transcriptase. This enzyme is capable of synthesis of DNA using RNA templates (the reverse of the 'natural' flow of genetic information).

Reverse transcriptase, in contrast to cellular DNA polymerases, is characterized by two further properties: it is not 'fault proof', i.e. it is unable to differentiate between nucleosides of closely related structure, and it lacks error correcting attributes. These qualities have been utilized in the development of the principal drugs used for the treatment of HIV infection. The ability of the virus to continually modify its antigenic structure and thus elude the body's immune mechanisms and develop drug resistance can also be explained on the basis of these properties of reverse transcriptase (for further details about this unusual virus, refer to Beyond core: more about HIV).

Pathogenesis

Transmission of the virus occurs through intimate contact with an infected (HIV-positive) person or

---

BEYOND CORE

MORE ABOUT HIV

Structurally, HIV type 1 is characterized by a lipid envelope and transmembranous glycoproteins surrounding a protein casing that contains the viral RNA and several molecules of reverse transcriptase. Two classes of transmembranous glycoproteins of different molecular weight are recognized: gp40 and gp120. The latter interacts with specific receptors on the surface of CD4 human lymphocytes, the main target for the virus.

In addition to reverse transcriptase and structural proteins, the viral RNA codes for a protease. This enzyme is crucial for the assembly of the different components of the virus (which are produced by the machinery of the infected cell) into a new viral body.

The virus is sensitive to heat and to a range of chemical agents. It is unable to survive long outside the host.

exposure to untreated contaminated blood and blood products. In adults, unprotected homosexual and heterosexual intercourse as well as intravenous drug abuse are the usual settings for virus transmission. Transfusions of blood and blood products have become much less of a threat in the developed world since the mid-1980s, as a result of the rigorous testing of donors and the introduction of safeguards for blood handling and pretreatment of blood products by heat or other means.

The principal group of children at increased risk of acquiring the virus are infants born to HIV-positive mothers. It is now clear that a substantial number of these infants become infected during labour and the immediate postnatal period. Transplacental transmission of the virus is possible, particularly in the third trimester. Breast feeding is also a potential risk. The overall rate of vertical infection is estimated at 20–40%. Adolescents engaged in reckless sexual practices and intravenous drug abuse are also at increased risk for acquiring the HIV virus. This is a rapidly growing group, particularly in large cities.

In the host, the virus is capable of entering a number of different types of cells, but the main target is CD4 T lymphocytes. Initially, there is only low-grade virus multiplication, and the infection mostly stays 'dormant' for a variable length of time, but it is passed from cells to their progeny. At a certain point, under the influence of various immune modulators, the infected CD4 lymphocytes are stimulated, and the infection is reactivated. As a result, large-scale multiplication of the virus occurs, and the infected cells disintegrate.

Most of the sequelae of HIV infection can be explained in terms of loss of function of the CD4 cells. These cells normally display helper, cytotoxic and immunoregulatory activities, and the loss of these functions results in disregulation of the immune response and immunodeficiency. Opportunistic infections and malignancies, the hallmark of AIDS, follow.

In infants and young children, several features characterize the course of HIV infection:

- The phase of 'dormant' infection, which is associated with little or no clinical features, is relatively short.

- Many infections in this age group represent primary infections and tend to be severe. Severe bacterial and viral infections are major features of paediatric AIDS. Disease due to opportunistic agents such as *Pneumocystis carinii* and *Candida* can also be devastating, since the first exposure occurs in the absence of a normal immune response. Similarly, in adults with AIDS, disease due to the herpes viruses or tuberculosis frequently represents reactivation of previously acquired infections while, in infants with AIDS, they are primary infections causing severe disease.

- In a large proportion of infants, when the viral load is not so overwhelming, the multiplication of the HIV virus evokes an immune response which is characterized by the lymphoreticular reaction. Clinically, this reaction manifests itself by lymphadenopathy and hepatosplenomegaly. In the alveoli, the lymphoreticular infiltration results in a special form of alveolitis: lymphoid interstitial pneumonitis (LIP). LIP is a common presenting feature of paediatric AIDS.

- Malignancies are generally a rare manifestation of paediatric AIDS.

✴ KEY DIAGNOSIS

AIDS

Clinical features
Infected infants manifest no specific clinical features in the early stages after acquiring the infection. After an indeterminate length of time, however, symptoms and signs of chronic multisystem infection begin to appear before more specific features of severe immunodeficiency or LIP ensue, thus signifying the AIDS phase of HIV infection.

Features commonly encountered paediatric HIV infection are:

- Chronic diarrhoea, failure to thrive and delayed development.
- Recurrent bacterial and viral infection, particularly otitis media. More severe infections occur as the course of HIV infection progresses.
- Lymphadenopathy and hepatosplenomegaly.

291

- Opportunistic infections; *P. carinii* pneumonia (PCP) and *Candida* oesophagitis are particularly troublesome.
- Respiratory distress, cough and hypoxaemia, together with bilateral nodular infiltrates on chest radiography, which fail to clear in spite of adequate antibacterial therapy (including that for PCP), characterize LIP in an HIV-positive child.

LIP, PCP and *Candida* oesophagitis are 'AIDS defining', i.e. in an HIV-positive child they signify the progression to the AIDS phase of the disease.

The list above is far from being comprehensive; there are numerous additional features, including neurological signs, the nephrotic syndrome and thrombocytopenia.

Diagnosis

The diagnosis of HIV infection depends on the demonstration of a specific antibody response or the detection of the virus or its components in the blood.

The presence of anti-HIV antibodies can be demonstrated employing the ELISA or Western blot techniques, both of which are highly sensitive and specific. In adults, there is usually a gap of around 2 months from the time of acquiring the virus to the appearance of detectable specific antibodies. Infants who are infected perinatally are thought to start to display an immune response, with production of their own specific anti-HIV antibodies, at around 4–6 months of age. The situation is, however, further complicated by the fact that maternal anti-HIV antibodies are transferred transplacentally to the fetuses of HIV-positive mothers, sometimes in very high titres. An uninfected infant born to an HIV-positive mother can thus test positive for anti-HIV antibodies for up to 12–18 months after birth.

Detection of the viral RNA is possible using the PCR. Detection of the various fractions of the viral proteins and isolation of the virus itself are also possible. These tests are generally of high specificity. Other laboratory findings include lymphopenia, with reduction of the CD4 lymphocyte count, and neutropenia. Anaemia and thrombocytopenia are frequently present. Total

serum immunoglobulin levels are usually elevated, reflecting disregulation of immune function.

Treatment

The aims of treatment are to decrease the viral load using antiviral agents, to enhance the immune function and to treat and prevent the infections which complicate the course of this condition.

Antiviral agents include AZT (zidovudine) and DDI (didehydroxyinosine). These are synthetic nucleotide analogues which cannot be distinguished from the naturally occurring nucleotides by the viral reverse transcriptase and are utilized in the building of the DNA molecule during reverse transcription. However, because these analogues lack the correct binding sites, their incorporation leads to termination of the viral DNA chain. Cellular DNA polymerase is not susceptible to this effect.

Other antiviral drugs include viral protease inhibitors and a host of other agents, many of which are still at the experimental stage. Because of the unusual ability of the HIV virus to mutate, several strains of the virus, including drug-resistant strains, are frequently encountered in the one patient. It is therefore necessary to use combination antiviral therapy. At present, the recommendation is to use triple therapy (AZT, DDI and a protease inhibitor) in patients with AIDS and also early in HIV-positive individuals, since this has been shown to slow the progression to AIDS.

Immunoglobulin transfusions are used for replacement if deficiency is demonstrated. Infections should be detected early and treated vigorously. PCP prophylaxis (co-trimoxazole three times weekly) is an important aspect of management.

Prevention

The rate of transmission of infection to infants from HIV-positive mothers can be significantly reduced by the administration of AZT to the mother during pregnancy and to the infant in the first 6 weeks of life, starting as soon as possible after birth.

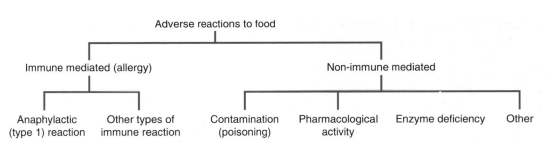

Figure 14.10   Adverse reactions to food

In the absence of a national HIV screening programme during pregnancy, it is likely that some women will continue to be unaware of their HIV-positive status until after delivery, and therefore after the window of opportunity to prevent transmission to the infant has closed. There is thus a strong case for establishing a screening programme, but issues such as confidentiality, eligibility for insurance and employment need to be considered.

ALLERGIC REACTIONS

The term 'allergy' refers to an acquired state of altered reactivity to a particular substance that is mediated by immune mechanisms and results in adverse physiological effects.

Any substance, whether inhaled, ingested or in contact with the body, has the potential to result in adverse physiological effects. Some substances (e.g. tobacco smoke and other irritants) are capable of causing physiological disturbances in any person exposed to them (non-specific); others may lead to adverse reactions only in a minority of people. If no immune mechanisms are involved in such abnormal reactivity, the term 'intolerance' rather than allergy should be used (see Ch. 5). A common example of such a state of affairs is lactose intolerance due to lactase deficiency, whether congenital or acquired. Figure 14.10 illustrates the various mechanisms involved in adverse reactions to food.

The immunological mechanisms which mediate allergy are largely the same mechanisms involved in body defences against infection and other immune functions. Whether an immune reaction

against a particular substance is viewed as allergic or part of a 'physiological' immune response depends on the context in which such a reaction occurs and on whether it makes physiological sense or not.

The type 1 allergic reaction (IgE-mediated, anaphylactic) is implicated in a number of common and important illnesses of childhood, including hay fever, asthma and a significant number of cases of food allergy. The role of IgE-mediated allergy in eczema is uncertain. Hay fever and eczema are discussed in Chapter 13, and asthma in Chapter 6. A brief outline of food allergy is provided here.

✴ KEY DIAGNOSIS

Food allergy

Allergic reactions to food are the cause of significant morbidity in children and occasionally may result in fatality. In clinical practice, anaphylactic (IgE-mediated, type 1) reactions are usually the underlying mechanism in a significant number of cases with acute presentation. In cases with a more chronic course (e.g. coeliac disease and some cases of cow's milk allergy), other immune mechanisms are operational.

Common food items implicated in the majority of reported cases of food allergy include milk, eggs, wheat, peanuts, nuts and fish. Reactions to peanuts have received a great deal of publicity of late and the frequency of reported cases seems to be increasing. Food allergies tend to worsen in the first few years of life.

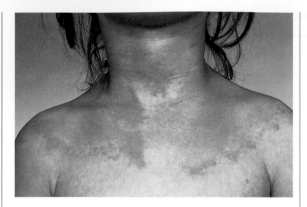

Figure 14.11 Urticaria in a child. Note the raised erythematous skin lesions of irregular shape

Clinical features

The principal clinical manifestations of IgE-mediated allergy to food include:

- Urticaria/angio-oedema
- Laryngeal/bronchial obstruction
- Anaphylactic shock.

Urticaria (Fig. 14.11) is the typical skin manifestation of IgE-mediated allergy. In food allergy, the urticarial rash is usually generalized, and consists of erythematous raised skin lesions of irregular shape and size. It results from dilatation and increased permeability of the capillaries in response to the action of histamine released as result of the interaction of the antigen with the mast cell-bound IgE. Angio-oedema results from swelling of deeper layers of skin. Severe swelling of the face and nasopharynx may compromise the airway.

Laryngeal oedema and bronchial obstruction result in the croup syndrome (see Ch. 6) and asthma-type attacks, respectively, and may occur together in the same patient. Laryngeal oedema and bronchial obstruction may be severe enough to cause serious respiratory embarrassment. These syndromes can occur in isolation (as the sole manifestation of the allergic reaction), as part of anaphylactic shock or with other allergic manifestations.

Anaphylactic shock results from generalized vasodilatation in response to histamine and other allergic mediators. The resulting relative hypovolaemia leads to hypotension and poor perfusion. Clinically, the initial symptoms are tingling around the mouth, tightness in the chest and apprehension. The skin is flushed, and there is usually increased sweating. Stridor and wheezing are frequently present. The pulse rate is variable but is usually increased. As the condition progresses, the patient becomes hypotensive, and consciousness is lost.

Treatment

Allergic reactions resulting in anaphylactic shock and/or severe respiratory distress are paediatric emergencies. Adrenaline is the life-saving treatment, and should be given as soon as possible. The dose is 0.1 ml/10 kg of the 1:1000 solution (10 mcg/kg) subcutaneously or intramuscularly. This can be repeated at 15–20 min intervals if necessary. Securing the airway by endotracheal intubation (if possible) or tracheostomy may be required. Intravenous fluids should be given for persistent hypotension. Antihistamines and steroids are useful, but they are second-line drugs. Since the allergic reaction may outlast the action of the initial therapy, careful observation in hospital for at least 24 h after improvement is necessary.

Nebulized adrenaline is the treatment of choice for less severe allergic laryngeal oedema (which accounts for some cases of spasmodic croup, see Ch. 6). The treatment of bronchial obstruction is along the lines recommended for asthma. Inhaled or intramuscular adrenaline is also indicated in cases of urticaria/angio-oedema accompanied by respiratory embarrassment. Antihistamines alone are effective in most cases of acute uncomplicated urticaria.

Avoidance is the key to long-term management of children with food allergy. However, this aspect of management frequently proves difficult: children's eating habits are difficult to control, and continuous supervision is not possible. Moreover, food labelling is often inadequate, and many food products contain items beyond what is declared on the label. The involvement of a paediatric dietician is frequently necessary, and the efforts of the family need to be coordinated with those of the school or nursery.

Because of the fulminant nature of the severe anaphylactic reactions, children with a documented history of anaphylactic shock or respiratory embarrassment following exposure to unavoidable or ubiquitous allergens (e.g. insect stings, peanuts), should be supplied with ready-to-inject adrenaline via a device such as the Epipen. It comes in two strengths: 0.15 mg of adrenaline 1:1000 for children aged over 7 years and 0.3 mg for children aged below 7 years (in the same volume of 0.3 ml). The indications and method for its use should be carefully explained and demonstrated to the parents and other care providers, including school teachers when appropriate.

Drug reactions

Beyond the neonatal period, adverse reactions to drugs are less common in children than in adults. This reflects the relative infrequency of renal or hepatic impairment in children and the fact that children are less likely to be on multiple-drug therapy.

As with food, drug reactions can be mediated by immune or non-immune mechanisms. In the case of drugs, the majority of the observed reactions are non-immune in nature and related, in one way or another, to the pharmacological activity of the drug (toxicity, side-effects, idiosyncratic reactions, interaction with another drug).

Immune-mediated reactions to drugs (i.e. drug allergy) can also be in the type 1 (anaphylactic, IgE mediated) category or due to other immune reactions. Figure 14.12 illustrates the main categories of drug reactions, with some common examples.

FURTHER READING

Behrman R E, Kliegman R M, Arvin A M 1996 Nelson textbook of pediatrics, 15th edn. Saunders, London
David T J 1993 Recent advances in paediatrics – 12. Churchill Livingstone, Edinburgh
David T J 1994 Recent advances in paediatrics – 13. Churchill Livingstone, Edinburgh
Davies E G, Elliman D A C, Hart C A, Nicoll A, Rudd P T 1996 Manual of childhood infections. Saunders, London

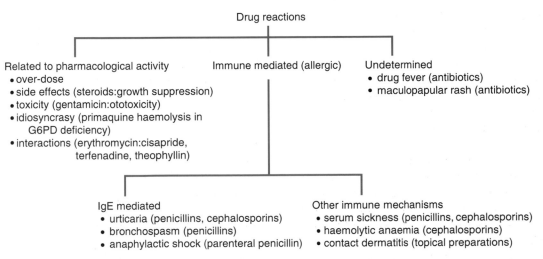

Figure 14.12 Drug reactions

CHAPTER 15

Accidents

A. Habel

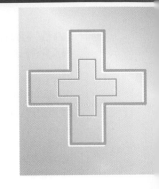

CORE PROBLEMS OF ACCIDENTS

CORE PROBLEM	KEY DIAGNOSIS	RELATED TOPICS
• Road traffic accident	Head injury	Other road traffic accident injuries
• Thermal injury	Scald	Flame burns and smoke inhalation Contact and electrical burns Disfigurement
• Drowning	Freshwater drowning	
• Swallowed foreign bodies		Inhaled foreign bodies
• Poisoning	Paracetemol ingestion	Tricyclic antidepressants, iron and aspirin Household substances Plants and berries
• Cot death	Sudden infant death syndrome	Near miss or acute life-threatening experience

ESSENTIAL BACKGROUND

INTRODUCTION

In the developing world, 97% of childhood deaths are caused by infection. In contrast, the developed world's epidemic is accidental injury (Table 15.1). It is the commonest cause of death from the end of the neonatal period to early adult life, and is a leading cause of disability, years of life lost, and health services costs. Each year in the UK about 500 children die and probably 10 000 suffer long-term consequences to their health.

Comparing all leading causes of child trauma in the UK they are, in rank order, road traffic accidents (RTAs), drowning, non-accidental injury and burns.

Throughout the world, but particularly in the developing world, exposure to weapons results in major indiscriminate injury, and is of increasing international concern (see Ch. 20). Landmines became the focus of media attention in 1997 through Diana, Princess of Wales, and are a significant cause in areas of recent armed conflict. The USA has witnessed a 60% increase in childhood firearm injuries (mainly accidental) over the past decade.

Table 15.1 Deaths from accidents in children under 15 years (UK, 1995)		
Type of accident	*Deaths*	*%*
Road traffic accidents	244	49
Home:		
Suffocation, submersion, choking	110	23
Burns, fires	69	15
Poisoning	6	3
Other	51	10
Total	486	100

Age distribution: 40% under 5 years, 25% 5–9 years, 35% aged 10–14 years

WHY UNINTENTIONAL INJURIES HAPPEN AND TO WHOM

The processes of development in physical growth, intellectual curiosity and behaviour present new opportunities and hence new hazards to the child.

Up to the age of 4 years most accidents take place in the home. They result from exploratory behaviour, without a sense of danger having yet developed. Examples include sources of heat (e.g. fires, irons, scalding hot water, ovens) and ingestion of untried substances such as tablets or caustic cleaning materials. In addition, young children have little perception of time and space as, for example, they step off a moving merry-go-round or in front of a swing.

Over 5 years of age there is increased risk taking. RTAs predominate, mainly as pedestrians. Children appear unable to interpret the direction, speed and contrary streams of traffic. Their small size prevents them being seen easily and, whereas an adult is hit in the leg, a small child may suffer head or neck injury.

In adolescence, peer pressure and desire to conform to the group increases the risks of alcohol and substance abuse and sexual activities. Self-poisoning may result from depression or acting-out behaviour. Boys generally take greater risks, and so have twice as many accidents as girls.

Although the term 'accident-prone child' has little scientific validity, unintentional injuries are more frequent in children with attention deficit and impulsive behaviour. However, if adequate resources are available to provide the necessary supervision for these children and to improve the safety of their surroundings, both the frequency and severity of accidental injuries can be reduced. Poverty, on the other hand, increases the likelihood of accidents, both in the home and while playing in the streets. Unintentional injuries are more frequent among emotionally deprived and disorganized families.

Despite ample legislation aimed at increased safety protection, and perhaps because of educational initiatives which are more likely to be taken up by the professional classes who tend to live in safer environments, the gap in mortality rate from accidents between the better

off and worst off in society has widened over the past decade.

The cause of an injury must always be assessed: was it unintentional, deliberate or from negligence? The term 'non-accidental injury' not only means deliberate acts which present as burns, organ damage, bruising or fractures, but should also include persistent neglect, i.e. failure to protect the child from the hazards he or she normally faces.

MORBIDITY AND MORTALITY DUE TO ACCIDENTS

Morbidity

Short-term morbidity in Britain

There are 2.2 million attendances at accident and emergency departments annually. Of these, 1 million are from home and 1.2 million from road, garden or playground accidents and sportsfield injuries. For accidents in the home, the order of frequency is being hit by an object > cuts > foreign body > burns and scalds > poisoning. Over 125 000 injured children are admitted annually to hospital for further treatment.

Long-term morbidity

Permanent injury, with loss of function and hence skills to society result in a drain on the community's resources. Probably 10 000 children are disabled in this way annually.

Mortality

Injury prevention

Mortality has been reduced by a fifth in the last decade as a result of a variety of strategies.

Most successful strategies for injury prevention are automatic (passive) strategies, e.g. safety caps on medication bottles and fire alarms. A change in behaviour, or active strategy, needs acceptance and compliance each time, e.g. wearing a bicycle helmet. Warning labels on medicines and poisons are far less effective than safety caps.

Legislation plays an important part in enforcing change, e.g. fire retardant in furniture fabrics and fillings decreases mortality in house fires by 80%, while seat belt legislation for rear seat passengers lowers mortality by over 50%. Injury prevention strategies can be primary, secondary or tertiary.

- *Primary prevention*: avert injury by preventing the accident from happening; anticipatory guidance, warning parents of dangers and telling them what action to take, are shown to be effective in infancy. Examples of successful interventions include:
  - Stair and fire guards
  - Safety caps for medicines, which reduced salicylate ingestion by 85% within 3 years
  - Traffic calming and reducing speed from 40 to 20 mph cuts mortality from 100 to 5% for pedestrian children
  - Reducing tap water temperature from 60°C, which causes a full-thickness scald in 2 s, to 50°C, which scalds after 10 min
  - Successful local initiatives in which a health visitor does a home safety check.
- *Secondary prevention*: reduce severity of injury to the individual, e.g. car seat belts, bike helmets, and safe landing areas in playgrounds.
- *Tertiary prevention*: minimize the lasting effects, e.g. improved emergency resuscitation, and rehabilitation.

CORE PROBLEMS

ROAD TRAFFIC ACCIDENTS

Injuries and death resulting from RTAs occur predominantly in pedestrians, with the UK rate among the highest in Europe, then car occupants and cyclists. Boys are nine times more at risk of injury than girls.

Children often sustain both head injury and multiple trauma. If multiple trauma is present the BBBB rule should be used to assess carefully **b**reathing, **b**leeding, **b**rain, **b**one in conjunction with the ABC of **a**irway, **b**reathing and **c**irculation, which applies in all emergency situations.

✱ KEY DIAGNOSIS

Head injury

Head injury is relatively more common in children than adults, and should always be suspected if any of the following are observed or reported: loss of consciousness (however brief), vomiting, headache, diplopia, inappropriate drowsiness, seizures and coma.

Assessment and management principles

Signs of central herniation through the foramen magnum include neck stiffness, slow pulse, raised blood pressure and irregular breathing. Brain herniation through the tentorium causes unilateral dilatation of the pupil, inability of the eye to move medially and hemiplegia. Cervical spine injury may have occurred, and must be assumed until fully assessed.

Primary brain damage from tears and contusion should be prevented from progressing to secondary damage by early recognition and treatment of hypoxia, ischaemia, loss of homeostasis, hypoglycaemia and convulsions.

Central to management is the fact that cerebral perfusion pressure is equal to mean arterial pressure minus mean intracranial pressure. Young children are particularly vulnerable to cerebral hypoperfusion because their blood pressure is normally lower than adults, while the intracranial pressure is the same. A drop in the perfusion pressure of blood to the brain will reduce the oxygen supply, and thus tend to extend tissue damage. Acute brain swelling, i.e. cerebral oedema of any severity, needs neurosurgical consultation and mechanical ventilation to stabilize the P_{CO_2} between 3.5 and 4.2 kPa. This procedure reduces dilatation of the cerebral circulation and thus reduces the movement of water into brain tissue (see Ch. 10).

Whilst making every effort to maintain normal blood pressure, fluids should be restricted in head injury to 70% of normal in order to limit brain oedema, which may be exacerbated by the syndrome of inappropriate antidiuretic hormone (SIADH) secretion.

Monitoring the level of consciousness is standardized by applying the Glasgow Coma Scale (GCS), modified for children under 4 years of age, to assess for responsiveness to commands, interaction with surroundings, consolability, and for emergence of decorticate (abnormal flexion to pain) or decerebrate (abnormal extension to pain) postures.

Children may have a subdural collection of blood without a fracture, and hence a routine skull radiograph is of limited value. A brain computerized tomography (CT) scan should always be considered if the GCS is significantly reduced and head injury likely, irrespective of whether external injury is evident or not.

Other RTA injuries

In addition to head injuries, other life-threatening injuries include crush injuries of the abdomen and pelvis, traumatic amputation of a limb and massive open long bone fractures. Complications which should be anticipated include pneumothorax, hypovolaemic shock from fracture sites, torn blood vessels or ruptured organs, ileus and pneumoperitoneum from ruptured intestine, acute kidney failure from shock, and rupture or massive muscle damage releasing myoglobin (which may aggravate renal damage).

Management

Close monitoring of the circulation is necessary. Appropriate fluid therapy should be initiated in order to maintain adequate blood pressure and normoglycaemia. Blood transfusions may be required to correct anaemia from blood loss. Pain can significantly worsen shock, and effective analgesia must be given if indicated. Investigations include urgent blood count and cross match, radiography of the skeleton, and radiography and ultrasound for intra-abdominal intestinal and organ injury.

Prevention

- In the car: mandatory use of baby seats, seat belts in front and back seats
- Pedestrians: road safety training, reflective clothing at night
- Cyclists: helmet (approved design) and cycling proficiency courses

THERMAL INJURY

Assessment of thermal injuries

Immediate action on coming upon an incident is as follows: do a primary survey; resuscitate; once the child is stabilized, do a secondary survey.

Primary survey

The primary survey concentrates on the basic functions necessary for life. First of all establish whether a thermal airway injury is evident by history, deposits around the mouth and nose, or carbonaceous sputum. The whole body should be examined. This should be complete but rapid to prevent heat loss, which can be swift in burnt children.

Assess ABC:

- *Airway and cervical spine*. Ensure the airway is unobstructed. Take precautions to avoid further possible cervical spine injury until such injury has been excluded. Log roll and apply a cervical collar. Intubation and ventilation may be indicated.
- *Breathing*. Look for chest movement, listen for breath sounds, feel for breath on your cheek. Give 100% oxygen by face mask if available.
- *Circulation*. Feel for the carotid artery. Since infants tend to have short fat necks, the brachial artery may be more easily palpated.

Inadequate or absent respiration or pulse requires immediate initiation of resuscitation procedures. Drowsiness or coma or may be due to shock, head injury or smoke inhalation causing hypoxia.

Secondary survey

The secondary survey detects other problems needing attention. Additional injuries, such as those sustained from a fall while escaping a fire, or falling objects, as well as the burn area and depth, should be assessed at this stage.

Assess the burn. Is it superficial/partial thickness, with blistering and pink or mottled skin and sensation intact, or full thickness with white or charred skin and absent pain sensation, or a combination of the two? Does it involve areas with special management needs, e.g. the face, hands (scarring causing loss of function) and perineum (prone to infection).

What is the extent of the injury? Express the area as a percentage of body area (Fig. 15.1). The relative surface area of the head and limbs varies with age, and the adult rule of nines only applies

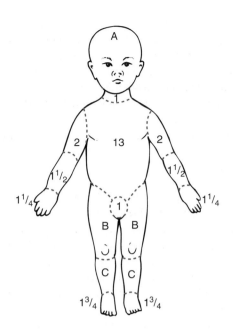
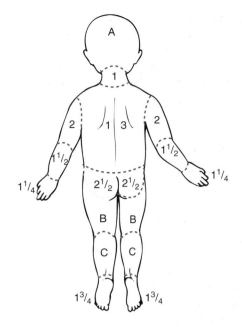

Relative percentages of areas affected by growth						
Area	Age 0	Age 1	Age 5	Age 10	Age 15	Adult
A = $^1/_2$ of head	$9^1/_2$	$8^1/_2$	$6^1/_2$	$5^1/_2$	$4^1/_2$	$3^1/_2$
B = $^1/_2$ of one thigh	$2^3/_4$	$3^1/_4$	4	$4^1/_4$	$4^1/_2$	$4^3/_4$
C = $^1/_2$ of one leg	$2^1/_2$	$2^1/_2$	$2^3/_4$	3	$3^1/_4$	$3^1/_2$

Figure 15.1 Percentage assessment of extent of burns in a child

over 14 years of age. In younger children use age-appropriate charts. Alternatively, use the child's own hand, which equals 1% of the surface area.

Essentials of general management

- Pain relief must be effective. Morphine is often best for everything other than minor burns.
- Fluid. Initially to support the circulation, then replacement of fluids exuding from the burn. Monitor blood pressure and urinary output to prevent prerenal failure from inadequate fluid therapy.
- Haemoglobin replacement. Anaemia results from red cells being destroyed in the injured tissues.

- Temperature monitoring is essential as children can quickly lose heat by evaporation from extensively damaged areas. Raise the environmental temperature with heaters.
- Occlusive dressings to protect the damaged areas from infection. Analgesia may be needed when changing dressings. Tight Tubigrip or special elasticated garments worn for months help reduce scar formation.
- Watch for signs of infection, take swabs and prescribe antibiotics appropriately.
- Skin grafting may be necessary. Split skin is suitable for most purposes, and full-thickness grafts over pressure points and for some cosmetic situations.

* KEY DIAGNOSIS

Scald

Scalds are far and away the most common form of thermal injury in children. Hot water or oil from a cup, kettle or cooking pot in the kitchen or dining area account for the majority of such injuries. Bathroom scalds occur in preschool children. Beware of deliberate immersion, characterized by glove and stocking distribution on the limbs, or 'doughnut' scald in which injury occurs from hot water around the lower back and upper thighs, sparing the buttocks, which are protected by being pressed against the cooler bathtub wall.

First aid and prevention

Immerse the affected part in cold/iced water for 10 min to reduce or contain the extent of tissue damage. Cover with a dry dressing, but do not apply creams. Blisters should not be pricked or de-roofed. Preventative measures include the use of cooker guards, keeping pot handles to the back or side, the use of coiled kettle flexes and avoiding hot drinks or smoking while holding a child. The bath temperature should be checked with the elbow, running in cold water first. Water heater temperature, which is usually set at 60–70°C in the UK will not scald if reset at the lower temperature of 50°C.

Flame burns and inhalation

Half of all fires in the home are caused by cigarette smoking. Respiratory injury results from hot gases, showing as sooty or singed nasal hairs or carbon particles in the sputum. Carbon monoxide poisoning results from incomplete combustion in a household fire or a faulty gas appliance, and accounts for a third of deaths associated with burns. Combustion of older fabrics containing cyanides causes sudden death in about a half of deaths from house fires. Respiratory failure results from airway obstruction, bronchoconstriction, asphyxia, and the toxic effects of poisonous gases. Treatment is with oxygen, airway care, early intubation and ventilation.

Preventative measures include installation of smoke alarms and the use of flame-retardant furniture and fabrics; keep matches and candles out of reach; check gas heaters are adequately ventilated. Parents should avoid smoking in bed.

Contact and electrical burns

These occur from coming in contact with hot surfaces, e.g. a cigarette, hot plate, toaster, iron or radiant heater. The possibility of non-accidental injury should always be considered. A distribution over the buttocks, hands and feet makes deliberate injury more likely. Examination of the edge of a burn may help in cigarette burns – an irregular margin is likely from an accidental brush whereas a clearly circular edge suggests abuse from a deliberate stubbing action.

Mouthing of a live connector or poorly insulated cable produces lip and mouth burns; insertion of fingers or metal implements into sockets causes hand burns. Both may result in electrocution.

BEYOND CORE

CARBON MONOXIDE POISONING

Haemoglobin has 200 times the affinity for carbon monoxide compared with oxygen. The half-life of the carbon monoxide–haemoglobin complex, carboxyhaemoglobin, is 2–5 h.

Acute poisoning causes coma, convulsions, and death when carboxyhaemoglobin comprises more than 50% of the total haemoglobin. The appearance is often pale, but venous blood looks arterial. Ischaemic changes and extrasystoles appear on the electrocardiogram.

Treatment is 100% oxygen, or hyperbaric oxygen (located at designated hospitals and Royal Navy diving schools).

Chronic exposure to low concentrations causes headache, flu-like symptoms, or symptoms similar to those of food poisoning.

Disfigurement

The child may have to come to terms with being visibly different. In the process, behaviour difficulties, teasing, and absence from school for treatment contributing to poor academic performance may be problems. The experience of James Partridge, burnt in a house fire at 18 years of age, led him to set up Changing Faces, a charitable foundation dedicated to helping the social adjustment of such individuals. A valuable insight is given in his and others recounting of their experiences of congenital and acquired facial disfigurement in *Visibly Different, Coping with Disfigurement* (see Further reading).

DROWNING

This is the third commonest cause of accidental death after RTAs and burns. The location (with declining frequency) is an unsupervised bath at home, garden ponds, private swimming pools, occasionally lakes and rivers, and the sea. It is commonest in the preschool child, then adolescent boys.

✳ KEY DIAGNOSIS

Fresh water drowning

Pathophysiology
Sudden immersion in very cold water results in the diving reflex found only in young children – apnoea, and shunting of blood to the head and heart. Eventually gasping leads to inhalation, finally hypoxia and cardiorespiratory arrest. Very little water may actually enter the lungs.

Freshwater drowning is exacerbated by hyperkalaemia due to hypo-osmotic lysis of red blood cells, which may cause cardiac arrhythmias; salt water death is slower, by asphyxia due to the hypertonic sea water (approximately 500 mOsm/l) pulling water from the circulation into the lung lumen.

Resuscitation
The duration of resuscitation attempts has special significance if drowning occurs in cold or icy water as hypothermia protects the brain against hypoxia. It should continue for at least an hour, even if initially the pupils are fixed and dilated, and until the core temperature is greater than 33°C. Heart arrhythmias are common during the rewarming process. However, cold-water drowning has a better prognosis than warm-water drowning; half of so-called 'lifeless' children survive following cold-water drowning, with only a small number severely brain damaged.

Investigations
These should include electrolytes, looking for hyperkalaemia, which is likely in freshwater drowning, blood gases reflecting the degree of acute hypoxia and chest radiography for lung changes due to water aspiration.

SWALLOWED FOREIGN BODY

- Preschool children can swallow such objects as stones, coins, ring pulls of drink cans and mercury cells. Ulceration, perforation and stricture can occur. Oesophageal hold-up requires urgent endoscopy.
- Sharp and long objects are the most likely to cause perforation. Abdominal pain and tenderness and failure of an object to progress radiologically in 24 h are each independent indications for surgery.

Inhaled foreign body

Problems relating to the inhalation of foreign bodies by children are discussed in Chapter 6.

POISONING

Although poisoning as the cause of death in the UK is mainly due to tricyclic antidepressants, thousands of children with suspected poisoning are brought to accident and emergency departments every year. Just over half of ingested poisons are medicines, while household products comprise most of the remainder. Plants and seeds make up the rest, and rarely cause serious problems. In contrast, kerosene (paraffin) is the single most important ingestant in developing countries, and deaths due to aspiration pneumonia and its complications are not uncommon.

Among medicines, tricyclic antidepressants and opiates have replaced salicylate, iron and barbiturates as the most important causes of morbidity and mortality. Tricyclic antidepressants (e.g. for enuresis) should not be prescribed to children who are, or have siblings, under 5 years of age. Child-resistant containers have been largely responsible for the observed reduction in deaths in the UK over the past 20 years. However, since 1 in 5 preschool children can open them, new solutions are still required.

Clinical features

Poisoned children may present with a history of ingestion or with other suggestive features:

- Sudden inexplicable illness
- Repeated encephalopathic illness with change in conscious level or seizures
- 'Drunk' or in coma from substance abuse, either inhaled or ingested
- The unexpected finding of medication in body fluids.

Where there are suspicious circumstances surrounding the poisoning in a child, particularly if of a repeated nature, the 'Munchausen by proxy' syndrome should be suspected. This is a form of child abuse in which an adult deliberately inflicts harm on a child in order to get attention, medical or otherwise, for him- or herself.

Management principles

Examination may elicit specific clinical signs indicating the type of poison, if previously unknown, its severity and the degree of urgency required for drug elimination, antidotes and other treatments.

Confirmation from the history and/or examination of a drug ingestion which has a specific antidote may be an indication for its use, depending on severity. Examples include naloxone for opiates, acetylcysteine for paracetamol (protection from liver injury, see later), Digibind, a ligand for digoxin poisoning, and chelating agents such as deferrioxamine, specific for iron ingestion. Regional poison information centres have a wealth of information and advice to give, and should be contacted.

Methods of drug elimination

Stomach emptying

There is little evidence that stomach emptying is beneficial and, in the majority of cases of poisoning, most of the ingested substance has already passed into the small intestine by the time the child reaches hospital. Furthermore, stomach emptying is associated with the risk of aspiration; this is particularly true in cases with depressed sensorium or impaired cough reflex. Some

---

BEYOND CORE

EFFECTS OF METABOLIC DIFFERENCES IN CHILDREN

Metabolic responses to excessive amounts of chemical substances, including drugs, do not just depend on size but on the maturation of metabolic processes. These may act to the detriment of the child, for example by prolonging the half-life of drugs such as theophylline, or increasing metabolic acidosis in salicylism. In paracetamol poisoning, however, the young have greater protection than older children and adults from its toxic effects because of their greater production of glutathione, which conjugates with paracetamol.

Hypoglycaemia may occur in alcohol poisoning in children by inhibition of gluconeogenesis. Some children, particularly those who are underweight or slim built, may be excessively susceptible to this effect of alcohol; profound hypoglycaemia has been documented in such children following exposure to a small amount of alcohol, such as a sip of a parent's drink or a leftover cocktail. The ataxia, slurred speech and loss of coordination induced by the hypoglycaemia may be misinterpreted as drunkenness.

substances pose far greater risks to the child if inhaled than if ingested, because of their potential to damage the lungs. For example, hydrocarbons are associated with little systemic toxicity unless ingested in a large amount (which is unlikely because of the unpleasant taste). Aspiration of hydrocarbons, however, may lead to severe respiratory failure.

Corrosives are another class of substances which, should stomach emptying be performed following ingestion, may cause further damage on their second passage through the oesophagus. The risks of aspiration and irritation of the nasopharynx and upper airways are also substantial. Stomach emptying should not generally be attempted if the child is seen more than 2 h following ingestion (longer in cases where normal gastric emptying is expected to be hindered such as in cases of ingestion of drugs with anticholinergic activity, e.g. antidepressants, or those causing stomach irritation, e.g. salicylates).

In summary, the decision to attempt stomach emptying should be based on the balance between the possible benefits and potential risks in each individual case. Stomach emptying can be achieved by ipecacuanha syrup BP if conscious or gastric lavage with water or antidote if unconscious, taking suitable precautions to protect the airway.

Activated charcoal

One gram of activated charcoal has a surface area of 1000 m² for adsorption. Its modes of action are threefold: immediate contact and adsorption in the gut; interruption of the enterohepatic circulation of drugs secreted in bile (e.g. tricyclics); gut dialysis against the rich capillary network in the intestine. It is useful in mild to moderate aspirin poisoning, and is especially effective against tricyclic antidepressants. It should ideally be given within 2 h of ingestion.

Peritoneal or renal dialysis

This may be useful in certain cases, e.g. severe salicylate poisoning.

Investigations

Blood testing for specific substances, e.g. salicylate, paracetamol, and serum iron, should be arranged.

If the presenting illness suggests poisoning, especially if abuse is likely, urine and blood for toxicology screen should be saved. An electrocardiogram (ECG) can be very helpful if tricyclic antidepressants have been ingested, as it may detect tacchyarrhythmias, heart block, and slurred QRS complexes. Psychiatric referral is indicated if deliberate self-poisoning has occurred.

✱ KEY DIAGNOSIS

Paracetamol ingestion

The increased use of paracetamol because of the association of aspirin with Reye's syndrome (see Ch. 10) has resulted in more accidental ingestions in preschool children, as well as in adolescents who deliberately self-poison. However, unlike adolescents and adults, liver failure is rare in children under 6 years because they conjugate more of the drug and metabolize less via cytochrome P450 which, when swamped, produces a hepatotoxic intermediate metabolite.

The stages of paracetamol poisoning are:

1. Minor nausea, vomiting, and sweating in the first 24 h
2. Feeling better in the next 24 h
3. Onset of liver failure at 2–4 days
4. Death or resolution by 7 days.

Management

In addition to general measures of emesis, gastric lavage and activated charcoal, acetylcysteine, an antidote which metabolizes to glutathione, is given intravenously. This conjugates with the paracetamol in the liver, rendering it harmless. Acetylcysteine must be given within 16 h of ingestion to be effective, but is indicated only if the blood level taken at least 4 h after ingestion displays toxic levels.

Tricyclic antidepressants

This class of medication can be associated with severe toxicity and carries a high mortality risk. Tricyclic drugs influence the body's autonomic functions with prominent anticholinergic activity. The main consequences of overdose are cardiotoxicity and neurotoxicity.

Anticholinergic effects (dilated pupils, delirium, tachycardia) are the earliest features and cardiac conduction delay and arrhythmias occur. Hyper- or hypotension are important features. Convulsions, abnormal movements and coma are manifestations of the neurotoxic effects. In some cases, initially mild manifestations are followed by rapid deterioration.

Tricyclic antidepressants have a large volume of distribution and are extensively bound to tissue proteins and other cellular sites. Because toxic effects of these drugs are determined by tissue levels, plasma levels are of little value in predicting severity. Children with a history of tricyclic antidepressant ingestion who exhibit any manifestations of toxicity, however mild, should be admitted for observation and monitoring for at least 24 h regardless of blood levels. The ECG can be extremely helpful in making the diagnosis. Alkalization helps reduce the cardiotoxic effects. The arrhythmia may require drug treatment or cardiac pacing.

Iron

The effect of ingestion of iron tablets has four stages:

1. Local irritation: presentation within an hour with epigastric pain, vomiting, haematemesis and bloody diarrhoea. Hypotension and shock are present in severe cases.
2. A quiet period of apparent improvement for up to 16 h follows. This may induce complacency, but absorbed iron is accumulating in the tissues during this period.
3. Metabolic manifestations appear as mitochondrial and other cellular metabolic activities are disrupted. Hypoglycaemia and acidosis may occur. Severe liver necrosis may follow.
4. The final stage is one of scarring in the stomach and intestine causing obstruction severe enough to require surgery weeks or months later.

Iron tablets are radioopaque, and abdominal radiographs may be helpful in making the diagnosis. Leucocytosis is frequently present. The free iron level in plasma (calculated from total serum iron and iron-binding capacity) is helpful in the prediction of possible toxicity, but the presence of symptoms is an indication of toxicity, no matter what the free iron levels are.

Intensive support of the circulation and breathing may be necessary. The antidote desferrioxamine, a chelating agent, is administered intravenously in cases in which the iron blood level is sufficiently high, or significant poisoning is likely on clinical grounds.

Aspirin

This type of poisoning is now quite uncommon in children since recommendations against routine use were adopted because of an association with Reye's syndrome. It is included here because it illustrates important toxicology principles and age-related differences.

Pathophysiology and clinical features

- Central stimulating effects on the central nervous system cause anxiety, central respiratory stimulation, sweating, tachycardia, tinnitus, vomiting, progressing to delirium, convulsions and coma.
- Uncoupling of oxidative phosphorylation results in fever and increased respiration due to increased metabolic needs.
- Acid–base changes vary according to the time elapsed from the overdose. Initially, the direct stimulatory effect of salicylates on the respiratory centre leads to hyperventilation and respiratory alkalosis. Later, the inhibitory effect of salicylates on the Krebs cycle leads to metabolic acidosis. In young infants, the metabolic effects predominate whereas in adolescents, hyperventilation is prominent and may initially be misinterpreted as 'hysterical'.
- Other metabolic derangements include hypoglycaemia, hyperglycaemia and ketone body formation.
- Progression to hypotension, pulmonary and cerebral oedema, renal failure and death occurs in severe untreated cases.

Management issues

Delayed absorption is common, especially if enteric-coated tablets have been ingested. An early blood salicylate level at 2–3 h (usual time of peak concentration) can therefore be misleading. Salicylate serum levels at 6 h can be interpreted more confidently as to severity and likely outcome (mild poisoning, <2.9 mmol/l; lethal poisoning, >8.8 mmol/l).

Appropriate fluid therapy and correction of electrolyte and glucose abnormalities as well as other metabolic disturbances are crucial. Vitamin K should be given if the prothrombin time is prolonged.

As salicylate is retained in the stomach, removal should be attempted by inducing emesis or gastric lavage up to 24 h after ingestion, instilling sodium bicarbonate and activated charcoal. Elimination through the kidneys is enhanced by alkalization, which increases ionization of salicylate and inhibits its reabsorption in the tubules (in the non-ionized state salicylate is lipid-soluble, can cross the cellular membranes and thus be absorbed from the renal tubules). Dialysis or exchange transfusion is effective in severe cases.

Household substances (corrosives)

Mildly corrosive substances include bleach, ammonia and dishwasher powders. Drain cleaners are highly corrosive, containing sodium hydroxide or sulphuric acid.

Management

Attempts at stomach emptying are contraindicated. Copious water is used to wash the skin, and milk drunk to reduce the irritation. The pharynx should be checked for burns, and the child monitored for respiratory obstruction. Early diagnostic oesophagoscopy may be needed (perforation is more likely if this investigation is delayed). Antibiotics may be indicated, and gastrostomy may also be required if the oesophagus is burnt. The use of steroids is controversial.

Plants and berries

Frequently ingested, these rarely cause serious toxic effects. However, unless the plant can be identified as non-toxic, the usual interventions of removal by emesis, and reduced absorption of toxins by activated charcoal, should be initiated.

COT DEATH

The term 'cot death' refers to sudden unexpected death in an infant. Although the sudden infant death syndrome (SIDS) remains the commonest aetiology, this presentation can also be due to unrecognized but treatable covert disease, accidents, and infanticide by suffocation. Careful evaluation of the circumstances surrounding cot death is crucial, but a post-mortem examination which is carried out by a pathologist with special expertise in the field is essential for the true nature of the underlying cause to be revealed.

✳ KEY DIAGNOSIS

Sudden Infant Death Syndrome

Our ignorance as to the root cause of SIDS is captured in the definition: a sudden and unexpected death in a previously healthy infant 1 week to 2 years old, in whom a carefully performed autopsy fails to reveal an adequate explanation.

Research has found that the supine position, avoiding overheating, and parents not smoking are protective. Through a national education programme to increase awareness (the UK Government's 'Back to Sleep' campaign) the incidence has fallen from 2 to 0.7 per 1000 live births. Nevertheless, SIDS still remains the commonest cause of death in this age group (Fig. 15.2). As the incidence of maternal smoking and bottle feeding has not declined, despite the campaigns, there is thus potential for a further significant reduction in SIDS (see Beyond core: epidemiology of SIDS).

The tragedy of SIDS ensures that each new hypothesis, however tenuous, often receives disproportionate media coverage. Such hypotheses have included suspicion of arsine gas production by mould on changing mats, and induced narcosis from rebreathing carbon dioxide

EPIDEMIOLOGY OF SIDS

- Timing: peak incidence is between 6 weeks and 6 months of age. Prior to the recent fall in SIDS, the incidence was greater in winter, and in the early hours of the morning. Now we see a plateauing without marked peaks and troughs in timing.

- Those at risk: boys, low birth weight infants with chronic lung disease from prolonged mechanical ventilation, and offspring of a single parent.
- Modifiable risk factors which could yet respond to education: mother smoking during pregnancy, bottle feeding, babies sharing a bedroom with a smoking adult.

while lying in a head-down position on a soft mattress; neither theory has stood up to critical evaluation.

Management

Considerable sensitivity is required in dealing with the parents who often express feelings of guilt. They need time, to hold the baby, to say 'goodbye', and at follow-up when the results of the post-mortem will be discussed. The legal investigative process, which is there to ensure that infanticide has not occurred, must be explained. Social work support and contact with the Foundation for the Study of Infant

Deaths parent support group should be offered. Reminders for vaccination and screening attendance should be cancelled to prevent distress.

A programme aimed at preventing recurrence in subsequent pregnancies, known as CONI, Care Of the Next Infant, has proved effective. As the incidence of SIDS has fallen, CONI has been adapted to support those infants with risk factors but without necessarily having a previous family history.

Near miss or acute life-threatening episode (ALTE)

This describes an event in which sudden unexpected deterioration occurs in a previously well infant, usually with complete (apnoea) or partial cessation of breathing, cyanosis, and profound loss of tone ('floppiness') for a period of seconds to a few minutes. Full cardiopulmonary resuscitation may be needed.

ALTE is a final common pathway with many causes, and comprehensive assessment and investigation are usually required. The possibility of sepsis, anaemia, aspiration of part of a feed (which may be due to gastro-oesophageal reflux), seizure, cardiac arrhythmia or metabolic abnormality must be explored. If repeated episodes occur in the same child, or previously occurred in another of the family, the possibility of parent-induced episodes of suffocation, a form of Munchausen by proxy, should also be considered.

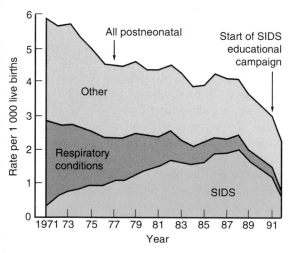

Figure 15.2 Postneonatal respiratory and SIDS mortality (rate per 1000 live births for 1971–1992, England and Wales)

'BACK TO SLEEP'

In the mid 1980s a link was postulated between Hong Kong's extremely low incidence of SIDS and the Oriental custom of laying babies in the supine position. At that time it was routine practice in the West to recommend lying prone. A clinical observation that SIDS babies often had raised core temperatures led to research showing that the prone position reduced heat loss. These facts encouraged New Zealand paediatricians to change their practice, to recommend laying babies on their backs, and avoid too many covering layers of blankets, etc. A significant sustained reduction in SIDS cases occurred, and the recommendations became national policy. Wherever the recommendations have subsequently been adopted, a fall in incidence followed.

FURTHER READING

Lansdown R et al (eds) 1997 Visibly different, coping with disfigurement. Butterworth Heinemann, Oxford
Towner E M L, Jarvis S N 1995 Unintentional injury prevention. In: David T J (ed) Recent advances in paediatrics 14. Churchill Livingstone, Edinburgh, pp 69–82

organ may have been arrested or misdirected early in embryonic development by some intrinsic abnormality. In others, normal development has been disrupted by external factors such as ischaemia or infection. Abnormal mechanical force may deform the developing fetus. Lack of amniotic fluid (oligohydramnios) may cause lung hypoplasia (see Ch. 6) and skeletal abnormalities such as hip dislocation or club foot (see Ch. 12).

Chromosomal abnormalities, single-gene disorders or environmental factors such as exposure to teratogenic agents (e.g. drugs, alcohol, radiation, maternal infection) each acting on their own may result in congenital malformations. Many of the most common congenital malformations, however, occur as a consequence of the interaction of multiple factors (both genetic and environmental).

Many relatives of children with congenital malformations and disabling or life-threatening illnesses will be concerned about the risks of the condition recurring in the family. The morbidity associated with some genetic disorders can be minimized with early detection and treatment. Couples at risk of having children with severely disabling conditions for which effective treatment is not available may seek prenatal diagnostic testing.

HISTORY AND EXAMINATION

A detailed history and clinical examination of affected family members is essential if such families are to be given useful advice about recurrence risks and therapeutic or preventive options. Nowhere in clinical medicine is an accurate diagnosis more important, for without it genetic advice can be totally misleading. For children with congenital malformations, any history of maternal illness or exposure to potential teratogens should be noted. A family history should be taken. Miscarriages, neonatal deaths, handicapped or malformed children and parental consanguinity may not be mentioned unless specifically asked about. At least basic details of both sides of the family should be taken, even in dominantly inherited disorders originating from one side, as unexpected findings may emerge. The

family history can often be most clearly and succinctly recorded by drawing a pedigree (Figs 16.2 and 16.3).

In some disorders, mental handicap or specific malformations are associated with characteristic dysmorphic features or appearances which may give important clues to the underlying aetiology of the patient's condition. In conditions with variable expression, careful clinical examination of apparently unaffected relatives may be required. Often key affected family members live elsewhere, in which case it may be necessary to seek confirmation of clinical findings from colleagues nearer their home with appropriate permission from the family. History and clinical findings may be supplemented with an increasing array of biochemical, cytogenetic and molecular

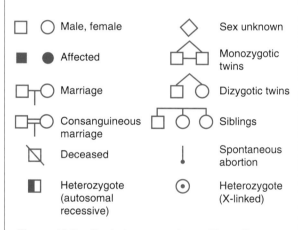

Figure 16.2 Symbols commonly used in pedigree drawing

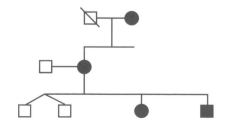

Figure 16.3 Pedigree of a family with neurofibromatosis type 1 illustrating vertical transmission of this autosomal dominant trait

genetic investigations where appropriate (see later).

CHROMOSOMAL ANALYSIS

The 22 pairs of autosomes and the X and Y chromosomes can be distinguished from each other during mitosis by their lengths and banding patterns when stained appropriately (Fig. 16.4). Cytogenetically detectable unbalanced chromosomal abnormalities, whether numerical or structural, involve relatively large chromosomal regions containing many genes with many functions and therefore have diverse effects on development. Numerical abnormalities involving the sex chromosomes tend to have milder phenotypic effects, but unbalanced abnormalities involving the autosomes are typically associated with multiple congenital malformations, with mental handicap being among the most consistent features.

Definitions

- *Non-disjunction*: failure of homologous chromosomes or sister chromatids to separate and migrate to opposite poles of the nucleus during cell division. This is the major mechanism by which monosomic and trisomic states originate (e.g. Down's syndrome). Non-disjunction occurring in meiosis will give rise to trisomy or monosomy, while non-disjunction taking place in mitosis in the early embryo will give rise to *mosaicism* (i.e. some cells display monosomy or trisomy while others have a normal karyotype).

- *Translocation*: transfer of genetic material from one chromosome to another (homologous or non-homologous). When there is a mutual exchange of segments with no associated loss of genetic material this is termed a *balanced reciprocal translocation*. Carriers of reciprocal translocations are usually phenotypically, normal since they have a full complement of genes. Children of such 'translocation carriers' will be abnormal if they receive only one of the two translocation chromosomes and thus become affected by an *unbalanced translocation* (Fig. 16.4).

- *Deletion*: one or more breakages occur along the chromosome with subsequent loss of the resulting fragment.

CORE PROBLEMS

CHROMOSOMAL DISORDER

✱ KEY DIAGNOSIS

Trisomy 21 (Down's syndrome)

Trisomy 21 affects about 1 in 700 live births. Most cases (95%) arise from non-disjunction during the first or second meiotic division, resulting in an egg or sperm containing an additional copy of the chromosome. In 85% of cases the extra chromosome is of maternal origin. The condition is more common in the offspring of older mothers. Thus the incidence at birth for a 35 year old mother is 1 in 380, rising to 1 in 50 for a 43 year old mother. Occasionally, a mitotic non-

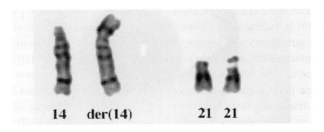

14   der(14)   21   21

Figure 16.4 Karyotype of a boy with Down's syndrome due to a centric fusion translocation involving chromosomes 21 and 14. The additional chromosomal material above the centromere of the derivative chromosome 14 (der (14)) is a third copy of chromosome 21.

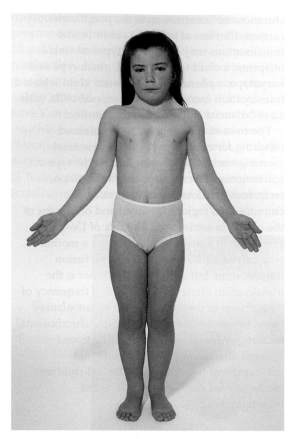

Figure 16.6 Classical phenotype appearance of a girl with Turner's syndrome (45X)

Turner's syndrome

Complete absence (45X0) or a mosaic pattern (46XX/45X) usually with defects (e.g. ring formation, partial deletion) of the X chromosome results in the phenotype (Fig. 16.6) described by Turner in 1938. The features are short stature, webbed neck, shield chest, valgus deformity of the elbow, congenital heart disease (classically coarctation of the aorta), and gonadal dysgenesis with delayed or absent puberty.

SINGLE-GENE DEFECTS

Although individually relatively rare, there are a very large number of conditions caused by faults in single genes or both copies of a pair of genes. Together they are a major cause of illness in childhood. These conditions segregate through affected families as mendelian traits, and it is therefore often possible to predict if relatives of affected individuals are themselves at risk or at risk of having affected children. Phenylketonuria (PKU), neurofibromatosis type 1 (NF1) and achondroplasia, discussed below, illustrate many of the key principles and problems involved in management of patients and families with single-gene disorders.

✳ KEY DIAGNOSIS

Phenylketonuria

Classical PKU is an autosomal recessive disorder caused by deficiency of the enzyme phenylalanine hydroxylase (PAH), which converts the essential amino acid phenylalanine to tyrosine in the liver. This deficiency results in the abnormal accumulation of phenylalanine, which damages the developing nervous system. Untreated, the condition results in severe mental retardation, but if affected infants are treated from early infancy by carefully controlled dietary phenylalanine restriction, they grow up to be virtually indistinguishable from normal (Fig. 16.8). Early detection and treatment of this condition, which affects about 1 in 10 000 children, is therefore essential.

A child with classical PKU has inherited a mutant copy of the PAH gene from both the mother and father. A single functional copy of the gene is all that is required for normal health. The parents will be symptomless carriers (heterozygotes), and are not usually identified as such until they have had an affected child. A couple who have had an affected child must both be carriers, and there will therefore be a 1 in 4 risk of the condition affecting any subsequent children. Males and females are equally likely to be affected. The risks for more distant relatives are low. A carrier related to an affected child would only be at risk of having affected children if his or her partner also happened to be a carrier. About 1 in 50 of the European population are carriers. Like many autosomal recessive traits, the frequency of the condition varies between populations. It is rare

BEYOND CORE

SUBMICROSCOPIC CHROMOSOMAL ABNORMALITIES

Children with unexplained mental handicap or multiple congenital malformations that do not form part of a recognized non-chromosomal syndrome should have chromosome analysis. Standard cytogenetic banding methods will detect most chromosomal deletions, duplications and rearrangements even when involvement of a specific chromosome or chromosomal region has not been anticipated on clinical grounds. However, the resolution of conventional banding techniques is limited. Increasing numbers of disorders are being recognized, involving deletion or in some cases duplication of chromosomal regions too small to be detected with conventional methods. Such microdeletions, which may result in loss of numerous adjacent genes, are often associated with recognizable clinical syndromes. When a child is suspected of having one of these disorders on clinical grounds,

specific molecular genetic or molecular cytogenetic confirmation of the presence of the associated microdeletion may be sought. In Figure 16.7 a microdeletion of chromosome 15q11–13 in a child with developmental delay, ataxia, seizures and electroencephalographic abnormalities confirms the diagnosis of Angelman's syndrome. Two fluorescently labelled DNA probes have been hybridized to spreads of mitotic chromosomes from the affected child. One, hybridizing at the lower end of the long arm of chromosome 15, helps to identify the chromosome; the other, which hybridizes nearer the centromere (at bands 15q11–13) tests for the presence or absence of the chromosome region containing the Angelman's syndrome gene (*UBE3A*). The deleted chromosome 15 lies at the bottom right-hand corner of the figure. The probe for the Angelman's syndrome region has not hybridized to the proximal long arm of this chromosome.

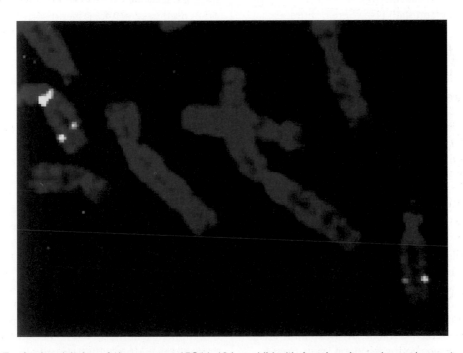

Figure 16.7 A microdeletion of chromosome 15Q11–13 in a child with Angelman's syndrome demonstrated by fluorescent in situ hybridization (FISH)

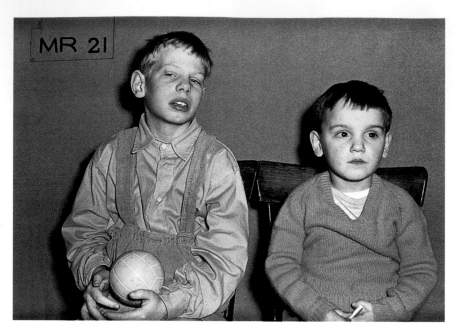

Figure 16.8   Two boys with PKU; the boy on the left has never had any dietary restrictions, and demonstrates the typical features of untreated PKU: severe mental handicap and lack of melanin. The boy on the right has been treated successfully. (Reproduced by courtesy of TALC)

in Ashkenazi Jews and Afro-Caribbeans but more common in Ireland than elsewhere in Europe.

Clinical featues

Infants with PKU are clinically normal at birth. In untreated children, mental retardation develops gradually, and may not be evident for several months. The urine is said to have a musty smell due to the presence of phenylacetic acid (derived from phenylalanine). Affected children are often blonder than unaffected siblings and are more likely to have fair skin and blue eyes (Fig. 16.8). Microcephaly and seizures can develop in untreated infants as they get older.

Diagnosis

Since neurological damage is likely to be irreversible by the time clinical signs of PKU are apparent, and since most couples at risk of having affected children will have no family history of the condition, all neonates in most developed countries are screened. Blood phenylalanine levels are estimated, usually using blood spots from a heel stab collected on a special filter paper

(Guthrie test, see Ch. 9). The same samples are often used to screen for other disorders such as congenital hypothyroidism and galactosaemia. Timing of testing is all important. Phenylalanine diffuses across the placenta, and so will not begin to accumulate in affected babies until after birth. Testing before the third day after birth increases the risk of missing infants with PKU.

For population screening to be appropriate and effective, the condition being sought must be relatively common in the population to be investigated, a cheap reliable screening test must be available and effective intervention must be possible for those families or individuals found to be affected. PKU screening fulfils these criteria in countries where it is common.

Management

Dietary phenylalanine levels can be controlled by the use of special low-phenylalanine dietary protein supplements and frequent monitoring of blood phenylalanine levels. Although most brain damage in children with untreated PKU occurs in early childhood, treatment should be continued

CARRIER DETECTION TESTS

Although children with PKU can be detected sufficiently early by neonatal screening to institute effective treatment, some couples want to know if they have a high risk of having an affected child before embarking on pregnancy. For some serious autosomal recessive disorders, such as sickle cell anaemia, thalassaemia, or Tay–Sachs disease, where cheap and reliable carrier detection tests are available, population screening for carriers enables couples at high risk of having an affected child to seek prenatal testing if they wish.

Population screening for carriers of recessive conditions is usually restricted to populations in which carriers, and therefore the associated conditions, are common. PKU carriers related to affected children can often be identified by tracking the mutated PAH genes through the affected family with polymorphic genetic markers within or adjacent to the gene (which lies on chromosome 12). Common detectable DNA sequence variations (polymorphisms) within the gene, which do not influence its function, can be used to distinguish between different copies of the gene within families. The copy of the gene that a carrier parent has transmitted to their affected child will almost always contain a mutation.

Detection of carriers without a family history of PKU is more difficult. Detection of heterozygous carriers by biochemical methods is complex and not completely reliable. The effectiveness of carrier detection by direct screening for mutations is also limited. The PAH gene has 13 exons and codes for a messenger RNA that is 2400 base pairs long. Over 60 different mutations have been identified in the gene of affected children in the UK. Some individual mutations are more common than others, but only 55–65% of carriers could be detected by testing for the six most common mutations in the UK. In contrast, four mutations account for about 85% of cystic fibrosis mutations in the UK, making genetic carrier screening for this disorder feasible in this population.

indefinitely as there is evidence of intellectual deterioration in individuals in whom dietary restriction is discontinued. Many women with PKU treated in early childhood are now of childbearing age. Affected women are only at risk of having children with PAH deficiency in the unlikely event that their partner is also a carrier. Despite this, they have a high risk of having handicapped children as a consequence of their condition. In affected women with poorly controlled phenylalanine levels, phenylalanine diffuses across the placenta, damaging the developing pregnancy and resulting in mental retardation, microcephaly and congenital heart disease. With adequate control of phenylalanine levels before conception and throughout pregnancy, these complications can be avoided.

Neurofibromatosis type 1

This is one of the more common autosomal dominant disorders, with an incidence of about 1 in 3500. It is characterized by pale brown pigmented macules (café au lait patches) and freckles in the axillae which first appear in infancy or early childhood with subsequent development of benign subcutaneous tumours of peripheral nerves (neurofibromata, Fig. 16.9) from adolescence onwards.

Café au lait spots are only considered to indicate that a child has NF1 if six or more spots over 5 mm in diameter are present. Small orange brown pigmented spots in the iris (Lisch nodules) are also very common in affected children. NF1 has almost complete penetrance. Virtually all individuals carrying a single neurofibromin (NF1 gene) mutation will have some signs of the disorder by the time they are about 5 years old. Expression of the condition is, however, very variable. In the family illustrated in Figure 16.3, several family members are affected but only two have major complications of the disorder.

About 30% of affected individuals have learning difficulties. Fortunately, moderate and

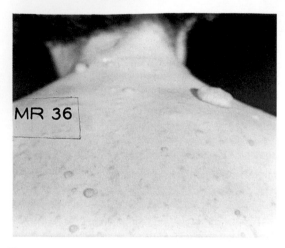

Figure 16.9 NF1 with cutaneous fibromata, patches of increased and decreased pigmentation, and neurofibromata of peripheral nerves. Epilepsy and mental retardation are frequent associations. (Reproduced by courtesy of TALC)

severe mental handicap only occurs in about 3%. Other serious complications include plexiform neurofibromata, which typically present as large soft subcutaneous swellings often first noted in infancy. These lesions may erode and displace adjacent structures and can be associated with hypertrophy of adjacent tissues. Very occasionally they undergo malignant transformation. Optic nerve gliomata (which rarely cause visual symptoms), renovascular hypertension, phaeochromocytoma (a catecholamine-secreting tumour), seizures, scoliosis and pathological fractures of the tibiae (leading to pseudarthroses) may also occur. Neurofibromata of the spinal nerve roots may cause nerve root compression and muscle weakness, sensory impairment or pain. Many affected children have relatively large heads (macrocephaly). This does not usually correlate with learning difficulties, mental retardation or structural abnormalities of the brain but occasionally macrocephaly is due to hydrocephalus. Only about 35% of affected individuals will have one of these more serious complications. The reason for the variation in severity within affected families is unknown. All affected individuals within an affected family will carry the same neurofibromin mutation.

Diagnosis

Awareness of the possible complications of the disorder and early detection and treatment can be facilitated by regular clinical examination of affected children. It is usually impractical to remove all of the cutaneous neurofibromata in affected adults, but lesions that are troublesome or disfiguring can often be excised.

Individuals with neurofibromatosis have one normal and one defective copy of the neurofibromin gene. When they have children there will be an even chance that they will pass on either the normal or the mutant copy of the gene to each of their children. Although there is a 1 in 2 risk of the condition affecting the offspring of an affected individual, the risk that they will develop a severe complication is lower. Since the life expectancy of mildly affected individuals is normal and the condition does not have a large effect on their chance of reproduction, the condition can segregate through many generations of an affected family (see Fig. 16.3).

The disorder can vary greatly in severity within families. Mildly affected individuals unaware that they have the condition may be at risk of having children with severe complications. It is therefore important to determine if other family members are affected when the condition has been identified in a family. Despite rapid advances in DNA mutation analysis, the diagnosis of neurofibromatosis and many other genetic diseases is still based primarily on clinical history, including family history, and physical examination. An adult from an affected family with no ocular or cutaneous signs of neurofibromatosis is very unlikely to be carrying a mutation in the neurofibromin gene, and will therefore be very unlikely to have affected children.

In approximately 50% of affected children the condition arises as a consequence of a new mutation. In such cases neither parent will have clinical signs of the disorder, and the recurrence risk in any other children that they have will be low. The new mutations are usually of paternal origin, and as is the case with other autosomal dominant traits, new mutations are more common in the offspring of older fathers.

Genetic testing

The neurofibromin gene is large, and most families with NF1 will have their own unique mutation somewhere within the gene, and so routine diagnostic testing by mutation detection is not possible at present. Direct mutation testing is feasible and effective for other conditions where the same or similar mutations occur in most affected families. In some NF1 families it is possible to use molecular genetic methods to determine if the offspring of affected individuals are affected in early infancy before the disorder is clinically apparent. DNA sequence polymorphisms within or lying close to the neurofibromin gene on chromosome 17 can be used to track the mutated gene through families in which more than one individual is affected already. This can help to determine which children require clinical follow-up. The same methodology can be used for prenatal testing, but this is infrequently requested because of the relatively mild clinical problems experienced by the majority of affected individuals. At present it is not possible to predict the severity of the condition.

Achondroplasia

This is the commonest form of congenital bone dysplasia (incidence 1 in 20 000), resulting in short-limbed short stature. It may be inherited as an autosomal dominat trait or arise as a new mutation. Affected children have short upper and lower limbs, with classical shortening of the upper arms and legs (spondylometaphyseal dysplasia). The head is large but spinal growth is normal (Fig. 16.10). The children are of normal intelligence, and have no difficulties in physical performance other than that related to their short stature.

X-LINKED INHERITANCE

X-linked disorders are caused by defects in genes on the X chromosome. Just as there are dominant and recessive autosomal traits there are X-linked dominant as well as recessive X-linked traits. Females with these conditions tend to be less severely affected than affected males. X-linked dominant conditions are very uncommon; some are incompatible with survival of an affected male pregnancy to term and so are only seen in females, with a 50% risk of transmission from affected women to their daughters.

Duchenne muscular dystrophy and haemophilia A (see Ch. 11) are examples of X-

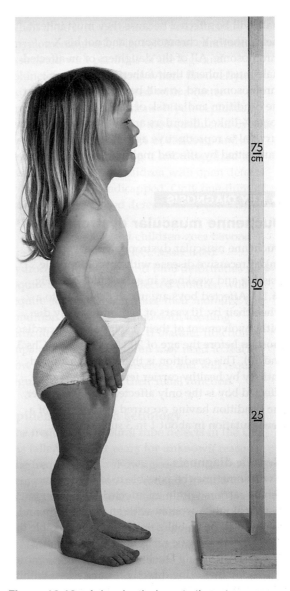

Figure 16.10 Achondroplasia: note the extreme shortening of the upper segments of both the upper and lower limbs

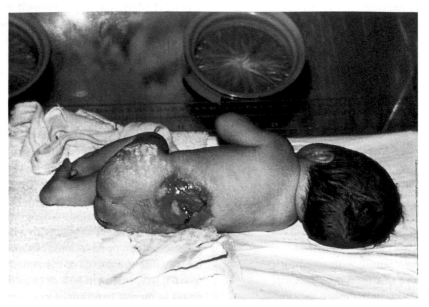

a

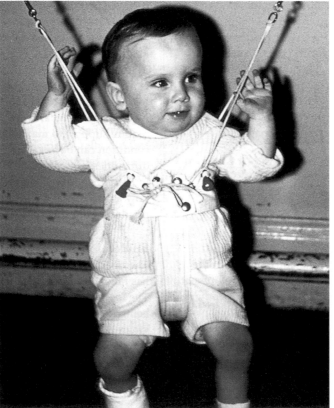

b

Figure 16.12 Myelomeningocele. **a** A newborn baby with a meningomyelocele with herniation of the spinal cord tissue and covering membranes through the bone and skin defects. There is a high risk of infection, and early surgery is essential for survival. **b** These children frequently have paralysis of the lower limbs, hydrocephalus and skeletal malformation of the lower limbs secondary to the neurological defect (note the Plaster of Paris boot on the right leg). (Reproduced by courtesy of TALC)

diabetic mothers and mothers taking the anticonvulsant sodium valproate during early pregnancy. The great majority of cases, however, are of multifactorial aetiology. Having excluded other causes, the recurrence risk after an affected pregnancy (or for the offspring of an affected individual) is 1 in 25–33. The recurrence risk rises to 1 in 10 for a couple who have had two affected children. Asymptomatic isolated bony neural arch defects (sometimes associated with a hairy patch in the overlying skin) involving three or more vertebral arches are termed spina bifida occulta, and are associated with an increase in risk similar to that for first-degree relatives of symptomatic spina bifida. Defects involving one or two arches from L_1 to S_2 are common, and are not associated with increased risk.

Less efficient utilization of folic acid in various metabolic processes in either the embryo or the mother may be associated with an increased risk of neural tube defect. The recurrence risk after an affected pregnancy is reduced to 1 in 100 with maternal folic acid supplements (4 mg/day) taken before conception and during the first 12 weeks of pregnancy. Preconception supplementation is essential because neural tube closure is complete before most women are aware that they are pregnant.

Antenatal diagnosis

Prenatal diagnosis is possible with detailed ultrasound scanning, and open lesions can be detected by measuring amniotic fluid levels of AFP and acetylcholinesterase that leak from the fetus through the open defect. Maternal serum AFP levels may also be increased in affected pregnancies.

Cleft lip and palate

Epidemiology and aetiology

The medial nasal and maxillary processes have normally fused to form the upper lip by the 35th day after conception. Fusion of the palatal shelves normally occurs at 8–9 weeks. Failure of these processes may result in isolated cleft lip or both cleft lip and palate (Fig. 16.13). About 1 in 1000 births are affected. The condition may be unilateral or bilateral.

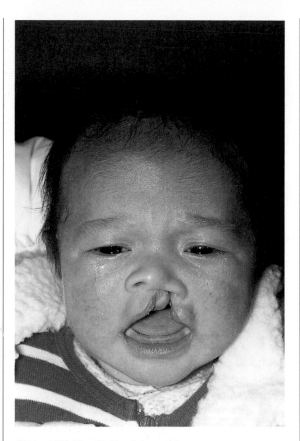

Figure 16.13 Cleft palate and lip

Cleft lip and palate occur as a feature of many single-gene disorders, and can be associated with chromosomal abnormalities such as trisomy 13. Most infants with one of these disorders will have other associated malformations or dysmorphic features or may have other affected relatives. Cleft lip and palate has a multifactoral aetiology in the majority of affected children. There is a 1 in 50 recurrence risk for a couple who have had a child with unilateral cleft lip. The recurrence risks are higher where the proband is more severely affected, rising to 1 in 20 where the affected child has bilateral cleft lip and palate. The malformation can sometimes be detected during pregnancy with detailed ultrasound scanning.

Management

Cleft lip is usually repaired within a few months of birth, with repair of the palatal defect at around 1 year. Breast feeding may be difficult particularly in children with a large palatal defect. Feeding can be aided with the use of plastic obturators or specialized teats. Recurrent otitis media and hearing loss are common, and must be recognized and managed appropriately should they occur. Speech defects may be present or persist even after good anatomical closure of the palatal defect due to impaired function of pharyngeal and palatal muscles. Due to the many facets of the condition, many specialists including speech therapists, and plastic, dental, and ear, nose and throat surgeons are likely to be required for optimum care of affected children.

Congenital dislocation of the hip

In this condition the hips are not usually dislocated at birth but are 'dislocatable' due to under-development of the cartilagenous acetabulum and laxity of the associated ligaments.

Epidemiology and aetiology

Hip instability usually occurs in otherwise normal infants but may be secondary to other conditions such as neuromuscular disease and disorders where external constraints limit fetal movement such as oligohydramnios.

About 1 in 1000 children have a dislocated hip, while 4–7 in 1000 have an unstable joint. The condition is six times more common in females than males. The risk of recurrence in siblings is 1 in 20.

Clinical features and management

When detected at birth, maintenance of the unstable hip in flexion and abduction for 1–2 months using appropriate splints or orthoses prevents hip dislocation and allows time for tightening of the ligamentous structures supporting the joint. If diagnosis is delayed, surgical reduction of the dislocated hip may be necessary, and the risk of irreversible damage to the joint is increased (see Ch. 12).

Routine screening for hip instability by means of the Barlow and Ortolani manoeuvres (see Ch. 4 and Fig. 4.1) can greatly reduce the morbidity associated with this condition. Hip stability and acetabular development can also be assessed with ultrasound scanning and radiography (see Fig. 12.5). If not detected at birth or in early infancy,

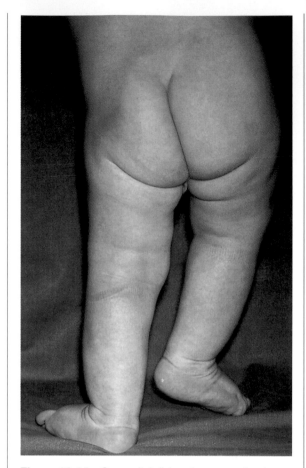

Figure 16.14 Congenital dislocation presenting in an older child with limping and obvious shortening of the left leg. (Reproduced by courtesy of the Wellcome Trust Photographic Library)

congenital hip dislocation may present as a pain-free limp with apparent shortening of the affected limb (see Fig. 16.14 and Ch. 12).

Talipes equinovarus

In infants with congenital talipes equinovarus, the sole of the foot faces medially (Fig. 16.15). The heel is small and high (equinus) and the metatarsal region is adducted (varus). The deformity is maintained by tightness of the tendons, ligaments and joint capsules.

Epidemiology and aetiology

As with congenital hip dislocation, talipes may occur in a wide range of neuromuscular diseases

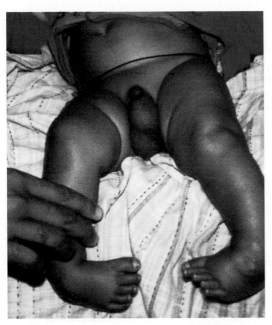

Figure 16.15 Severe congenital talipes of the equinovarus type – 'club foot': plantar flexion with inversion and abduction of both the heels and forefoot. Early orthopaedic intervention is required in this condition. (Reproduced by courtesy of TALC)

(including many single-gene disorders), chromosomal disorders and as a result of constraints on fetal movements in utero associated with problems such as oligohydramnios. In most cases, however, no precipitating factors are apparent. The condition is present in about 1 in 200 live births, with 1 in 1000 being severely affected. It is bilateral in about 50% of cases. The condition is twice as common in males as it is in females. The recurrence risk in siblings of a male proband is 1 in 50, but 1 in 20 if the proband is female. Families with several factors (either genetic or environmental) are more likely to have affected female family members.

Correction of the deformity can usually be achieved by manipulation of the foot towards the correct position and the application of plaster casts or splints to maintain the foot in position. In some cases surgical correction is necessary.

Hypospadias

Clinical features

Hypospadias is a congenital malformation of the male genitalia in which the urethral opening may lie anywhere along the ventral surface of the shaft of the penis, or, in severe cases, may open into the perineum. Fibrous bands within the penis (chordee) may result in ventral curvature of the penis. The foreskin usually has a ventral defect resulting in a hooded appearance. Hypospadias can be associated with undescended testes and inguinal hernias. Mild hypospadias is usually repaired for cosmetic reasons, but in more severe cases surgery is essential if an affected boy is to urinate normally and have normal sexual function. Repair is usually undertaken in infancy.

In its more severe forms, and when the testes are not palpable, the sex of an affected child may be ambiguous (see Ch. 9). Chromosome analysis will establish the genetic sex of a severely affected child and may detect associated sex or autosomal chromosome abnormalities. Some cases may be difficult to differentiate clinically from disorders such as congenital adrenal hyperplasia (see Ch. 9) in which there is virilization of female pregnancies. Isolated hypospadias is not usually associated with upper urinary tract abnormalities, but renal malformations are common in boys in whom hypospadias is associated with other malformations such as imperforate anus or spina bifida. Renal and other upper urinary tract malformations can be detected with ultrasound scanning.

Epidemiology and aetiology

Hypospadias affects about 1 in 500 newborn boys. It can occasionally occur in association with chromosomal abnormalities or as part of syndromes determined by single-gene defects. However, the great majority of cases have a multifactorial aetiology. Where hypospadias occurs as an isolated malformation, the risk of the condition affecting the siblings or children of an affected male is around 1 in 10.

SPORADIC CONGENITAL MALFORMATIONS WITHOUT FAMILIAL CLUSTERING

Some congenital malformations and malformation syndromes occur sporadically with no apparent clustering in families. Parents of children with these disorders can be reassured that the risk of recurrence is low.

✳ KEY DIAGNOSIS

Capillary haemangioma (strawberry naevus)

Capillary haemangiomata are cutaneous vascular lesions which usually appear in early infancy (Fig. 16.16). They have a brief period of growth, with endothelial proliferation followed by fibrosis and regression that is total. They present as raised, red and often lobulated masses, which may be disfiguring initially when they occur on the face. Parents can be reassured that the great majority of these lesions regress spontaneously without surgical intervention, leaving little or no trace. The lesions may sometime become ulcerated or infected. Laser treatment or cryotherapy may

sometimes be indicated in such cases or if the lesion is in a location which may cause complications (e.g. the eyelid, leading to amblyopia). Superficial capillary haemangiomata may overlie cavernous haemangiomata (vascular lesions deep in the dermis consisting of large dilated thin-walled vessels). Such lesions may very occasionally be so large that they cause haemodynamic disturbance, resulting in heart failure, or thrombocytopenia due to platelet consumption.

Although strawberry naevi occasionally occur as part of recognizable familial syndromes, the great majority are sporadic.

FURTHER READING

Connor M, Ferguson-Smith M 1997 Essential medical genetics, 5th edn. Blackwell Science, Oxford
Gelehrter T, Collins F, Ginsburg D 1988 Principles of medical genetics, 2nd edn. Williams and Wilkins, Baltimore

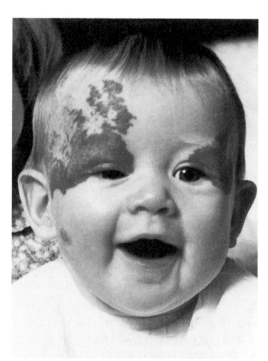

a

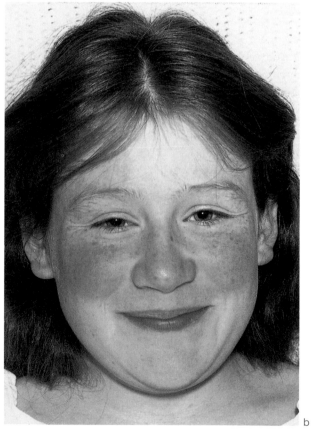

b

Figure 16.16 a An extensive capillary haemangioma above the right eye. **b** Spontaneous resolution of the same child, aged 12 years

Community and social paediatrics

H. Hammond

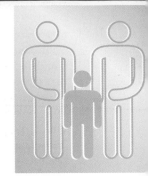

ESSENTIAL BACKGROUND

INTRODUCTION

The need for a community-based child health service and, in particular, a school health service was first recognized at the time of the Boer War, when the recruits were found to be in a very poor state of health. At that time the main problems were the result of malnutrition and chronic and recurrent infections, and many of the conditions would have been readily curable if identified and treated. The early community child health doctors were called medical officers, and were responsible to their medical officer of health, who was employed by the local authority. It was not until 1974 that community medical services were brought into the National Health Service and the role of the medical officer of health more clearly defined as a director of public health responsible to the area health authority or health board.

COMMUNITY CHILD HEALTH SERVICES

Community child health services differ from primary care and hospital-based services in their population-based approach. In other words, the service seeks to ensure that all children are reached by surveillance and immunization programmes and that through these programmes children with significant health and developmental problems may be identified at an early stage. Over the last 15 years the responsibility for offering surveillance and immunization services to preschool children has largely moved into general practice, allowing the community child health service to develop a more specialist role, meeting the needs of children with identified medical problems and disabilities. In almost all parts of the country the community child health service is led by consultant paediatricians working closely with their hospital secondary services aiming to provide a seamless service to children and their families, particularly those with complex disabilities.

A typical team consisting of paediatricians, community and school nurses and specialized therapists will cover a population of approximately of 100 000 people with approximately 20 000 children aged between 0 and 16 years. To be effective, this secondary care service needs to be very well integrated with general practitioners and health visitors, who remain the primary link to health care for young people. Developing the service in this way allows community paediatricians to target resources to the most needy children. These children can be regarded as falling into two main categories: vulnerable children and children with special needs, as described in Figure 17.1.

Vulnerable children are described as those with health needs resulting from deprivation or abuse. Children with special needs are all those children who require additional health input as a result of chronic illness or disability. Both these groups include children and families with very wide-ranging problems, and are not of course mutually exclusive. Many youngsters with disability live in deprived circumstances with families who struggle to meet their physical and social needs. Research studies have clearly demonstrated that children who live in deprived circumstances have a higher incidence of health problems, e.g. glue ear, and respiratory and gastrointestinal infections.

LEGISLATION

Recent years have seen the enactment of new legislation both in England and in Scotland concerning the care of children. In 1989 the

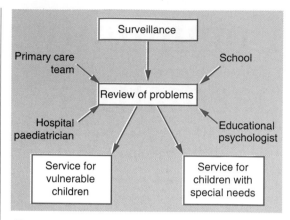

Figure 17.1 Overview of the community child health service

Children Act (England and Wales) came into effect, and in 1996–97 the Children (Scotland) Act 1995 was fully implemented. These acts build on previous legislation and incorporate the principles of the UN Convention on Human Rights. Within them the rights of children and the rights and responsibilities of their parents and carers are more clearly laid down. This is of particular importance in the growing climate of litigation, and as we try to refine our systems for child protection and for children with special needs. It is helpful to remind ourselves of the essential principles of the act which are clearly laid out in the regulations and guidance in *Scotland's Children: The Children (Scotland) Act 1995*, volume 1, *Support and Protection for Children and their Families* (Table 17.1).

Table 17.1   Children (Scotland) Act 1995 – essential principles
• Each child has a right to be treated as an individual
• Each child who can form a view has the right to express those views
• Parents should normally be responsible for the upbringing of their children and should share that responsibility
• Each child has the right to protection from all forms of abuse, neglect and exploitation
• So far as is in the child's best interests the public authority should promote the upbringing of children by their families
• Any intervention by a public authority in the life of a child must be properly justified and supported by services from all relevant agencies working collaboratively.

Child protection

Guidance for the improvement of the child protection services has been given within the Department of Health documents initially *Effective Intervention* in Scotland and *Working Together* in England. These reports were influenced by major enquiries into the handling of cases of child abuse in Orkney and Cleveland in the late 1980s. All the reports, guidelines and legislation emphasize the importance of close interagency working in child protection.

Children with disability

Meeting the needs of children with disability in our community has also been the subject of many government reports and working parties, again emphasizing the importance of multidisciplinary working, with all the involved professionals and agencies coming together to plan to meet the child's needs. The Court Report (*Fit For the Future*, 1976) set out the fundamental principles of this approach, and the Education (Scotland) Act 1981 laid down basic principles of practice and established the record of needs process in Scotland, with its English equivalent the statement of needs process. This legislation has been extremely important in ensuring that a child with significant problems of any kind receives a comprehensive health and educational assessment, leading to clear identification of his or her special needs in an educational setting and makes clear recommendations about how these should be met.

Record of needs

In drawing up a record of needs (e.g. for a child with cerebral palsy), the medical report is written by a senior paediatrician based on a full examination and developmental assessment and detailing all aspects of the child's presentation, abilities and difficulties, and describing the nature and amount of input (e.g. physiotherapy, medication, special equipment, help with toiletting) that the child would need in order to attend school. Education staff draw up a similar assessment of the child's cognitive ability and educational needs in a school setting, and these are then taken together with the parent's views and views of any other involved professionals (e.g. nursery school staff) in completing a record or statement of the child's needs and making a recommendation on school placement. Increasingly, children with disabilities are being integrated into mainstream education. For many children with normal intellectual and social development but significant medical problems or disabilities, this represents huge progress in enabling them to benefit from the full educational and social opportunities available to their peers. However, for some children their degree of disability and dependence on adult care or their degree of learning difficulty makes this impractical and ineffective in meeting their physical or educational needs.

INFORMATION SYSTEMS

In the past a great deal of effort has been placed on routine assessment of children, both through preschool surveillance and the school health programme, but it has been difficult to measure the success of these programmes in terms of early identification of problems or measurement of health gain through early intervention. Computerized child health information systems are now being established throughout the UK, enabling us for the first time to undertake audit and gather important population information, e.g. health problems in relation to demographic data. Hopefully this information will allow more effective targeting of resources by discontinuing activities which are not shown to be useful but also, and perhaps more importantly, to provide important information for local authority and central government on which to base plans for reducing adverse factors in our local communities and promoting health.

Computerized systems have been developed to call and recall children for immunization, preschool surveillance, school surveillance and assessment of special needs, to collate the data into a computerized individual health record and to produce regular outputs for monitoring and audit of the health processes.

Parent- and child-held health records

The introduction of parent-held records was a very important initiative to encourage parents to be more actively involved in the health care of their children, and has provided a vehicle for health education and health promotion. Work is currently ongoing to introduce a follow-on record for youngsters themselves, recognizing that children mature at an earlier age and are ready and able to take more responsibility for their own health as they develop through adolescence. Student health questionnaires, which have been in use in a number of areas for several years, demonstrate that young people have clear views and concerns about their health and are well able to indicate what further information and advice they would value. Again, the parent/child-held record offers the opportunity to disseminate important health information about contraception, HIV and drugs, for example.

A record particularly designed to meet the needs of children being 'looked after' by their local authority has also been designed. These children are the most vulnerable in our society and among the most difficult to reach in terms of health services. Frequently they miss out on the school health education programmes because of frequent moves, truanting, etc. They find it particularly difficult to seek health advice from professionals, regarding them as authoritarian and unsympathetic. Of course, parent- and child-held health records are only of benefit if hospital and community doctors, general practitioners and other health professionals are prepared to take the time to read and complete them.

POPULATION AND SURVEILLANCE AND SCREENING PROGRAMMES

Nationally recommended core programmes of surveillance and immunization have been agreed and are carried out in an increasingly uniform way across the country (Table 17.2). It is important to remember that surveillance is a much wider process than screening, and involves the sharing of parents concerns, developmental assessment and health promotion as well as specific examinations which fulfil the criteria for screening. A test can only be regarded as a tool for population screening if it fulfils certain criteria: it is a simple and reproducible with low false-positive or false-negative results that can be offered to the whole population and for which appropriate intervention/treatment is available (see also Ch. 16).

Within preschool child health surveillance, examination for undescended testes or congenital dislocation of the hips clearly meets the criteria for screening tests. Assessments of hearing and vision, examination of the heart for congenital heart disease and the eyes for cataracts would also be included in this category, where early intervention clearly improves outcome. In contrast, developmental assessment would not generally be regarded as meeting the criteria for screening since it is hard to prove that intervention alters outcome. However, there is growing evidence that where developmental delay results primarily from social deprivation, early intervention improves educational outcome in the early years. Providing speech therapy to children with significant language delay is another area where early intervention has been shown to improve prognosis.

There is little doubt, however, that in terms of the family's ability to cope and respond to the child's difficulties, early identification of developmental and physical problems does improve outcome by providing early support and reassurance and putting parents in touch with key professionals, support groups and voluntary agencies.

Growth

Growth is the best single indicator of a child's well being, physical and emotional, during childhood (see Ch. 2). Most paediatricians and general practitioners with an interest in surveillance believe it should be measured and carefully recorded at each surveillance point. Although most parents with children with significant short stature requiring investigation will eventually take their child to their general

Table 17.2	Preschool surveillance and immunization schedule		
Age	*Surveillance programme*	*Immunization*	*Comments*
11 days	Health visitor first report		
6–8 weeks	General practitioner and health visitor examination		
8 weeks		Diphtheria Tetanus Pertussis *Haemophilus influenza* b Polio (oral)	First dose
3 months		As above	Second dose
4 months		As above	Third dose
7 months	Hearing examination		
8–9 months	General practitioner and health visitor examination Hearing result		
12–15 months		Measles Mumps Rubella	
21–24 months	Health visitor development check		
39–42 months	General practitioner and health visitor examination		
4–5 years	Health visitor preschool check and report	Diphtheria Tetanus Polio (oral) MMR	Booster Second dose
11–14 years		BCGa	
13–18 years		Diphtheria Tetanus Polio (oral)	Booster

a BCG may be given in the neonatal period to babies with a high risk of tuberculosis

practitioner, this may result in a late referral with a less effective outcome in terms of eventual height. Children with underlying medical problems, e.g. chronic renal insufficiency, may be detected through poor growth before specific signs and symptoms develop. Growth charts can also provide the only medical evidence that children are being abused or neglected. Growth also provides a good monitor of the adequacy of management of a known chronic medical problem, e.g. asthma, and of effective intervention in a serious social problem such as child abuse. It is well recognized that failure to grow is a very important sign of emotional abuse, and population studies have shown that social deprivation is a much more common cause of growth failure (see Ch. 9) than an unrecognized endocrinological or medical problem. When assessing the growth of infants or very young children, it is important to measure all of the three following parameters: weight, height (or length) and head circumference. In older children it is acceptable simply to measure height unless there are obvious concerns about weight and/or development. At all ages, precise technique is of great importance in obtaining accurate reproducible measurements. Measurements are meaningless unless plotted on a growth chart allowing the child's pattern of growth to be followed (see Fig. 2.5).

Immunization

Preventing illness by carrying out a population immunization programme is regarded as a key element of surveillance, using that term in its broadest sense. Table 17.2 shows the current immunization programme. In order to achieve adequate herd immunity a population uptake rate of over 90% is necessary. In promoting uptake, direct discussion between parents, health visitors and general practitioners, and sharing information through the parent-held record, are all of great importance. There continues to be a need to counter the myths about contraindications to immunization such as a concurrent upper respiratory infection or a family history of epilepsy. Health staff need to be very well informed on the current views on contraindications, which are regularly reviewed by the Joint Committee on Vaccination and Immunization, which is responsible for overseeing the National Immunization Programme and produces a manual ('The Green Book') on a regular basis.

The Green Book gives guidance on recommended routes and time intervals for immunization as well as detailing the different vaccines available and their indications and contraindications. The current recommendation on the route of administration is the use of the muscle or deep subcutaneous tissue of the anterolateral aspect of the thigh or the deltoid muscle in the upper arm. This avoids the risk of damage to the sciatic nerve by injecting into the buttock. Very young infants often have poor deltoid muscle bulk, and therefore the anterolateral thigh has become the favourite route, particularly since the introduction of the accelerated schedule of primary immunization starting at 8 weeks of age. This was put in place to try to reduce the incidence of whooping cough (pertussis) in young infants, where the risk of morbidity and mortality is high. Currently, immunization is only contraindicated if the child has an acute febrile illness, has had a previous significant reaction to that vaccine or, in the case of pertussis immunization, has an evolving neurological problem, or in the case of polio immunization, suffers from immune deficiency.

Like surveillance, immunization is now almost completely carried out within primary care by general practitioners or health visitors, apart from the BCG and booster diphtheria/tetanus and polio programmes, which are carried out in secondary schools by school doctors and nurses. Where doubt exists about whether or not a child should be immunized, general practitioners are encouraged to seek specialist help rather than withholding immunization. Children who have not been immunized owing to clinical contraindications earlier in their life are vulnerable to infectious diseases, and it is important to review the appropriateness of immunizing them later. This is particularly relevant in children who have a neurological problem, e.g. cerebral palsy, who should be reconsidered when their condition has stabilized.

School health service

Improved primary health care and preschool surveillance services have reduced the need for routine surveillance within the school age population. The school health service is becoming steadily more selective, offering comprehensive health assessment and intervention for children with recognized problems. School surveillance has been cut back to a minimum with, in most areas, school nurses offering the first tier surveillance screening for growth, vision and hearing problems and offering health promotion initiatives. School doctors see children with recognized chronic medical or developmental problems and those referred by school nurses, teachers or hospital colleagues with newly emerging concerns.

An important group of new referrals are those children whose performance either educationally or socially is not coming up to the expected level or has deteriorated without any obvious explanation. It is vital that, even where there is no reason to suspect a medical cause, a full assessment by health as well as educational staff is carried out.

Children may begin to fail academically or show significant behaviour problems as a result of previously undiagnosed medical problems such as increasing visual or hearing difficulties (not being able to see the blackboard or hear the teacher), developmental difficulties such as dyspraxia or dyslexia, or mental illness (particularly depression). Equally, a fall-off in school performance may be the only sign that a child is being bullied or abused. Children in difficulties of any of these kinds may become increasingly withdrawn or act out, displaying attention-seeking or even aggressive behaviour. A careful history and examination will enable any health problem to be identified. It is also important to remember that a relatively minor problem, for example a mild conductive hearing loss, may become much more significant in terms of the functional difficulty it produces if the child has associated problems such as a degree of learning difficulty.

Where children have problems identified, school doctors play a key role in their physical and developmental assessment and advice on the implications of the problem both to the families in terms of the child's home management and to the education staff in terms of their school programme. School doctors and nurses are involved regularly in multidisciplinary case conferences where children's difficulties and needs are discussed by everyone involved and a plan put in place to try to ensure that, whatever the child's problems, access to the full educational curriculum including physical education and all social opportunities are available to the child.

The school health team also takes responsibility for ensuring that the child has completed his or her preschool immunization programme, the BCG programme to prevent tuberculosis and programmes for booster immunization against diphtheria/tetanus and polio, which are offered during secondary school years. A variety of health promotion initiatives including increasing opportunities for teenagers to self-refer for specific advice, e.g. contraceptive and drug information, are increasingly being made available, and are part of the overall objective to encourage greater participation of young people in their own health care.

CORE PROBLEMS

DISABILITY

Successful management of the disabled child in the community depends on a comprehensive assessment of the child's health and development within the context of his or her family and community and the setting in place of a well-coordinated plan of management involving not only health services but services from other departments and agencies such as social services, the education department, housing, transport, and the voluntary agencies. The child's medical diagnosis provides only a very small contribution to this overall package of information which is required. The *International Classification of Diseases* (ICD) describes problems in terms of impairment, disability and handicap, and this is very helpful in beginning to build up a picture of the child's needs:

Impairment	Disability	Handicap
Pathology and neurology, e.g. brain damage leading to hemiplegia	Loss of function, e.g. difficulty walking cannot run and kick a ball	Social restriction Cannot walk around school Cannot play football 'Not one of the gang'

- *Impairment* is the child's actual medical problem, e.g. a hemiplegia or severe hearing loss.

- *Disability* is the extent to which the child cannot perform functions which other children of the same age and status would perform. For example, the child with a hemiplegia being unable to run or climb the stairs, or the child with a hearing loss unable to hear the teacher in the classroom.

- *Handicap* is the extent to which the disability limits the child and family in terms of overall daily life within their family, school and community, e.g. the hemiplegic child unable to go to his local school in a Victorian building with many steps situated at the top of a hill or the child with a hearing loss unable to walk safely to school on her own because she cannot hear the traffic or finds it hard to cope in school because of being teased about her hearing aid. Within the ICD classification, disability and handicap are described as being mild, moderate, severe or profound, giving further help in the description of the child's difficulties.

In considering the child's difficulties and needs, it is not just the diagnosis itself that is important but also the resulting disability and handicap coupled with the family's and the local community's ability to respond to them. This depends on a large number of factors, including the child's personality, the family and community expectation, the extended family relationship, and the support which is present within the family and local community. Other factors include how well adapted the local environment (schools, swimming pool, etc.) is to disability and how motivated and well-resourced the local education and social work departments are to meeting the needs of handicapped children in their local schools and community. Good multidisciplinary care depends on the proper consideration of all these factors and a well-coordinated team approach to the management of the child. Many areas now have child development centres which act as an important focus for assessment and services for children with disabilities. Parents greatly value the 'one stop' approach to care, and can offer each other a great deal of support and encouragement in these settings given appropriate guidance.

Multidisciplinary working

The setting up of teams of professionals including representatives from health, education, social work and the voluntary agencies to coordinate the management of children with significant handicaps was first described within the Court Report, and has been recommended in numerous reports subsequently. Not only does this approach lead to better use of limited resources but also improves communication and reduces misunderstanding and confusion, where from the parents' perspective different professionals seem to have a different view of their child's problems. Regular review within such a multidisciplinary team can also help to identify the family's particular needs at a given time, which will change as the child grows and develops. For example, initial assessment may highlight the child's needs for additional therapy input or input from the home visiting preschool teacher, whilst a subsequent review might identify the need for professionals to give the family a little more space as they cope with the death of a grandparent or difficulty within the parents' own relationship.

Within the multidisciplinary team, a key worker is identified to provide the most frequent support and provide a link to the other services if new needs should emerge. In the early stages the health visitor frequently fulfils this role, but as the child progresses through school the family may choose a member of teaching staff, and as the child approaches school leaving, a member of the social work team. The key worker will help the family to identify their own needs and wishes and help to communicate these directly to the relevant professionals.

✳ KEY DIAGNOSIS

Cerebral palsy

The child with severe cerebral palsy (see Ch. 10) affecting all four limbs and accompanied by severe learning difficulties and perhaps a degree of sensory impairment places huge strains on the capacity of a normal young family to care. Such a child may have had a very stormy neonatal period, during which the parents may have anticipated the child's death. They have subsequently come to terms with the loss of the normal child they were expecting and the huge problems and needs of the child that they have in its place.

Parents of a child with cerebral palsy will have to learn to handle the child in particular ways, positioning it carefully for feeding, for dressing and for sleep. Feeding may take long periods of time, perhaps up to $1^{1}/_{2}$ h as the child pushes the spoon or bottle away with increased tongue thrust because coordination of the basic functions of sucking or chewing and swallowing are disordered. The child's sleep pattern is frequently very disturbed due to discomfort and an inability to move around in the bed in a normal way. On top of this the child may be very demanding of attention, being unable to occupy itself in any way. The family will be expected to take the child to seemingly endless clinics – paediatric, neurological, orthopaedic, eyes, ear, nose and throat – and to sessions with the physiotherapist, occupational therapist and the speech and language therapist. It is very difficult for them to have time for themselves or each other, and they may be very reluctant to leave the child with other people given the very high level of specialist care required.

In making plans for a child like this it is important to hear from the parents what their main problems in day to day life with the child are. Frequently they will point to the large number of clinics, and attempts need to be made to coordinate better clinical services. Often poor sleep patterns and problems in feeding are the next areas of difficulty, and trials of medication and other ways of feeding, e.g. through gastrostomy, may need to be considered. The provision of respite care, allowing the parents and carers some time to themselves, is of great importance. In most areas a range of respite care facilities is now available, including provision of 'sitters' to come and care for the child in his or her own home or 'side by side' families who will care for the child in their home for periods of hours, weekends, etc., or the use of residential or even hospital facilities for the more profoundly disabled children.

Sequelae of extreme prematurity

Survivors of extreme prematurity and very low birth weight are a newly emerging group of youngsters who may have significant disability (Table 17.3). Many of these children will have been discharged from hospital with the label 'miracle baby', where parents have been through weeks of agonizing waiting through a stormy neonatal course. Having lost the early period of bonding and interaction, they take home a baby who seems to them to be extremely fragile and difficult to handle normally. Difficult attention-seeking behaviour often follows, with the children demonstrating very brief attention spans, and as they progress into the early years of primary school specific learning difficulties, particularly due to visuoperceptual problems, may begin to emerge. It is also well recognized that there is a higher incidence of abuse among these children. It is extremely important that there is a full discussion with the parents about the possible difficulties the child may present before he or she leaves hospital. Careful monitoring by hospital and community paediatricians should then help to identify any problems early and give appropriate guidance. Again, support from other parents who have been through a similar experience is very helpful.

Dyspraxia

The management of the child with specific learning difficulty such as dyspraxia (difficulty in

Table 17.3 Problems of low birth weight survivors
Neurodevelopmental problems
Central motor impairment
Cerebral palsy
Clumsy child
Language delay
Perceptual problems
Visual impairment
Hearing impairment
Learning difficulties
Behaviour problems

planning and execution of motor tasks) requires a multidisciplinary approach with a comprehensive health assessment and detailed assessment by the therapists. In a child with one area of learning difficulty it is important to ensure that there are not associated difficulties in other areas and that the child does not have a visual or hearing impairment compounding his or her difficulties. Although a relatively mild problem in the overall spectrum of disabilities, children with unrecognized dyspraxia can present with major problems in a classroom situation. As a result of their difficulties they may become withdrawn and reluctant to attempt new tasks; equally they may become disruptive as a result of their frustrations, or even aggressive in a classroom or playground setting. They may become the butt of jokes due to their difficulties with writing, their slowness changing for gym and problems keeping up with their peers in activities requiring good coordination (e.g. playing football).

Attention deficit hyperactivity disorder (see Ch. 18)

Children with attention deficit hyperactivity disorder are a poorly understood group of children presenting enormous difficulties in the classroom setting. Even those responding to medication continue to experience difficulties. Again, a careful multidisciplinary approach to their assessment and diagnosis and input in the classroom and at home in order to enable these children to achieve their potential educationally and socially is required.

Autism (see Chs 3 and 18)

This condition is characterized by general and profound failure to develop social relationships, language retardation, and ritualistic and compulsive behaviour. Children with autism or other forms of pervasive, social and communication disorders place great strains on their families. In some ways this is worsened by the apparently normal appearance of these children, who are therefore expected by the extended family and members of the local community to behave normally. This area of disability also presents problems to doctors in terms of explaining the nature of the problem to parents and the uncertainty of the prognosis. Well-coordinated multidisciplinary management is particularly important in this context. Appropriate educational placement with specialist teachers and speech and language therapists is vital to the ultimate outcome. Provision of respite services is just as important as in the severely physical disabled child, allowing these parents to spend time together and with any other children without the continuous need to adapt the situation around the disabled child.

DEPRIVATION

Despite the relative affluence of Britain there are still pockets of deprivation in all our cities and large towns, and indeed areas of deprivation within some rural communities. Young families may be trapped in a cycle of poverty, poor educational opportunity, unemployment and bad housing, in communities where disillusionment and distrust of professional agencies make access to the available services difficult. Children growing up in these communities have a higher incidence of common health problems such as glue ear and respiratory infections, associated at least in part with damp housing and a high level of smoking. Their families are often poor users of primary care services. A higher proportion are developmentally delayed through lack of stimulation and opportunity rather than genetic or medical factors.

    Health factors may also in themselves lead to a lack of appropriate stimulation and care of the child. For example, parents who are suffering from a physical illness, the effect of drugs or alcohol abuse or mental health problems may find it difficult to have the time and energy to relate appropriately to their child. Such parents are also limited in their ability to take the child out to enjoy normal preschool opportunities such as a playgroup or nursery or a trip to the swimming pool. Health visitors play a key role in monitoring the well-being of these children, visiting them at home, advising on feeding, clothing, physical

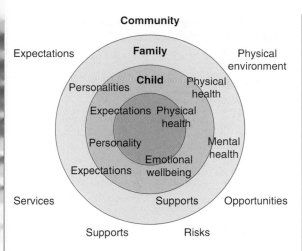

Figure 17.2 Factors in family disturbance

safety, and stimulation and encouraging the parents to take the child for surveillance and immunization and to consider preschool opportunities.

If the health visitor and general practitioner are concerned that the level of deprivation is threatening the long-term health and development of the child, or indeed his or her immediate safety, a referral to the social work department and community child health department will be made for further assessment. The child then requires comprehensive health assessment, including full physical examination, growth measurements and a developmental assessment. A case conference will be convened to assess the child's situation, looking carefully at all the relevant factors in the child and family situation and at the community setting before reaching a recommendation on how best to help the child and family. Figure 17.2 illustrates the many factors which affect a child and their family's response to health and development problems.

✱ KEY DIAGNOSIS

The 'looked-after' child

Where deprivation is a major factor in the child's environment, every attempt is made to input services to the family to help them to care for their child. However there are situations where the level of deprivation or actual abuse is such that the child needs to be removed from the family, at least for a period of time, so that work with the family can be undertaken prior to a decision being taken about the long-term placement of the child. Children in this situation are placed in substitute families and are described under the new legislation as being 'looked after'. If in the long term it appears that rehabilitation back to the natural family is going to be unsuccessful, a decision will be made to place the child in a substitute family on a permanent basis. The child can then be referred to the fostering and adoption panel, which will decide on the basis of extensive reports whether the child should be placed for adoption or long-term fostering. Long-term fostering is usually the choice for an older child who, despite all difficulties, will have significant ties to his or her natural family and wishes to continue to have regular contact. Trying to place a child in those circumstances for adoption is likely to lead to disruption due to attachment difficulties. For the very young child, or the child with significant special needs where a family wishes him or her to be placed in an alternative family, adoption allows the child to be fully 'claimed' by a new family, and is the preferred choice.

Many children received into care through family difficulties present very significant emotional and behavioural problems to their new carers. These may range from extreme withdrawal, soiling and bed wetting, abnormal eating behaviours, sleep disturbance to aggressive and sexually provocative behaviours. Foster carers receive quite extensive training before children are placed with them, and require a great deal of ongoing support from the social work department and from health and education professionals to enable the children to settle and begin to make progress again.

Issues around HIV and hepatitis infection may also be raised where children are placed as young children of intravenous drug abusers or following sexual abuse. Because of the difficulties associated with testing for HIV infection, all foster carers have now been advised that they should treat all children as potentially infected and to have in place a high standard of health and hygiene within their household which will reduce any risk of infection. There is no evidence currently that HIV infection can be transmitted horizontally to the household of an infected child, but anxieties are still raised, and families and foster carers need appropriate advice and reassurance.

CHILD ABUSE

Definition
'There are many definitions of child abuse; a reflection perhaps of society's difficulty in identifying and coming to terms with the problem.'

> **Definition of child abuse**
> Abuse of children is human-originated acts of commission or omission, and human created or tolerated conditions that inhibit or preclude unfolding and development of the inherent potential of children

This statement by David Gill is particularly useful in that it emphasizes the significant incidence of 'abuse by omission', in other words failure to provide adequate care for children, as well as deliberate ill-treatment of children. It encompasses not only the ill-treatment of children within their family or immediate community setting but also the abuse of children caught up in war or famine (see Ch. 20).

Patterns of referral
It remains impossible to quantify the exact extent of abuse. Referrals of children and prosecutions have steadily risen over recent years, but this is in the main due to an increasing awareness of the problem within society and improved systems for referral and investigation. Table 17.4 shows the main types of abuse which are fairly typical across the country. Well-recognized patterns of age at presentation are emerging.

Confidentiality
Child abuse cases regularly raise issues around confidentiality, particularly for doctors working in general practice where the parents are also patients of the practice. Recent General Medical

Table 17.4 Types of abuse
Physical abuse
Physical neglect
Non-organic failure to thrive
Emotional abuse
Sexual abuse
Multiple abuse

Council guidance issued in 1995 makes it clear that where a practitioner suspects that a child may be being abused, the circumstances 'usually require' referral on to another agency. Some leeway is left in this advice in order to allow professionals, particularly those in the Mental Health Services, to prepare a patient for referral where a child is not considered to be currently at risk (e.g. if an adult patient reports previous abuse by a father with whom she is no longer living). Of course care must be taken in deciding to delay referral as the alleged perpetrator may have access to other children.

Consent
Consent also raises anxieties which have been clarified to some extent by the recent Children Act legislation. In 1991 the Age of Legal Capacity (Scotland) Act clarified the position in Scotland by making 16 years the age at which all young people have the ability to give their own consent, but made it clear that prior to that age any child who was felt competent to understand the significance of the examination and treatment should be asked to give his or her own consent. It also established that it is the doctor's responsibility to make a decision as to whether or not the child is competent to give consent.

Where the doctor decides that a child is competent, the child's consent must be sought, and the parents no longer have a right to make the decision for the child, although they would be expected to give the child appropriate guidance and support in reaching a decision. The nature and circumstances of the child's medical condition has an important bearing on whether or not he or she is competent to give consent. For example, a child of 10 years might be felt able to give consent for his fractured arm to be put in plaster under general anaesthetic but not to give consent for open heart surgery. Giving his or her own consent for an examination for sexual abuse, which might lead to the imprisonment of a parent, raises much more complex issues about a child's ability to consent and the meaning of the phrase 'understanding the implications'.

✳ KEY DIAGNOSIS

Non-accidental injury

Presentation

Children present in a wide variety of ways with possible abuse. Frequently concerns are raised by health visitors, general practitioners or nursery or school staff, particularly where a child presents repeatedly with inadequately explained bruising. Sometimes children may be referred anonymously by neighbours or will be brought by another member of the family. Older children are now encouraged to refer themselves, either through telephone help lines (e.g. Childline) or through disclosing to a trusted adult, particularly a guidance teacher in secondary school. Prevention programmes in primary and special schools have an important role.

Children may present directly to the health services, either by being brought to the accident and emergency department or through attendance at the outpatients department with vague symptoms such as abdominal pain. In any injured young child presenting to casualty but without an adequate explanation it is very important to consider abuse among the differential diagnoses. A number of alerting signs can be recognized, and are shown in Table 17.5.

In children under 2 years of age where an accidental cause of injury is given, it is important to consider carefully whether the child is at a developmental stage at which such an accident is possible. For example, children are frequently brought in with a number of fractures, and described as having 'climbed out of their cot'.

Table 17.5 Alerting signs of abuse
Unexplained delay in presentation
Changes in the details of the history as reported
Evasiveness/anger when details are sought
Inconsistency between the history and clinical findings

In a child under 9 months of age who is not yet pulling to stand this cannot be the correct explanation. Parents giving a false explanation for injury frequently change their story or the details of their story when pressed, particularly if interviewed separately. It is therefore extremely important that all explanations given are noted in detail in the contemporaneous notes, and clearly signed and dated so that such discrepancies can be preserved. This may be crucial to the success of any subsequent legal proceedings and therefore to the long-term protection of the child.

Types of abuse

Five types of abuse are recognized and these are shown in Table 17.4, together with a sixth category of multiple abuse. It is very important to remember that in many instances the child may have been subject to more than one form of abuse. For example, a physically abused child may also be being neglected or emotionally abused; a sexually abused child is by definition also emotionally abused. There are some recognized associations in patterns of abuse, e.g. sexual abuse accompanied by cigarette burns, particularly to the lower body and injuries from restraining the child such as bruising to the inner thighs or ligature marks to the ankles.

The term 'physical abuse' covers a wide spectrum from hitting or striking (see Fig. 11.11), deliberate burning or scalding, the breaking of bones from rough handling (Fig. 17.3) or non-accidental falls, to brain injury through shaking or striking the head against a hard surface.

In court, paediatricians are often asked to comment on the age of bruises. Research has indicated that this should be done with great care, as bruising of all different colours may appear

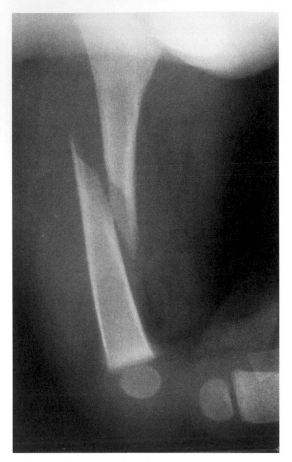

Figure 17.3 Femoral shaft fracture in a non-weight bearing young child highly suspicious of non-accidental injury

falling off a swing. This is a further reminder of the importance of very careful documentation of the nature and exact site of all injuries.

Interpretation of fractures is another area of difficulty where defence experts may attempt to maintain that a child has an underlying abnormality of bone metabolism predisposing him or her to fractures as a result of trivial force. Similarly, in children where intracranial injury from severe shaking is diagnosed, pre-existing congenital brain abnormality or perinatal brain damage may be asserted by medical experts for the defence. Such pre-existing conditions are, in reality, rare occurrences.

History and clinical examination

The examination of a child who may have been abused should follow the same format as any other clinical examination. It should be preceded by a full history of the child's health, development, and family and social situation, and a complete physical examination, including measurement of growth and a brief assessment of development, leading to a differential diagnosis and a plan of necessary investigations to exclude or confirm possible alternative explanations for the child's presentation. It must be meticulously documented, including accurate quotes of any explanation given by the adult or child. The examiner must be very careful to use open-ended questions.

Investigations and initial management

Investigations which should be considered in causes of possible physical abuse and/or sexual abuse are blood film and clotting studies and a skeletal survey. Children referred to as abused have been found on investigation to have idiopathic thrombocytopenic purpura or haemophilia (see Ch. 11). Rarely, children may present with a suspicious pattern of repeated fractures with inadequate explanation and found to have osteogenesis imperfecta.

Where suspicions that the child has been abused are high, the paediatrician will examine the child jointly with a police surgeon, who will take responsibility for the gathering of forensic

rapidly after serious injury, and the speed with which the blood products within the bruise begin to break down, giving the yellow to green coloration as bruises age, is also very variable. The colour changes depend very much on the force of impact and underlying surface to the skin, i.e. whether it is over bone or over soft tissue such as the abdomen. What is clear is that where bruises are red the injury has occurred within 24–48 h and that the yellowing discoloration seen as the blood products start to break down is not seen before 18–24 h. However, of much more importance is the description of clear variation in the age of bruising on a child where all the injuries are described as occurring due to a single accidental injury, such as

specimens. This is particularly important in cases of alleged sexual abuse where the taking of specimens may enable identification of the alleged perpetrator through DNA found in semen on vaginal swabs or from saliva from swabbing round breasts or bite marks. He or she will also oversee the taking of photographs to be used in any subsequent criminal proceedings. The recent introduction of the colposcope, providing illumination and magnification, for the examination of children who may have been sexually abused has been of great benefit in allowing a more detailed assessment. It also makes it possible to record the findings by still photography or video for use in court and avoids the child having to be re-examined by defence medical experts. Genital injuries heal very rapidly and diagnostic findings may well have disappeared by time any subsequent examination is carried out.

Following the examination and investigation, the paediatrician is responsible for the immediate ongoing care of the child, and may decide to admit the child for observation if there are any concerns about significant head injury or internal bleeding in an acutely injured child. Admission can also be very useful in the neglected child, where rapid weight gain and developmental progress (particularly in social and play skills) can be very valuable additional evidence when the case reaches court.

Interagency process

In approaching the investigation of a child who may have been abused or neglected, the medical history, examination and investigation are frequently crucial. However, such assessment will only be effective if it is carried out carefully within the context of an interagency investigation with social workers and the police, so that all previous information and knowledge about the child and family will be brought together, including whether there have been previous suspicious incidents, or whether one of both parents has a criminal record or perhaps mental health problems. Where an accidental cause for the injury is alleged, a visit to the scene of the

incident may be vital in confirming or refuting the story. The medical evidence is therefore only one piece of the jigsaw used to build up a picture of the child and family. Put together, the information should lead to a conclusion as to whether or not the child has been deliberately abused and an assessment of likely ongoing risk to the child.

The case conference and legal process

Once the investigation is complete, a child protection case conference is called at which it is very important that the medical team present the medical evidence and discuss its significance. This evidence, taken together with police and social work evidence and information from the primary care team and the family itself, helps to establish whether or not abuse has occurred and the degree of ongoing risk to the child. Plans are then made for the future care of the child. The conference will decide whether or not to place the child on the child protection register and whether or not the child needs to be referred on for legal proceedings to ensure protection.

In Scotland, the children's hearing system decides whether or not a child needs a supervision order for monitoring in the home setting or in a substitute family placement. The police pass evidence to the Procurator Fiscal, who will decide whether or not legal proceedings against the alleged perpetrator should take place.

Where the child is placed on the child protection register, a child protection plan will be put in place, part of which is the ongoing health care of the child. Questions that should be addressed include:

- Does the child require further investigation in terms of the possibility of sexually transmitted diseases, such as hepatitis or HIV infection or pregnancy?
- Does the child require psychological or psychiatric care particularly in follow-up to sexual abuse?
- Does the child's basic growth and development require ongoing monitoring?

Responsibility for ensuring that the ongoing health plan is put in place usually falls to a senior community paediatrician. The health visitor is, of course, in a key position to offer ongoing support and monitoring to the child and family.

Evaluation of severity of abuse and risk of recurrence

One of the difficulties in the management of children who may have been abused is deciding whether or not the child has or is likely to suffer significant harm. This is a phrase embodied in the legislation, and is a very useful concept although there is no clear definition. However, considering two simple examples may be helpful. Firstly, it might be felt that where a confrontational teenager has deliberately stayed out 2 h later than expected, come home drunk and then been struck across the face by the father, this physical assault is provoked and not likely to cause a degree of significant harm in itself. In contrast, when considering fresh deliberate burns and severe facial bruising to a toddler, there would be no doubt that significant harm has occurred. It is clear then that even from the health viewpoint alone it is essential to consider the child's immediate presentation (irrespective of whether it is with severe physical injury or disclosure of sexual abuse) within the context of a comprehensive assessment which examines the child's growth, development, and social and emotional well being. In order to complete this picture, it may be necessary to ask for a specialist psychiatric or psychological opinion as part of the initial assessment, as well as considering the role of such specialists in the management of the child.

FURTHER READING

Hall D M B 1996 Health for all children, 3rd edn. Oxford University Press, Oxford

Hobbs C J 1999 Child abuse and neglect, 2nd edn. Churchill Livingstone, Edinburgh

Polnay L 1993 Community paediatrics, 2nd edn. Churchill Livingstone, Edinburgh

CHAPTER 18

Behavioural disorders

K. J. Aitken

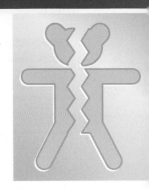

CORE PROBLEMS IN BEHAVIOURAL DISORDERS

CORE PROBLEM	KEY DIAGNOSIS	RELATED TOPICS
• Developmentally inappropriate behaviour	Enuresis	Soiling and encopresis Chronic constipation[5]
• Developmentally abnormal behaviour	Hyperkinetic disorder	Conduct disorder Sleep disorder Autism Other disorders of social and intellectual function
• Problems with psychosomatic component	Functional abdominal pain	Headache[10] Chronic fatigue syndrome Fibromyalgia[12] Hypothyroidism[9]
• Adolescent behaviour disorder	Eating disorder	Drug abuse Overdose and suicide attempts

Where the primary location of a topic is in another chapter, this is indicated by a superscript

ESSENTIAL BACKGROUND

INTRODUCTION

Difficulties encountered in coping with children's behaviour are amongst the most common reasons for parent consultations with the general practitioner and for subsequent referral on to secondary paediatric services. The range of conditions which deserve coverage is considerable – fears and phobias, tics and Tourette's syndrome, depression, eating disorders, effects of abuse and of parenting skills problems. Quoted rates for specific disorders vary widely, but Table 18.1 gives an idea of the population prevalence in children of some of the more commonly referred behaviour problems.

Many childhood behaviour problems, such as temper tantrums, are naturally transient. The 'terrible two's' is a real phenomenon; there is a phase where the normal child is physically able to do a wide range of things which parents and other caregivers are unable to see as appropriate or acceptable but where their child's language comprehension is not sufficient to accede to or accept the setting of limits by adults.

The vast majority of behavioural difficulties will show improvement or disappear completely within a fairly brief period of time. Non-compliant behaviour, food refusal, temper tantrums, enuresis and encopresis ('elimination problems') are all likely, in the majority of otherwise developmentally normal children, to remit without clinical intervention. Other problems are less tractable. For example, without systematic clinical intervention, childhood sleep difficulties are likely to remain relatively unchanged over a lengthy period. For certain conditions, such as conduct disorder, the evidence suggests that clinical intervention is unlikely to effect significant improvement. Neurodevelopmental problems of behaviour are also often less amenable to change. Some of these conditions have distinct somatic

Table 18.1 Prevalence of common behavioural disorders	
Disorder	Prevalence
Sleep disorders	Night terrors: 100–400/10 000 preschool children Settling problems: 800–1200/10 000 preschool children Night waking: 1000–2100/10 000 preschool children
Temper tantrums	Most days: 1100–1800/10 000 preschool children
Enuresis	980/10 000 at age 7 years
Phobias	500/10 000 (age 7–12 years)
Encopresis	150/10 000 (age 7–8 years) 80/10 000 (10–12 years)
Depression	200/10 000 of school age children (male = female) 800/10 000 (4 to1 male to female) by 17 years
Anorexia nervosa	90/10 000 in girls (age 0–15 years) 10/10 000 in boys (age 0–15 years) Peak age of onset 14–15 years
Autism	4.5–21.1/10 000 (age 0–15 years)
Asperger's syndrome	28 /10 000
Tourette's syndrome	0.7–21/10 000 (age 7–16 years)
Schizophrenia	Very rare, but similar in presentation and course to adult-onset schizophrenia

features, and when association between these features and the pattern of behaviour is strong, we can describe it as a 'behavioural phenotype' (see Beyond core: abnormal behaviour phenotype).

Most frequently, difficulties are encountered by parents in attempting to deal with behaviours which they see as either developmentally inappropriate or unpredictable. Often parental concerns are appropriate, but on some occasions parents are unduly concerned about a behaviour which is developmentally normal, and they should be reassured on this point. To be able to provide such reassurance, it is clearly important for the clinician to have a firm working knowledge of normal developmental processes and of the ages at which certain problems are most common.

To optimize clinical effectiveness we, therefore, need knowledge of what is developmentally appropriate for a given child at a given age (see also Ch. 3) and a means of analysing problem behaviours in a manner which will highlight key features of those behaviours.

HISTORY TAKING

Basic component

There are two crucial components in working effectively with behaviour disorders, whatever the nature of the referred problem: a detailed developmental history and a functional analysis of the behaviour problem. Reduced to its simplest form, it is essential to identify whether a problem is due to:

- Lack of development of a particular skill or function (a problem of omission) or
- The presence of a specific behaviour in the context of more appropriate alternatives (a problem of commission).

In the situation where the behaviour problem is predictable on the basis of the underlying condition and the age of the child, it is still important to ensure that other factors are neither contributory nor a primary causal factor. Medical teaching still veers towards the concept of differential diagnosis and of mutually exclusive

ABNORMAL BEHAVIOUR PHENOTYPE

It is important to identify medical conditions in which abnormal behaviour is a known and predictable component. They include:

- Lesch–Nyhan syndrome (Hypoxanthine–guanine–phosphoribosyltransferase deficiency): single gene abnormality leading to an obligatory and severe form of self-injurious behaviour.

- Fragile-X syndrome: fragile chromosome site on the long arm of X chromosome, resulting in macro-orchidism, dysmorphic facial features (long face, prominent jaw and large ears), gaze aversion and stereotypies. This condition, which is the commonest form of mental retardation in males, gives rise to a range of behavioural patterns, including attention deficit–hyperactivity disorder (ADHD).

- Prader–Willi syndrome: neonatal hypotonia, childhood obesity and the associated abnormal behaviour of hyperphagia, short stature, hypogonadism, mental retardation and chromosome 15 abnormalities.

- Williams syndrome: dysmorphic facies with round face and full lips, supravalvular aortic stenosis, hypercalcaemia, chromosome 7 abnormalities and mental retardation. These children exhibit a peculiar behaviour, 'cocktail party chatter', which is the result of a low IQ combined with enhanced social use of language.

causes, whereas child psychiatry has become more comfortable with the idea of comorbidity (more than one diagnosis being given to the same individual at the same time). Thus, several different factors (which may be variously social, constitutional, infective or other) might be viewed as having equally significant impact on an individual at the same time and together contribute to the manifestation of a given behaviour.

Developmental component

A critical element in arriving at a diagnosis is that the behaviour being shown is developmentally inappropriate. It is important that any developmentally anomalous behaviours are clearly described and also that they are compared to what would be seen as developmentally appropriate behaviour for a child of the same age and background. The background history needs to contain information on a number of areas which may be pertinent:

- Pregnancy, labour and delivery
- Early milestones
- Language development
- Social development
- Development of self-care skills (feeding, dressing, toileting)
- Motor development
- Academic progress
- Any significant medical history.

Accurate information on behaviour abnormalities is best obtained in the form of a 'functional analysis', and typically requires prospective diary keeping by the family and/or school to gain an acceptably detailed picture. A functional analysis is an assessment of the behavioural problem by systematically examining various aspects that are potentially critical to its maintenance. It is possible to effect major changes in the presentation and severity of many disabling behavioural disorders through identifying and intervening to alleviate the effects of maintaining or exacerbating factors. A functional analysis tries to identify any pattern in the presenting problem behaviour by firstly recording what leads up to it (its antecedents), secondly noting the form and concomitants of the problem itself (the behaviour) and lastly looking at what happens once it has occurred (its consequences) – the ABC approach.

The most important component of the functional analysis is the information obtained about the behaviour itself. This is of two types:

the typology (detailed description) of the behaviour and the setting in which the behaviour occurred.

The typology of the behaviour

Features which may be relevant are:

- Its frequency: how often (per day/week/year) does the problem occur?
- Its severity: how severe is the problem when it does occur? (If we take the example of hand biting, is the skin marked/broken/has the child drawn blood/removed tissue?)
- Its duration: within any particular episode, how long did it last?
- Any aspects which can be counted, e.g. number of hits/bites/encopretic episodes (these measurements can form the basis for simple means of monitoring interventions).
- Any clustering or cyclicity to the problem.

The setting of the behaviour

Features which might be relevant include:

- Who was present?
- Where did the behaviour occur?
- At what time did it happen?
- Was anything else happening in parallel with the problem?

What one is attempting to identify is any clear pattern to the behaviour, whether there is:

- A sequence of predictable events which, if not interrupted, leads into the problem
- Something about the behaviour itself which appears to be rewarding
- A consequence of the behaviour which appears to maintain it.

A condition which exemplifies all three aspects of the behaviour is breath-holding attacks (child's perception: 'When I hold my breath like this I get what I want').

Occasionally, the keeping of a diary will highlight an association with other factors that had previously gone unnoticed such as maternal pre-menstrual tension or parental migraine. Equally, dietary factors such as rebound hypoglycaemia to

refined sugar intake can emerge as a component in preschool behavioural difficulties such as non-compliant behaviour and temper tantrums.

CORE PROBLEMS

DEVELOPMENTALLY INAPPROPRIATE BEHAVIOUR

✱ KEY DIAGNOSIS

Enuresis

Developmentally inappropriate incontinence of urine was first described some three and a half millennia ago in the Eber's Papyrus, and continues to be one of the most commonly referred refractory problems seen in childhood.

> **Diagnostic criteria for non-organic enuresis**
> - The child has a chronological and mental age of at least 5 years
> - Voiding of urine into bedding and/or clothes at least twice monthly under 7 years of age or once monthly over 7 years
> - The problem has been present for at least 3 months
> - The problem is not due to epilepsy, other neurological disorder or structural abnormality of the urinary tract
> - There is no evidence of any other psychiatric disorder
> - Enuresis can be further subdivided as follows:
>   - Nocturnal enuresis only – no daytime accidents but wet at night
>   - Diurnal enuresis only – daytime accidents but dry overnight
>   - Nocturnal and diurnal enuresis – wet both by day and by night

Prevalence and epidemiology

It was not so long ago that most mothers expected their children to achieve bladder control within the first year of life, with many starting training within the first 6 months. In reality, most children are not continent of urine by day until 3–4 years of age. A recent Scandinavian study provides the best epidemiological data to date on a large sample of several thousand 7 year old children. Overall, nearly 10% had a significant problem with wetting: the majority (6.4%) bedwetting and the remainder with daytime or both daytime and night-time problems. In respect of nocturnal enuresis, a rough estimate of prevalence is: 10% at 5 years, 5% at 10 years and 1% at 15 years. There are some emerging indications that the strong family histories of enuresis can be underpinned by genetic factors. A recent Danish study found an association between a chromosome 13q DNA polymorphism and dominantly inherited primary nocturnal enuresis.

Presentation and assessment

Frequently parents will consult their general practitioner when they are becoming concerned about difficulties in initial toilet training. The time of presentation varies widely in line with variations in parental expectation. As the child approaches school entry, parents tend to become concerned at persisting daytime wetting. However, as indicated above, clinical concerns should not be high in the child with a developmental level of under 5 years.

A detailed history of the problem is important:

- Is there any family history of similar problems?
- Is this a primary or a secondary problem (was there a period of control before concerns were raised or has the child always been wet)?
- Is there any suggestion of an intermittent urinary tract infection?
- Can any pattern be identified on functional analysis (see p. 349)?
- Is there any relationship with the setting (e.g. child wets at home but not when he stays with granny)?

Treatment

Treatment approaches to enuresis can be divided into behavioural and non-behavioural.

Behavioural

In general terms, behavioural treatments have proven highly effective with non-organic childhood enuretic problems, being successful in over 75% of cases. Behavioural treatment should be attempted first because it is generally more innocuous than pharmacological intervention. For nocturnal enuresis there are several approaches which may be used in combination.

Of these, the bell-and-pad and incentive (star) chart are the most common.

The *bell-and-pad*: is a proven and effective treatment strategy. Its effectiveness increases with age, and in general this form of therapy is reserved for children beyond 6 years. Urine from involuntary micturition soaks a pad and completes an electrical circuit triggering an alarm; the child wakes with the noise, thus 'learning' the sensations preceding the voiding, and is taken to the toilet, thus linking these sensations to the process of getting up and going to the toilet. If this approach is going to work, it should do so within a few weeks. In the absence of a significant response within 4–6 weeks it should be abandoned, leaving an interval of at least 6 months before trying again. The bell-and-pad can be used in conjunction with an incentive chart (see below), and there is some evidence that urine retention training (see below) as an adjunct is more useful than the bell-and-pad alone with children who have low functional bladder capacity. There has been a progressive move towards the use of pants alarms as opposed to sheets placed on the bed. These appear to be better tolerated by many children.

The *incentive chart* approach, which provides positive reinforcement with the 'reward' of stars for dry nights, can be used from 5 years upwards. A number of factors are important and often missed:

- The child must find the materials interesting – do not assume that blue or gold sticky backed stars have some magical quality
- Ensure that the child is rewarded at a reasonable rate – unless the child achieves a reward between 60–70% of the time, it is highly unlikely that a star chart will generate change in behaviour
- Try to encourage active collaboration – get the child to choose his or her stickers/pictures for the chart.

Other approaches, which can be linked to use of an incentive chart, include *urine retention training* (gradually building up the period between the urge to urinate and voiding), and *dry bed training* (lifting the child regularly throughout the night, gradually increasing the toileting interval; this is usually too much for all but the most motivated families).

For daytime/diurnal enuresis an additional strategy can be added: *bladder drill training*. This approach begins by establishing a routine of regular self-toiletting, usually every 90 min, with gradual build-up of the time between urination until a 4 hourly schedule is attained.

Non-behavioural

Several drug therapies have been evaluated, but only two found to be useful in the treatment of childhood enuretic problems:

- *Desmopressin acetate (DDAVP)*. This is clinically useful, albeit transiently. DDAVP seems to be more effective with older children, providing temporary improvement in some 70% of cases but with relapse on cessation of treatment. It is at best only an adjunct to behavioural intervention, but often helpful when, for example, a child with persistent night time enuresis is attending a camp or staying with friends who are unaware of the problem.
- *Imipramine hydrochloride*. This acts via its anticholinergic effect, and has been used extensively in the treatment of enuresis. However, the overall success rate for continued continence on withdrawal of medication is no better than 25%, and in some studies less than 10%. Tricyclic drugs are an important cause of fatal accidental poisoning (see Ch. 15), and should not be prescribed if there are young preschool children at home.

Effective treatment of nocturnal enuresis leads to significant improvement in a child's self-esteem. Furthermore, there is evidence of an association between how the nature of persistent enuresis is viewed and the levels of reported associated stress. Thus, it is important to provide a full explanation about the nature of the condition; never simply recommend appropriate reading matter outlining an effective approach without support and discussion of the practicalities of the method. This can often do more harm than good, and some parents whose children fail to respond to such methods can be left with a feeling of incompetence and a reduced ability to cope with their child – 'I can't even get this right!'.

Soiling and encopresis

Chronic problems with toilet training and bowel habit affects 1% of children at some point, more frequently in males. The symptom of encopresis is the passage of faeces into inappropriate places at any age after bowel control should have been established. It is linked to social class and other behavioural difficulties. Organic causes are extremely rare.

Constipation and soiling may persist from birth onwards (primary, suggesting an organic cause such as Hirschsprung's disease; see Ch. 5) or develop after successful toilet training (secondary, indicating functional disorder). Chronic constipation may lead to faecal impaction with overflow, resulting in soiling, and if present for a significant time may result in 'psychogenic' megacolon.

In infancy, secondary constipation may arise during an illness, perhaps associated with dehydration, resulting in painful defaecation and subsequent retention. It is easy to see how a vicious cycle can be set up, but early effective intervention with laxatives is often very effective. In other cases, particularly in association with encopresis, complex psychological and family functioning issues are usually the basis of the problem and may require long-term supportive behavioural therapy. Similar approaches are required to those used in the treatment of enuresis, but the time-scale is nearly always increased. Drug therapy is used in addition to the behavioural approach. In children, combined therapy is usually given in the form of an osmotic laxative (lactulose) and stimulant laxatives (docusate sodium or senna). Potent stimulant laxatives such as sodium picosulphate may initially be required to clear the bowel area and occasionally enemas are required if faecal impaction has occurred. Manual evacuation is needed in the very severe chronic cases with secondary megacolon.

The stigma of soiling (e.g. in the classroom) may add to the underlying psychological problems driving this behavioural condition, but other aspects of psychological disturbance may persist. The outlook for the vast majority of children is good, with eventual acquisition of good toileting habits.

DEVELOPMENTALLY ABNORMAL BEHAVIOUR

* KEY DIAGNOSIS

Hyperkinetic disorder

Epidemiology and diagnosis

This group of disorders (which largely parallels the US diagnosis of attention deficit–hyperactivity disorder, ADHD) has apparently increased in prevalence in recent years. However, difficulties in diagnosis are considerable, and differences in interpretation of the condition exist both within the UK and between the UK and other countries.

UK diagnostic criteria for hyperkinetic disorder
- Core features: abnormal levels of inattention, hyperactivity and impulsivity are present :
  - Across situations (i.e. not just at home or at school)
  - Across time (i.e. not just at the weekends).
  The core features are required to have been present for at least 6 months and to an extent which is both maladaptive and inconsistent with the developmental level of the child.
- Age of onset should have been before 7 years of age.
- There should be clear information consistent with the criteria from more than one source (e.g. home and school). Additionally, the features observed cannot be better accounted for on the basis of a manic episode, anxiety disorder, pervasive developmental disorder or other psychiatric condition.

Of all children, 3% meet the diagnostic criteria, with a high preponderance of males over females (5:1). Reported rates in the USA are more than in the UK because of the broader diagnostic criteria used but, when like is compared with like, the reported prevalence figures are very similar.

Some evidence exists of a genetic basis to this disorder. A recent series of studies has identified a D_4 dopamine receptor gene abnormality in a high proportion of cases. However, the picture is undoubtedly more complex.

Presentation

Family concerns about the behaviour of children with hyperkinetic disorder are usually present from an early age, but it is unusual for there to be a clinical referral under the age of 3 years, unless there is a family history of similar difficulties which have heightened parental awareness of potential problems.

Assessment

It is crucial to take a detailed developmental history. From the perspective of a formal diagnosis, it is important to elucidate both the chronicity and pattern of emergence of reported difficulties. As regards current presentation, information needs to be collected from more than one setting (e.g. home, nursery or school) concerning the level of attention, hyperactivity and impulsivity; ideally by the use of both direct observation and a standardized assessment measure such as the Connor's Parent and Teacher Rating Scales. There are associations with a number of medical conditions, the best known being those with asthma, chronic otitis media, and abnormalities of thyroid function.

Treatment

The variety of associated difficulties experienced by children with hyperkinetic disorder indicates the need for multimodal and individualized treatment plans. Three main groups of treatment approaches are the focus of clinical and research attention, with medication and behavioural interventions seen as particularly effective in combination:

- *Medication.* There is an extensive literature on the role of medication in the treatment of overactivity, beginning with a report on the use of the stimulant medication benzedrine in 1937. Methylphenidate (Ritalin) is the best known, most successful to date, and most widely used in the treatment of hyperactivity.
- *Behavioural approaches based around strategies to improve function.* Behavioural work with this disorder began with attempts to improve attention and self-control, employing

psychometric tasks such as the Matching Familiar Figures Test as a means of monitoring treatment effects.

Current behavioural work largely adopts a threefold approach:

- Parent, child and teacher education about the condition, highlighting its combined effects on the child's social, emotional and academic development in the short and long term, and the need to develop a series of realistic treatment goals.
- Parent/teacher training in child behavioural management strategies, and classroom management.
- Direct work with the child, focusing upon developing self-control strategies (e.g. the child being trained to talk through the steps of solving a problem, choosing a solution on the basis of the best outcome rather than an impulsive decision) and social skills (e.g. how to accurately interpret the intentions of others, develop conversational skills and manage anger).

- *Dietary interventions.* The best known, but perhaps least effective approach is the 'Feingold diet'. This was much publicized as an approach that focused on the possible role of food colourings and additives such as the food colouring dye tartrazine (E102) on children's behaviour. Subsequent work has shown that such additives and colourants can be a significant factor, but only in a small group of such children.

Outcomes

While there has now been extensive research into the long-term outcome of hyperkinetic children reaching adulthood, failure to distinguish between the various subgroups and the existence of associated disorders (co-morbidity) makes interpretation of the outcome of hyperkinesis difficult. Comorbidity with other psychiatric disorders occurs in a high proportion of cases. From studies to date, 30–50% of cases are comorbid for conduct disorder (characterized by defiant, aggressive and antisocial behaviour); 35–60% for oppositional defiant disorder (can be considered as a subtype of conduct disorder seen more frequently in younger children); 20–30% for anxiety disorders; 30% for mood disorders; and 20–25% for learning disabilities.

Conduct disorder

Conduct disorder is characterized by non-compliance, aggression, poor personal relationships and disruptive behaviour. Early family relationships and the environment play a key role in the development of this disorder, and typically the family fail to provide appropriate and consistent socializing experiences for the child. As a consequence, the child's ability to resist temptation and empathize with others is compromised. It is a condition often associated with delinquency and school failure.

Conduct disorder has a greater prevalence than hyperkinetic disorder, although the two conditions can share similar features. Although the prognosis is poor, recent research indicates that behaviourally based parenting programmes have the best chance of effecting change.

Sleep disorders

These are common in childhood, and indeed for many children are part of normal development. Most difficulties with sleep are temporary and related to appropriate reactions (excitement, fear and anxiety). They may be an expression of concern over parental anxiety and conflict. Rarely, sleep disorders may be an expression of a hyperkinetic disorder or a behavioural phenotype (see above, p. 348). Adolescents may have difficulty in getting to sleep and/or early waking and underlying depression should be considered. Nightmares, night terrors and sleep walking occur relatively frequently, possibly in up to 15% of children.

Most sleep disorders are relieved by parental support, reassurance and encouragement. Occasionally drug therapy (e.g. light sleeping medication) is used to break the cycle and establish a normal routine.

Autism

In 1943, Leo Kanner first described autism as a 'biologically provided disorder of affective contact' (a position which is little different from our current view) and noted an 'inability to relate in an ordinary way to people and to situations' coupled with an 'anxiously obsessive desire for the maintenance of sameness'.

Most authorities agree that the following features are essential for the diagnosis:

- General and profound failure to develop social relationships
- Language retardation
- Ritualistic and compulsive behaviour.

In addition, these features must be manifest by 3 years of age.

Epidemiology and pathophysiology

Reported rates of autism have been steadily rising with studies giving variable rates between 5 and 20 per 10 000 children (see Table 18.1).

A variety of causal explanations are currently proposed in attempts to explain autism. A number of gene markers have been found. Most recently, two separate serotonin transporter gene abnormalities in two different populations have been identified. Some authorities argue that the data are most consistent with several affected genes (probably three or four but perhaps as many as ten) being both necessary and sufficient to cause autism.

Presentation

Typically, parents become aware that something is wrong sometime during the second year of life. This in some cases leads parents to suspect a link with inoculations such as the MMR (mumps, measles and rubella vaccine) which is currently given in the UK at 13 months of age. However, a recent review has established that there is no such link. Often the child is extensively assessed for problems such as hearing, speech and visual difficulties before an autistic diagnosis is suspected. Various features of early development give rise to parental concern, in particular, odd eye contact, limited use of pointing, inconsistent turning to parents' voice, extreme reactions to change in routines and limited initiation of activities with others.

Assessment

Early screening measures such as the Checklist for Autism in Toddlers (CHAT) hold much promise for early detection of autism. It can be administered by the health visitor at 18 months of age, and relies on the absence or distortion of three key areas of behaviour: lack of protodeclarative pointing (pointing in order to draw attention to something or someone as opposed to pointing in order to obtain something), lack of fantasy play, and abnormalities of eye contact.

Treatment

A wide variety of treatments have been advocated. These include:

- *Medication*. A variety of drugs have been tried in autistic children with no definitive benefit. A significant proportion of autistic children (some 30–40%) have sleep problems. Recent studies suggest that melatonin can be highly effective in a significant proportion of these, particularly in children who have difficulty in settling to sleep.
- *Behavioural interventions*. Several papers demonstrate statistically and clinically significant treatment effects of early intensive behavioural treatment. The most promising studies claim a high proportion of autistic children can be integrated into mainstream education; however, these findings lack independent replication.
- Other approaches which focus on early aspects of developmental process, in particular *video home training*, an intervention approach based on video feedback of family interaction, developed in Holland, which has achieved significant impact on recent European clinical practice.

Outcomes

Systematic longer-term follow-up work with autistic children is limited, in part because the condition was not widely recognized until the early 1970s. Studies suggest that the majority of autistic individuals will require residential or supported accommodation as adults and are unlikely to live independently or to hold down a job.

Other disorders of social and intellectual function

Several disorders show some clinical similarities to autism, and are important to identify as separable entities:

- *Tourette's syndrome* is a complex of vocal and motor tics, and other associated features including an increased frequency of concurrent obsessive–compulsive disorder and educational difficulties.
- *Asperger's syndrome* is a disorder which manifests with autistic social impairment with obsessional preoccupations (and commonly with clumsiness), in the absence of communication or intellectual deficits.
- *Rett's syndrome* is a disorder which exclusively affects girls. It is associated with developmental delay, acute regression of skills around 1–2 years of age, progressive microcephaly, loss of ambulation by the mid-teens and a high incidence of associated epilepsy.

PROBLEMS WITH A PSYCHOSOMATIC COMPONENT

✴ KEY DIAGNOSIS

Functional abdominal pain

Funtional abdominal pain is the most common diagnosis in children who present with recurrent abdominal pain (see Ch. 5).

Clinical features

Of school-age children (peak incidence 9 years), 10–15% suffer from functional abdominal pain, and many more suffer pain that does not disrupt normal activity. The pain is frequently periumbilical, worse in the mornings and may be associated with vomiting, dyspepsia or change of bowel habit. There is probably no single cause of functional abdominal pain. Affected children have a greater awareness of distension of their gastrointestinal tract, but not necessarily of painful stimuli elsewhere. Autonomic nervous system dysfunction, mucosal inflammation, and abnormal psychosocial background may all play their part in the genesis of pain. Lactose intolerance, *Helicobacter pylori* gastritis, and food additives are not responsible for the majority of cases, but are frequently blamed. A family history of abdominal pain is often present, and sources of stress may be found at school (e.g. bullying, or impending examinations), at home (e.g. parental arguments or moving house) or elsewhere (e.g. social clubs, sports).

Management

Management starts with a full history and examination. The parents should be given an explanation of functional abdominal pain which includes recognition that the pain is 'real' and originates perhaps in the child's greater awareness of normal gastrointestinal motility. The absence of pathology should be stressed, and the parents' specific worries identified and answered. Stresses known to cause the pain should be avoided, and reinforcement of the pain behaviour minimized. Normal attendance at school should be encouraged, and may require communication between physicians and school teachers. A high-fibre diet can sometimes be of benefit.

The prognosis is adversely affected by a family history of abdominal pain, male sex, age over 6 years, and symptoms lasting longer than 6 months before diagnosis. Symptoms resolve in up to 50% of affected children within 2 months of diagnosis, but many will have abdominal pain or other functional disorders as adults (e.g. headache and backache).

Chronic fatigue syndrome

Prevalance and epidemiology

Chronic fatigue syndrome is a condition which is encountered in children and adolescents, but prevalance rates, particularly in this age group, remain uncertain. Definitive treatment approaches and aetiology are yet to be established, and available evidence suggests that chronic fatigue syndrome is heterogeneous in nature and multicausal.

Presentation and assessment

The key features of chronic fatigue syndrome are continuous or recurring physical and mental fatigue of at least 3 months duration, associated with marked disability, unexplained by any recognized organic disease. The primary task of assessment is to exclude an extensive differential diagnosis of both physical and emotional disorders through taking a comprehensive history, thorough physical examination and investigation. Investigations might include: a full blood count, routine biochemistry and C-reactive protein measurement, urinalysis and culture. Hypothyroidism and Addison's disease, which can present with non-specific symptoms (including lethargy) should be excluded, not because these disorders are common but because they are eminently treatable if diagnosed.

Treatment

The reality of the child's symptoms have to be acknowledged whilst helping the family accept that a diagnosis of chronic fatigue syndrome warrants both physical and psychological diagnosis and management. This condition in childhood demands early intervention, and close liaison with all agencies in the child's care (i.e. family, school, psychological services and paediatricians) to help prevent other aspects of the child's emotional, social and academic development being compromised. The key treatment aim is to minimize disability, social isolation, and any reward the child might gain through illness (influence in family relations or school avoidance). Views differ on specific treatment strategies. However, there is strong evidence with adults that graded exercise and cognitive behavioural therapies are effective, and these should be considered for children although further research is warranted.

ADOLESCENT BEHAVIOUR DISORDER

Teenagers and their parents often need advice and help in differentiating between the normal discomforts of this period and the rare but distinct truly abnormal behaviour. Most aberrant adolescent behaviour is driven by cultural factors (poverty, ethnicity, gender issues, employment, religion) with no underlying pathophysiology. While specific medical problems are rare in the teenage years, certain clinical problems are emerging during this.

✳ KEY DIAGNOSIS

Eating disorder

Eating disorders include anorexia nervosa, bulimia nervosa, psychogenic vomiting and obesity (see Ch. 9). In the Western world they are most common in the young female population, and a common thread is a 'morbid dread of fatness'. There is probably a multifactorial aetiology: cultural pressures, family attitudes, individual psychodynamics and, possibly, genetic and biochemical susceptibility. Many teenagers have underlying depression, with a small number who have specific psychotic illness.

Criteria for diagnosis of eating disorders

Anorexia nervosa
- Body weight maintained at least 15% below expected for age and height
- Weight loss self-induced
- Restriction of intake
- Vomiting and or purging
- Excessive exercise
- Use of drugs (appetite suppressants, laxatives, diuretics)
- Morbid fear of obesity
- Self-set low weight threshold
- Primary or secondary amenorrhoea

Bulimia nervosa
- Binge eating followed by
- Counteractive measures to reduce calorie intake as in anorexia nervosa

Psychogenic vomiting
- Persistent vomiting where no other cause is found
- Body weight maintained 15% below expected for age and height

---

The management of these teenagers is a challenge. Negotiation of the treatment approach requires careful discussion with all involved parties, group and individual behaviour therapy and sometimes antidepressant therapy. Occasionally, inpatient therapy with supportive nutrition is required.

Drug abuse

The misuse of drugs is a problem for the whole of society and is not one that is specifically linked to adolescence. However, teenagers have a high profile in this area because of the change of practice from childhood into adolescence. Alcohol, smoking and recreational drug taking commonly feature in teenage disruptive behaviour. These factors should be considered in all situations where unexplained symptomatology is present.

Overdose and suicide attempts

These are often seen as a problem of teenage girls, but are not exclusively so. The majority are reactive (depression and mood swings) in relation to family and social difficulties and are more parasuicidal attention-seeking than true suicidal attempts. It is important to estimate and distinguish between lethality (the chance that the attempt could have resulted in death) and degree of intent (the seriousness with which the perpetrator attempted to kill him/herself). True underlying psychiatric problems may be present, and all cases should be referred to a specialist child and adolescent psychiatrist. Paracetamol, which is freely available without prescription, is particularly dangerous as an overdose. As little as 10 g (i.e. 20 tablets each containing 500 mg) can lead to severe hepatocellular necrosis. Patients who change their mind or did not wish to die in the first place (parasuicide) may nevertheless go on to develop encephalopathy and cerebral oedema within a few days and then die (see also Ch. 15).

FURTHER READING

Howlin P (ed) 1998 Behavioural approaches to problems in childhood. Clinics in Developmental Medicine 146

Lewis M (ed) 1996 Child and adolescent psychiatry: a comprehensive textbook, 2nd edn. Williams and Wilkins, Baltimore

Wolraich M L (ed) 1996 Disorders of development and learning: a practical guide to assessment and management, 2nd edn. Mosby, St Louis

CHAPTER 19

Paediatric surgery

R. Carachi

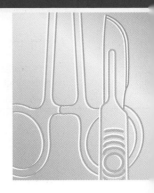

CORE PROBLEMS IN PAEDIATRIC SURGERY

CORE PROBLEM	KEY DIAGNOSIS	RELATED TOPICS
• Neck lump	Cervical lymphadenitis	Congenital cysts Malignancy
• Abdominal pain	Acute appendicitis	Mesenteric adenitis Intussusception Volvulus Meckel's diverticulum
• Groin/scrotal swelling	Inguinal hernia	Hydrocele Varicocele
• Painful scrotum	Torsion of the testis or its appendages	Epididymo-orchitis
• Absent testis	Cryptorchism	
• Painful foreskin	Balanitis	Phimosis Labial adhesions
• Abdominal mass	Constipation[5]	Hydronephrosis[8] Neuroblastoma[11] Nephroblastoma[11]

Where the primary location of a topic is in another chapter, this is indicated by a superscript

ESSENTIAL BACKGROUND

This chapter provides an overview of the commonest and most important surgical problems seen in children. The relevant physiological and anatomical considerations are discussed in the individual sections.

CORE PROBLEMS

NECK LUMP

Lumps in the neck are common in children, with enlarged lymph nodes being the commonest cause. Over 200 lymph nodes are present in the neck, and are a natural safeguard against infection entering the body through the oral or nasal cavities (see Ch. 11).

The swellings in the neck can be divided into those arising from the midline and those in the lateral aspect of the neck. Midline swellings include lymph node, dermoid and thyroglossal cyst. Lateral swellings include lymph node, branchial cyst, lymphangioma (cystic hygroma).

✱ KEY DIAGNOSIS

Cervical lymphadenitis

Following a sore throat or acute tonsillitis, enlarged jugulodigastric lymph nodes appear in the neck. These are usually sore to touch. With progression of the infection, the lymph node develops a reactive hyperplasia and, if the process is not aborted by the body's natural defences or by antibiotics, it may progress to abscess formation. Discoloration of the skin and fluctuation are not early features, as the glands lie deep to the deep cervical fascia. Abscess formation is usually caused by a penicillin-resistant strain of *Staphylococcus aureus*.

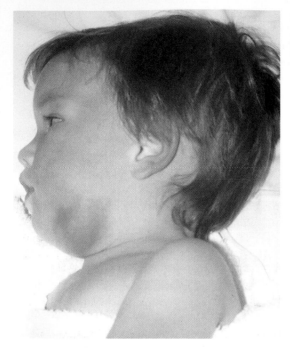

Figure 19.1 A young child with large cervical nodes consistent with cervical lymphadenitis

Evacuation of the pus is essential surgical treatment for this condition (Fig. 19.1).

Tuberculous and other 'atypical' mycobacteria should be considered when the swelling follows a more protracted course and signs of acute infection are not prominent. Rare causes of lateral swellings in the neck include lymphoma (Hodgkin's and non-Hodgkin's) and metastases from tumours elsewhere.

ACUTE ABDOMINAL PAIN

Acute abdominal pain is a common complaint in childhood. In small infants a characteristic pattern of behaviour helps to convey distress in spite of the lack of verbal communication. The crying is usually intermittent (reflecting the frequently colicky nature of the pain), and is accompanied by drawing up of the legs. Toddlers are frequently able to indicate the source of their irritability by pointing to the abdomen.

In many cases of acute abdominal pain, no specific underlying cause is found, and the term 'non-specific abdominal pain' is applied. In a significant number of cases, a 'medical' cause for the pain is diagnosed. Mesenteric lymphadenitis, food poisoning, gastritis, gastroenteritis and urinary tract infections are a few examples of such causes. The initial presentation of conditions resulting in chronic or recurrent abdominal pain (e.g. infantile colic, constipation, food allergy) are also included in the differential diagnosis (see Ch. 5). Pathology of a systemic nature or arising outside the abdomen, such as diabetic ketoacidosis, Henoch–Schönlein purpura, pneumonia or even meningitis/encephalitis may also have to be considered.

In some instances, acute abdominal pain may signify an underlying surgical emergency. One of the most helpful features pointing to a surgical cause is the accompanying presence of symptoms and signs of intestinal obstruction. Feeding refusal, bilious vomiting and abdominal distension should always call for urgent clinical and ultrasonographic/radiological assessment to exclude the presence of a surgical cause for the abdominal pain. However, in the early stages of some 'surgical' conditions, features of obstruction are frequently not prominent or may be absent. This is one of the main reasons for the delay in reaching a diagnosis in children with surgical emergencies. Such a delay may mean that more extensive surgery becomes necessary, with increased morbidity and mortality.

Features of peritonism, abdominal muscle guarding and rebound tenderness are also indicative of the presence of an abdominal surgical emergency. Peritonism is, however, usually a late feature, and every effort should be made to arrive at the diagnosis of a surgical emergency before the condition has progressed to that extent. Features of peritoneal irritation, particularly of a localized nature, can be present early in some cases (e.g. appendicitis), and are then helpful in reaching the correct diagnosis.

Even in the absence of features of intestinal obstruction or peritoneal irritation, there may be certain aspects of the abdominal pain which are specific to one or the other of the common surgical conditions and thus may allow a presumptive diagnosis of a specific pathology.

The following subsections outline the features of the common paediatric surgical abdominal emergencies. Only acute appendicitis will be discussed in any detail, but it provides an example for the approach to children with acute abdominal pain in general.

✳ KEY DIAGNOSIS

Acute appendicitis

Anatomy and pathology

There is a marked variation in the anatomy of the appendix. In childhood the appendix lies in a retrocaecal position in 70% of patients. Obstructive appendicitis is common in children; the obstruction being caused by a kink, a faecolith or the scar of previous inflammation. When inflammation occurs there is an accumulation of purulent exudate within the lumen, and a closed-loop obstruction is established. The appendix distends, and thrombosis of the appendicular vessels causes gangrene early on. Free fluid drains into the peritoneum and, within a few hours, this fluid is invaded by bacteria from the perforated appendix or from organisms translocating across the inflamed but still intact appendix wall. Peritoneal infection may be localized by adhesions between loops of intestine, caecal wall and parietal peritoneum. Administration of a purgative in these children is dangerous because it increases intestinal and appendicular peristalsis and, in this situation, perforation and dissemination of infection is more likely to occur.

Clinical features

Acute appendicitis is the most common pathological condition requiring intra-abdominal surgery in childhood. The disease runs a more rapid course in children, and it may generally present as uncomplicated acute appendicitis, appendicitis with local peritonitis, an appendix abscess or diffuse peritonitis.

In addition to variation according to the pathological stage of the disease, the clinical picture varies also with age. Thus, in adolescents and older children, the presentation of acute appendicitis resembles that of adults with shifting pain and right iliac fossa tenderness (maximal at the McBurney point). Such a picture, however, may not be obvious in the small child. The onset of symptoms in younger children is vague and initially may be of a general nature. Only one-third of younger patients are seen in hospital within 24 h of onset of abdominal symptoms, and in a high percentage of these young children the appendix has ruptured before admission.

Anorexia is common, and the pain is usually followed by vomiting and diarrhoea, but these are usually infrequent and of small volume. Unless complicated by peritonitis, moderate rather than high temperature elevation is frequently present. Psoas spasm from irritation of the muscle by the inflamed appendix may cause flexion of the hip resulting in a limp, thus distracting attention from the abdomen.

Further variation in the clinical picture may be related to variation in the anatomical location of the appendix. Thus, if the appendix is retrocaecal, abdominal pain and tenderness may be slight; if the child has a pelvic appendix, tenderness may be absent and elicited only on rectal examination.

In summary, although right iliac fossa pain, tenderness and muscle guarding remain the principal diagnostic features of acute appendicitis, it is important to be aware that these can be vague, subtle and difficult to elicit in young children. A high index of suspicion is required in order not to miss this diagnosis.

Investigations

These are more helpful in excluding other conditions than in confirming the diagnosis of acute appendicitis. A leucocytosis is frequently, but not always, present. Because of the anatomical relationship of the appendix to the right ureter, a urine analysis may show mild pyuria and haematuria, but no bacteria. The finding of a swollen appendix on ultrasonography supports the diagnosis, as does a distended small bowel or a 'mass effect' in the area of the caecum on plain or contrast radiographs. Computerized tomography is rarely indicated.

Differential diagnosis

There is a large number of conditions presenting with abdominal pain, fever and vomiting which could be included in the differential diagnosis of acute appendicitis. The extent to which these conditions should be investigated has to be decided on an individual basis. If the initial assessment reveals that appendicitis is highly likely, minimal additional investigations are required. On the other hand, if after such assessment the diagnosis remains uncertain, further evaluation including a period of observation is necessary. The conditions which frequently have to be included in the differential diagnosis of acute appendicitis are:

- Upper respiratory tract infection and mesenteric lymphadenitis: the presence of a common cold, sinusitis, acute tonsillitis, pharyngitis may all be associated with acute non-specific mesenteric lymphadenitis. This is the most common condition to be differentiated from acute appendicitis. The presence of enlarged glands elsewhere in the body accompanied by an upper respiratory tract infection may suggest this diagnosis.
  Fever may be absent or very high. The presence of abdominal tenderness is not as acute as that in appendicitis. It is usually more generalized and not localized to the right iliac fossa, and there is no rebound tenderness. Mesenteric lymphadenitis can sometimes be impossible to differentiate clinically from appendicitis. Ultrasound examination may be helpful.
- Gastroenteritis: vomiting usually precedes the abdominal pain, and diarrhoea is profuse. Abdominal pain and tenderness is often generalized rather than localized to the caecum. Other members of the family may have similar symptoms. Rectal examination can differentiate between a pelvic appendicitis and appendicitis with a pelvic peritonitis from gastroenteritis.
- Urinary tract infection: there may be heavy pyuria accompanied by proteinuria. The additional presence of bacteria in an adequately collected urine sample is strong evidence of this diagnosis.
- Pneumonia: the presence of cough, increased respiratory rate or other features of respiratory distress may suggest a respiratory infection. Routine examination of the chest is essential to pick up any signs of consolidation, since a right lower lobe pneumonia may result in referred pain to the right iliac fossa. A chest radiograph should be obtained if there are any respiratory symptoms or signs.
- Other surgical abdominal conditions such as strangulated hernia, intussusception and volvulus may present a picture similar to that of appendicitis. The addition of features of vascular compromise (pallor, tachycardia, haematemesis or melena) may point to this possibility. Inspection of the groins and examination of the scrotum and testes should be an integral part of the physical examination of any child with acute abdominal pain. The differentiation of these conditions from acute appendicitis is not always possible, and often the diagnosis is made at operation, which is the treatment of choice in most cases.
- Other conditions that may have to be considered are abdominal trauma, infective hepatitis, primary peritonitis, haemolytic uraemic syndrome, diabetic ketoacidosis, Crohn's disease, torsion of the testis and Meckel's diverticulum.

Treatment

Treatment of the child with acute appendicitis is prompt surgery. In the toxic child with peritonitis, time may be profitably spent in combating toxaemia and dehydration. It is important to resuscitate the patient and start intravenous antibiotics before surgery is undertaken. In such cases, metronidazole, together with ceftazidime or cefotaxime, should be given intravenously. Intravenous antibiotics given as three doses pre-, peri- and postoperatively, with peritoneal lavage, considerably reduce the incidence of postoperative complications.

Intussusception

Intussusception is the invagination of one intestinal loop into another, most frequently involving the ileocaecal region. It is the commonest cause of intestinal obstruction in infants and young children beyond 3 months of age, with a peak incidence at around 9 months.

The pathogenesis is frequently unknown, but in some cases may be related to gastrointestinal or other infection where hypertrophied lymphoid tissue within the intestinal wall stimulates intestinal peristalsis. Stimulation of peristalsis may also result from Henoch–Schönlein purpura, local lesions caused by trauma (haematoma), malignancy (lymphoma), or anatomical structures (Meckel's diverticulum). The invagination leads to mechanical obstruction as well as to interruption of the circulation of the affected part. Bowel gangrene and necrosis follow in the majority of cases, although spontaneous correction can occur.

Clinical picture

This is characterized by the sudden onset of paroxysmal colicky abdominal pain, which increases in frequency as the disease progresses. During these episodes of pain the child may appear to be straining, pale and sweating. In the initial stages, the child is typically well and comfortable in between bouts of pain. However, as the condition progresses, a shock-like state supervenes, with tachycardia and a weak thready pulse.

Vomiting is initially frequent and clear, but later becomes bilious and less frequent. Normal bowel motions may be passed initially, but there is constipation later on or only small stools passed. Blood is passed per rectum within the first 24 h in the majority of cases, usually in mucousy motions ('red currant jelly').

The onset of these symptoms commonly occurs on a background of a 'previously healthy' baby. However, sometimes there is a preceding upper respiratory tract infection or gastroenteritis. In the latter case the gastrointestinal illness may seem to take a biphasic course, with initial improvement followed by symptoms associated with intussusception.

A tube-like mass may be palpable in the right upper quadrant or centrally. Blood and mucus on the finger on rectal examination is a classic sign. The abdomen becomes tender and distended as the disease progresses.

Investigations

Plain abdominal radiography may show a dense mass in the affected area. Ultrasound scans may show a typical target or doughnut configuration. A barium (Fig. 19.2) or air enema may be required for diagnosis.

Treatment

Resuscitation measures, including fluid replacement, may first be required. Reduction of the intussusception should be arranged as an emergency. Hydrostatic reduction utilizing a barium or air enema, under fluoroscopic or ultrasonic control, should be first attempted in children presenting with symptoms of short duration. Surgical reduction is indicated in those in whom hydrostatic reduction has failed, as well as in children with advanced disease when there are features suggestive of shock, peritonism or perforation.

Malrotation and volvulus

Malrotation refers to failure of the normal rotation of the bowel in the fetus (see Fig. 5.1). The main consequence of this is that the bowel mesentery becomes attached to the posterior abdominal wall on a narrow pedicle instead of the wide base that normal rotation provides. The bowel mesentery thus becomes more likely to twist upon itself (volvulus), leading both to obstruction and interruption of the blood supply to the gut (Fig. 19.3). Malrotation may also result in bands that overlie the duodenum and which may also be a cause of mechanical obstruction.

This condition frequently presents in early infancy, and should always be included in the differential diagnosis of intestinal obstruction at this age. In some cases, however, volvulus and acute complete obstruction may not occur at an early age, and the malrotation may go unrecognized. Some of these children may suffer from varying degrees of mesentery twists and obstruction occurring intermittently, giving rise to a wide range of manifestations. The diagnosis of malrotation may be established by ultrasound examination or barium studies. Plain radiography may sometimes be helpful.

Meckel's diverticulum

A remnant of the yolk sac or omphalomesenteric (vitelline) duct, Meckel's diverticulum, is located

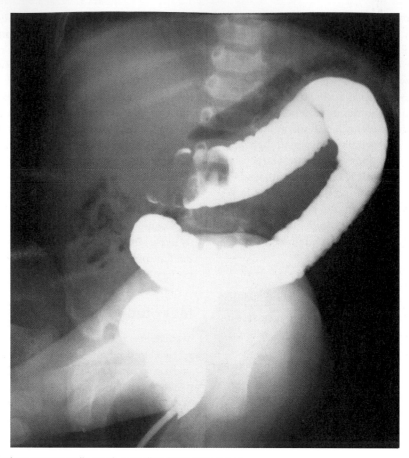

Figure 19.2   Barium enema radiograph revealing intussusception

at the antimesenteric border of the ileum. It is the commonest congenital anomaly of the intestine occurring in 2% of children. Meckel's diverticulum is about 2 inches (5 cm) in length and is located about 2 feet (60 cm) from the ileoceacal junction ('rule of two').

Meckel's diverticulum may become symptomatic if it contains acid-producing ectopic gastric mucosa and thus may lead to ulceration of the ileal mucosa, and bleeding. Alternatively, Meckel's diverticulum may act as a leading point for intussusception. It can also become inflamed (diverticulitis), resulting in an identical picture to appendicitis.

GROIN/SCROTAL SWELLING

The differential diagnosis of groin swellings in children is mainly limited to inguinal lymph node enlargement, inguinal hernia and retractile or undescended testis. Rarely, other structures or pathology may account for the swellings, such as haemangiomata or traumatic and inflammatory lesions. The differential diagnosis of scrotal swellings includes inguinal hernias, hydrocele, epididymo-orchitis, torsion of the testis and other testicular pathology.

✱ KEY DIAGNOSIS

Inguinal hernia

Inguinal hernia is one of the most common surgical problems in childhood, and it is invariably of the indirect type. Males are affected 10 times more commonly than females and, taking both sexes together, the incidence under 12 years of age is ten per 1000 live births. The right testis descends at a later date than does the left,

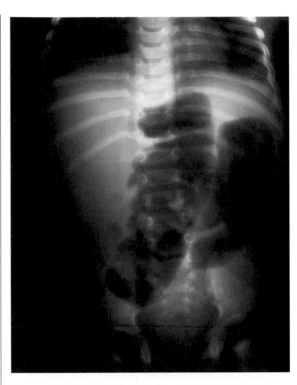

Figure 19.3 Plain abdominal radiograph revealing severe dilatation of intestinal bowel consistent with an acute volvulus

and accordingly the processus vaginalis is closed off later on the right side. This probably accounts for the greater frequency of right-sided inguinal hernia (right 60%, left 20%, bilateral 20%). The indirect inguinal hernia passes down the tract of the processus vaginalis to the inguinal canal, where it appears near the skin surface at the external inguinal ring. Inguinal hernia develops in 30% of premature babies.

Clinical features

The most important feature of hernias is that they are reducible swellings, sometimes appearing only on manoeuvres which increase intra-abdominal pressure, such as coughing, crying, straining or standing.

A hernia may be discovered at or shortly after birth, and a very large scrotal hernia may appear during the first week of life. Most commonly, hernias are first noticed during the second or third month following a period of coughing or crying. The hernia may be empty or it may contain intra-abdominal contents, especially bowel. The contents usually reduce spontaneously when the child ceases to cry or strain.

The hernia may be small and appear near the external ring or may be elongated and extend beyond the inguinal canal into the scrotum (Fig. 19.4). Examination of an older infant or child with an inguinal hernia is carried out bimanually. It is important to gain the confidence and cooperation of the child, and the scrotum should be inspected before touching it. If the child wishes to stand he may be allowed to do so, and coughing in the erect position may induce the hernia to bulge. The presence of an already visible bulge that is easily reducible is very suggestive of a hernia. The testes should also be palpated to show they are present and properly descended. An undescended testis may be mistaken for a hernia.

On occasion there may be a good history of recurrent swelling but no inguinal swelling can be found during the examination. The clinical findings may be only those of a thickened spermatic cord at the site of the hernia.

Complications and treatment

The two main complications of inguinal hernias are incarceration and strangulation. In incarceration, the contents of the hernia cannot be reduced back into the abdominal cavity. The intestine is usually the organ contained within the hernial sac, and features of intestinal obstruction develop. The hernia becomes tense, and the overlying skin oedematous with some erythema and tenderness, although not to the degree seen in strangulated hernias (see later). The infant becomes irritable, and may cry inconsolably.

Prompt reduction is indicated for incarcerated hernias, and this can be achieved without resorting to emergency surgery in the majority of cases. The use of sedatives (e.g. chloral hydrate) and placing the infant in the head-down position are helpful. Gentle pressure is applied when the child is quiet. Surgical repair is indicated 24–48 h after successful reduction, when tissue oedema has settled.

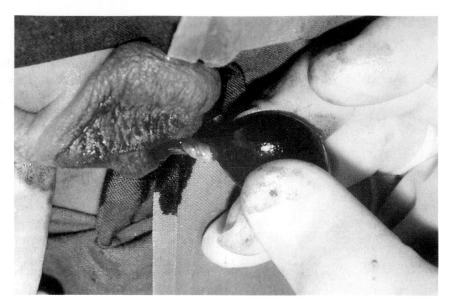

Figure 19.6 Torsion of the testis; operation revealed a swollen and gangrenous testicle which required removal

occur if they remained in the peritoneal cavity. Bilateral undescended testes and impalpable testes need ultrasound and laparoscopy for diagnosis. Some of these patients have chromosomal disorders which need to be investigated. Ectopic testes account for 10% of undescended testes; they descend normally in the inguinal canal and then get pulled into unusual locations, e.g. the perineum. Treatment (see also Highlights and Hypotheses: cryptorchism – when, why and how to treat?) is by orchidopexy, which is easy to perform because the testicular vessels are on a long leash.

The retractile testis is a normal physiological variation. Testes are retractile in small children due to the strong 'cremasteric reflex'. Under warm conditions, testes can be coaxed into the scrotum and remain there. There is no need for any further treatment or follow up in these cases.

PAINFUL FORESKIN

✳ KEY DIAGNOSIS

Balanitis

During the period when the child is incontinent in nappies, the glans is protected by the prepuce.

Despite this protection, it is easily traumatized. Less than 5% of foreskins are retractable at birth, and it is only gradually, over the following decade that the foreskin becomes freely retractable. In about half of all infants, the foreskin cannot be retracted to display the external meatus of the urethra or the glans, but the infant has adequate space to pass urine. This situation can be regarded with equanimity in the preschool child unless the smegma which forms and collects around the coronal sulcus becomes infected, causing balanitis, which is sometimes associated with retention of urine. Treatment with baths, analgesics and antibiotics usually quickly settles the child. When a second attack of balanitis occurs, retraction of the foreskin and clearing out of retained smegma should be performed under anaesthesia after treatment of the infection. Circumcision may also be performed to guarantee freedom from recurrence.

Phimosis

In this condition there is a tight prepuce which does not allow retraction of the foreskin and in severe cases may obstruct urinary flow (Fig. 19.7). Forceful retraction of foreskin in early life may

CRYPTORCHISM

When, why and how to treat?

Ninety-seven per cent of full term infants and 79% of premature infants have normally descended testes at birth. During the first year there is a further incidence of complete descent in over 99% of male infants. Thereafter the prevalence remains the same.

Even though its incidence has changed only slightly over the years, the number of orchidopexies for cryptorchid testes has tripled! The inevitable conclusion is that inappropriate operations for retractile (i.e. normal) testes are being undertaken. Surgeons and physicians appear reluctant to admit to having difficulty in defining a retractile testis. Prevention of the cremasteric reflex which causes retraction of the testis requires the careful examination of a relaxed child in a warm room. In difficult cases, the scrotum should be examined with the child in a squatting position to increase intraabdominal pressure and thus coax a reluctant testis into the scrotum. Several examinations should be undertaken before finally accepting the diagnosis of cryptorchism.

As indicated above, surgical treatment is usually advised before 3 years of age. Some studies have suggested very early surgical treatment under 1 year, but this may be technically difficult. Hormone therapy (gonadotrophins either by spray or injection) is used commonly on the Continent, and may be successful in inducing descent of the testis in a proportion of cases. Gonadotrophin therapy is indicated in known cases of central pituitary cryptorchism.

---

cause fissuring of the meatus of the foreskin, with scarring and progression to phimosis. True phimosis is rare in early childhood, and usually occurs in the 5–10 year old age group. If a tight prepuce is retracted, it may constrict the base of the glans and cause oedema of the glans: paraphimosis. In such cases, a general anaesthetic may have to be administered and a small dorsal slit performed in order to return the prepuce to its normal position. The definitive treatment is circumcision.

Labial adhesions

Rarely at birth, the labia may appear to be fused. In early childhood, this is relatively common and probably related to local inflammation associated with the hypo-oestrogenic state prior to puberty. The child's genitalia are otherwise normal. Treatment is by topical oestrogen application, and surgical separation is required only rarely.

ABDOMINAL MASS

The differential diagnosis of abdominal mass in children includes the following:

- Faecal masses of a loaded colon associated with constipation (see Ch. 6). This is probably the commonest explanation for a palpable abdominal mass in children. Two helpful features in making the distinction from other aetiologies are that the mass(es) are indentable and they disappear or change in size and position following bowel evacuation.
- A full bladder may also be mistaken for a mass. The 'mass' is in the lower abdomen although its upper edge may reach the

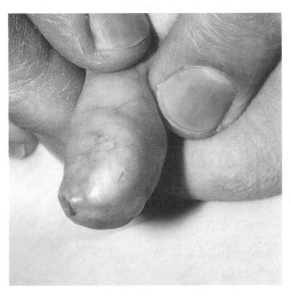

Figure 19.7 Phimosis of the penis with a tight prepuce preventing retraction of the foreskin

umbilicus; it disappears on emptying the bladder.

- A true abdominal mass in children is most frequently accounted for by one of the following:
  - Hydronephrosis (see Ch. 8)
  - Neuroblastoma (see Ch. 11)
  - Nephroblastoma (Wilm's tumour, see Ch. 11).

FURTHER READING

Cockburn F, Young D G, Carachi R, Goel K N 1996 Children's medicine and surgery. Edward Arnold, London

MacMahon R A 1991 An aid to paediatric surgery. Churchill Livingstone, Edinburgh

CHAPTER 20

International child health

A. Costello

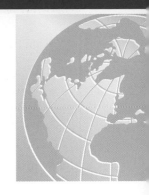

CORE PROBLEMS IN INTERNATIONAL CHILD HEALTH

CORE PROBLEM	KEY DIAGNOSIS	RELATED TOPICS
• Perinatal problems	Intrauterine growth retardation	Neonatal tetanus Asphyxia[4] Septicaemia[4]
• Malnutrition	Protein–energy malnutrition	Micronutrient deficiency Overnutrition
• Infectious disease	Acute respiratory infections	Diarrhoea Tuberculosis Malaria HIV Common childhood illnesses
• Children in difficult circumstances	War	Child abuse[15]

Where the primary location of a topic is in another chapter, this is indicated by a superscript

ESSENTIAL BACKGROUND

GLOBAL TRENDS IN HEALTH

The past few decades have seen the most dramatic improvements in the health and welfare of human populations in history. The increase in life expectancy and the decrease in fertility over the past 40 years (see Ch. 1) have been greater than during the past 4000 years. The proportion of children who die before reaching the age of 5 years is now less than half the level of 1960. Immunization and diarrhoea control programmes introduced in the past two decades save 4 million lives annually.

But we cannot be complacent; 1300 million people still live in absolute poverty, and 900 million have no access to even basic health services. There are 200 million children under 5 years who suffer from malnutrition and anaemia, 8.1 million maternal and perinatal deaths annually, and 2 million deaths due to vaccine-preventable diseases. At least 30% of the world's population have no access to safe water, and sanitation systems, and 120 million couples are without access to modern family planning methods.

New threats to health and welfare, especially for mothers and children, include the HIV pandemic, the resurgence of tuberculosis and the spread of drug-resistant malaria. Some immunization programmes have collapsed in the poorest countries, or as a result of economic problems: in Russia a decline in immunization coverage in the 1990s led to large epidemics of diphtheria (Fig. 20.1) and whooping cough. Finally, civil unrest and warfare currently affect over 80 conflict zones around the world.

THE NATURE OF POVERTY

In approaching the core problems in international child health we need to be aware of the nature of poverty and vulnerability. Poverty seems an intuitively straightforward issue, but there is much disagreement about how it should be

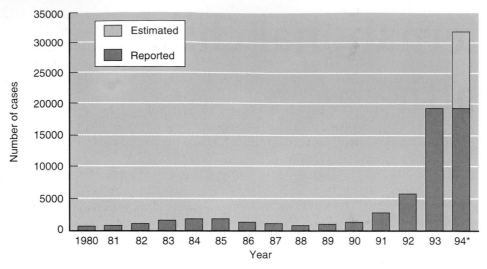

Figure 20.1 Epidemic of diphtheria following the break up of the Soviet Union

defined, measured or alleviated. A hierarchy of poverty is recognized (Chambers 1997):

- *Survival.* For the absolute poor, the essential problem is ensuring sufficient consumption of food, or generation of income to enable basic needs to be met. Many of the poorest people consume diets deficient in calories and essential micronutrients. They have no savings or safety nets should crops fail, or for wage labourers, incomes may cease through unemployment or sickness. In its most extreme form, poverty may lead to starvation or famine. Famine does not usually arise because there is an absolute lack of food, but rather because the most vulnerable lack the resources or entitlements to gain access to food. The relationship between poverty and famine is brilliantly laid out in Amartya Sen's classic text, *Poverty and Famines.*
- *Vulnerability.* Basic needs (food, shelter, water, primary education) are met for most families, but their security is in jeopardy through lack of savings, limited assets and no access to social security safety nets. A crisis, such as a family illness or loss of employment, can quickly lead to extreme poverty and the inability to meet basic needs.
- *Self-esteem.* For many people in the industrialized world, basic needs are met, and social security systems ensure that basic needs will be provided during periods of unemployment or other crises. But they may suffer from relative poverty: stress and a lack of self-esteem; living in polluted, crime-ridden inner cities in substandard accommodation; labelled as an under-class; vulnerable to drug abuse, prostitution and gambling as a way out of their predicament; victims of the 'inverse care law', whereby those that need services most use them least and those that need them least use them most.

THE VULNERABILITY OF CHILDREN

It is generally accepted that the group most vulnerable to the effects of poverty, war and famine are children and their mothers. Vulnerability varies at different stages of childhood. The perinatal period, from the last trimester of pregnancy until the end of the postpartum period (6 weeks after birth) carries the highest risk of mortality for both mothers and infants.

In infancy, acute respiratory infection and diarrhoeal disease leading to dehydration are the commonest causes of death. Malaria is a major cause of death in affected areas, mainly in sub-

Saharan Africa. In the past decade, HIV infection in children has increased dramatically. In many hospitals in southern Africa, over half of all paediatric admissions are HIV related.

Fully breast-fed infants grow as well as their developed world counterparts until the weaning period (about 6 months) even if suckled by relatively malnourished mothers. After weaning, there is an increased risk of infection through contaminated food or water and often an inadequate intake of calories. Those under 5 years of age have the greatest risk of protein–energy malnutrition. Micronutrient deficiencies during this period, such as of vitamin A, iron, zinc and iodine, may have effects on survival, growth and cognition.

School age children are at lower risk of death from infection or of protein–energy malnutrition, but their school performance and attendance may be affected by hunger, protein–energy or micronutrient malnutrition, and parasite infection such as by worms, malaria and schistosomiasis. In the adolescent period, sexually transmitted disease and early pregnancy become significant problems; in urban areas, drug abuse and crime rates are increasing.

At any age, warfare or civil unrest increases greatly the risks of malnutrition and infectious disease. In the 1990s, perinatal mortality rates more than trebled during the Bosnian war in Europe, and in Somalia half the population aged under 5 years died during the civil war.

INTEGRATED MANAGEMENT OF CHILDHOOD ILLNESS

Every year some 12 million children die before the age of 5 years. Of these deaths, 70% are caused by five common preventable or easily treatable childhood conditions: pneumonia, diarrhoea, measles, malaria and malnutrition. Developing countries have extremely low health budgets, many spending less than US$3 per head annually on health services. Effective, high-coverage mother-and-child health services which are low-cost, deprofessionalized and integrated can be provided by clinics and community health workers for those under 5 years of age, but

depend upon good management, and well-trained and well-motivated staff.

In developing countries, disease-specific vertical control programmes, such as those targeted at diarrhoea and acute respiratory infections, have been criticized by planners for their bureaucratic duplication and by doctors who recognize that health workers often deal with children whose symptoms have overlapping causes or for whom a single diagnosis may not be appropriate. For example, cough and tachypnoea may be caused by pneumonia, but also by severe anaemia or malaria. A 'very sick' young infant may have pneumonia, septicaemia or meningitis, or more than one diagnosis. Many health workers continue to misdiagnose: research in Kenya showed that only 8% health workers correctly classified severe pneumonia.

To improve the prevention and management of childhood illness, the World Health Organization (WHO) and UNICEF have developed a new strategy, the 'Integrated Management of Childhood Illness' (IMCI). IMCI has three components, and activities have already been initiated in more than 60 countries, mainly in Africa and Latin America.

> **The IMCI strategy**
> - Improvements in the case management skills of health workers through the provision of locally adapted guidelines and training activities to promote their use
> - Improvements in the health system required for effective case management of childhood illness, especially essential drug supplies
> - Improvements in family and community practices in relation to child health

The third component of IMCI, improvement in family and community practices, is especially important, with practical interventions needed to help mothers respond promptly to childhood illness. Some ideas such as the sick child home visit, communication skills training for health workers, and media health promotion campaigns will need evaluation for cost-effectiveness.

Essential newborn care is an integral part of a safe motherhood programme. School health interventions, e.g. deworming or micronutrient supplementation programmes, have the advantage of achieving a high coverage quickly, and are potentially cost-effective. In practice, however, services directed towards the newborn, the school-aged child and the adolescent are generally absent or rudimentary in developing countries.

CORE PROBLEMS

PERINATAL PROBLEMS

In the poorest countries, where access to emergency obstetric care is severely limited, maternal mortality rates may be as high as 500–1000 per 100 000 births. Taking into account an average fertility rate of perhaps six pregnancies per woman gives an overall lifetime risk of a maternity-related death of as much as 1 in 15–20 in some settings. Stillbirths account for over 60% of the perinatal mortality rate (stillbirths plus first week deaths per 1000 total births), and neonatal mortality (neonatal deaths in the first 28 days per 1000 livebirths) accounts for over 60% of all infant deaths (those occurring up to 12 months).

✳ KEY DIAGNOSIS

Intrauterine growth retardation

In the UK, 6% of newborn infants are low birth weight (born weighing less than 2500 g) usually because they were born prematurely. In developing countries such as India and Bangladesh, 30–40% of newborn infants are born with a low birth weight for different reasons; these are usually full-term infants who have suffered malnutrition during pregnancy through intrauterine growth retardation (see Ch. 4). There are many contributory causes to intrauterine growth retardation, including maternal nutritional status, especially height, before pregnancy, young age at conception, poor diet during pregnancy, anaemia, heavy physical exercise during agricultural and domestic work, and infections such as malaria and gastroenteritis.

Neonatal tetanus

Worldwide more than 5 million newborns die in the first 4 weeks of life, two-thirds in the first week; 98% of these deaths occur in developing countries. Low birth weight infants are especially vulnerable, particularly if they are premature. In the industrialized world up to 95% of infants born before 32 weeks of gestation will survive; in the poorest countries, survival rates are below 10%. Neonatal tetanus, caused by infection with the anaerobic bacterium *Clostridium tetani*, often as a result of poor hygiene in cutting the cord, is still a problem in many areas. Active immunization is highly protective but, although cases have declined over the past 20 years due to the expanded programme of immunization for mothers and children, mortality rates are still high. Symptoms result from a toxin, tetanospasmin, causing spasms of skeletal muscles and inability to feed.

Asphyxia accounts for a quarter of perinatal deaths (see also Ch. 4). Many of these deaths could be prevented by identification of high-risk mothers in the antenatal period, prevention of anaemia through better diet, iron supplements and treatment of malaria, and better access to safe obstetric services. Poor hygiene increases the risk of neonatal septicaemia, which may be rapidly fatal.

Newborn care need not be expensive – in practice good perinatal care can be achieved with limited resources and appropriate technology:

The principles of newborn care
- Resuscitate when necessary and maintain an airway
- Maintain warmth and avoid hypothermia
- Good hygiene for delivery and cord care
- Treat newborn diseases such as infection, jaundice and hypoglycaemia
- Early breast feeding
- Keep newborns with their mothers when possible and involve mothers in the special care needed for high-risk and premature infants

MALNUTRITION
✳ KEY DIAGNOSIS

Protein–energy malnutrition

Children may present with severe malnutrition from 6 months onwards up until 5 years of age, after which it is uncommon. The prevalence of cases increases considerably at the time of weaning the infant off the breast.

Malnutrition arises through a combination of poor diet and infection, which interlink through what is called the malnutrition–infection cycle. For example, well-nourished exclusively breast-fed infants in poor rural villages in Bangladesh are often weaned at six months of age on to a low energy rice diet, deficient in fats and micronutrients. The frequency of feeds may be too low because of other demands on the mother's time. The food may be prepared in unhygienic circumstances, stored without refrigeration, and both food and water may be contaminated with gastrointestinal pathogens. Diarrhoea or dysentery may ensue, causing fever (which increases metabolic rate) and exposing the infant to the risks of dehydration. The infectious illness reduces appetite (anorexia) and food intake further decreases. The result is rapid weight loss leading to a state of protein–energy malnutrition. Among infections, persistent diarrhoea, tuberculosis, measles, pertussis and HIV are all important as precipitating causes of malnutrition.

Clinical features

Severe malnutrition occurs as the clinical syndromes of kwashiorkor (malnutrition with swollen face or limbs due to oedema fluid in the tissues), marasmus (a thin and wasted child) or marasmic kwashiorkor (a mixture of the two syndromes). Kwashiorkor was first described by the British paediatrician Cicely Williams who worked in Ghana in the 1930s, and is derived from a local expression for malnutrition. There is no clear evidence why one child develops kwashiorkor and another marasmus.

Clinical characteristics of moderate or severe malnutrition
- Skin changes: scaly, scalded skin characteristically associated with pale brown hair
- Dehydration
- Hypoglycaemia
- Severe infection
- Anaemia
- Oedema (kwashiorkor)
- Hypothermia
- Anorexia and apathy
- Vitamin A and zinc deficiency

Severe malnutrition occurs when the weight for age is below 60% of an internationally defined standard value or if oedema is present. Even moderate degrees of malnutrition are associated with an increased risk of death and serious infection. Mortality rates, ranging from 0 to 20%, will be affected by the stage of malnutrition, the availability of staff with skills in nutrition rehabilitation and the necessary resources to feed frequently and treat infection. Many malnourished children have associated clinical or subclinical infections.

Management

Children with severe malnutrition may be treated in a hospital or nutrition centre, as an outpatient attending at day care nutrition rehabilitation centres, or through nutrition rehabilitation in the home. The strategy chosen will depend upon the circumstances of the child, his or her family, and the availability of local services. Rates of recovery are slightly slower in day centres or at home compared with hospital residential treatment. It is important to involve parents in the nutrition management regimen.

A diet containing 100 kcal/kg per day should be provided. In marasmus this can be built up to 200 kcal/kg per day within a few days; however, this high intake should only be given to kwashiorkor children once their oedema has cleared. Feeding up to eight times a day is necessary to achieve satisfactory rates of growth. Often children will take 3–5 weeks to obtain a target weight for height. Home-based nutrition rehabilitation can be achieved with support from experienced workers if there are suitable foods available locally. Weekly weighing and careful attention to recognition and treatment of infection is essential. Vitamin A supplements should be given orally.

Long-term prevention

Health workers do not hold the key to long-term prevention. The most important preventive measure is to improve the economy and welfare of families in the society, which is to do with politics, economics and international development. Health workers can certainly identify and treat individual malnourished children and assist the family and community to address some of the underlying problems that cause malnutrition. Health promotion to encourage mothers to attend under-five clinics, immunization days and to seek treatment for problems quickly can help to reduce the prevalence of malnutrition.

Micronutrient deficiencies

The major micronutrients which cause clinical problems through deficiency are iodine, iron and vitamin A.

Iodine deficiency

Deficiency of iodine may arise among people living in areas where the soil is deficient in iodine, usually mountainous regions far from the sea such as the Himalaya, the Andes, parts of inner China and the highlands of east Africa. The risk increases if a population does not consume foods fortified with iodine or iodized salt. Iodine deficiency causes a reduction in the production and blood levels of thyroid hormones, and a compensatory increase in the size of the thyroid gland, causing a neck swelling 'goitre'. Thyroid hormone deficiency may in turn cause an increased risk of miscarriage and perinatal death, neurodevelopmental problems such as cretinism (a syndrome in infancy with developmental delay and characteristic facial and skin changes), deaf mutism, thyroid dwarfism, spastic diplegia and learning difficulties.

Cretins may present with a large tongue, slow psychomotor development and protruberant abdomen. WHO Goitre Grades may be used to assess the prevalence and severity of endemic goitre. Urinary iodine is a good estimate of dietary intake. The proportion of children with urinary iodine levels of below 50 μg/dl is an important indication of the severity of the prevalence of iodine deficiency disease in a community. Normally such levels occur in 1% or fewer children but, in severely deficient areas, low levels may occur in over 50% of children. Blood hormone profiles show characteristic low T_4 and high thyroid-stimulating hormone levels.

Strategies for preventing iodine deficiency disease are listed below:

Prevention of micronutrient deficiencies
Iodine deficiency
• Iodination of salt or water supplies
• Iodized oil injections for women of reproductive age
• Iodized poppy seed oil capsules
Vitamin A deficiency
• Vitamin A supplementation to children in deficient areas, and all measles cases
• Reduction of infectious disease
• Food fortification
• Nutrition education
Iron deficiency
• Iron supplements in pregnancy
• Nutrition education

Benefits from reducing iodine deficiency disease include decreased reproductive losses, improved birth weight and improved intellectual function of children.

Vitamin A deficiency

This was first recognized as a cause of eye disease and blindness (xerophthalmia) in developing countries, but recent studies have shown an important effect of vitamin A deficiency on immune response in childhood, susceptibility to infection and the overall risk of mortality. Vitamin A deficiency is most prevalent among children aged from 6 months to 6 years, and is commoner among infants who are not breast fed. Precipitating factors include measles, pneumonia, septicaemia and malaria, persistent diarrhoea, intestinal parasites (including *Giardia*, *Ascaris* and *Trichuris*) and severe protein–energy malnutrition. Prevention of vitamin A deficiency can reduce mortality in young children from 6 months to 5 years by up to 20%.

Clinical signs of xerophthalmia include dried heaped up areas of the conjunctiva, nightblindness and severe corneal lesions. Children may also have low levels of plasma retinol.

The principles of managing vitamin A deficiency are:

- A dietary intake of carotene-containing foods with sufficient oil to absorb the carotene.
- Prevention (see above) and early treatment of infectious disease
- Treatment of established cases by oral vitamin

A, 100 000 IU below 1 year of age and 200 000 IU above 1 year of age
- Vitamin A supplementation for all children with measles.

Overnutrition

Excess intake of calories relative to energy requirements and imbalanced intake of other nutrients (generally excess fat and insufficient fibre) are small but growing problems, particularly in middle-income and poor urban areas. Obesity and lack of exercise in childhood may increase the risk of ischaemic heart disease, hypertension and diabetes in later life.

INFECTIOUS DISEASE

✳ KEY DIAGNOSIS

Acute respiratory infections

These are infections of less than 30 days duration affecting any part of the upper or lower respiratory tract. Acute respiratory infections are a major cause of mortality, especially in infants less than 2 months of age. Risk factors include low birth weight, young age, lack of breast feeding, vitamin A deficiency, overcrowding and exposure to air pollution.

Pneumonia causes more than two-thirds of deaths from acute respiratory infections and, in developing countries, is predominantly bacterial. *Streptococcus pneumoniae* and *Haemophilus influenzae* are the most common causes. Since young infants can die quickly with pneumonia, suspected cases should be referred to hospital and not treated at home. For children above 2 months of age, tachypnoea, cough, fever, head nodding and chest recession are the most important diagnostic features (see also Ch. 6). Children may be treated effectively using appropriate antimicrobials such as amoxycillin or trimethoprim. The WHO has produced standard guidelines for the diagnosis and management of acute respiratory infections by community health workers to improve the coverage and cost-effectiveness of treatment in communities where rapid access to hospital is difficult.

Diarrhoea

Diarrhoea is defined as the too frequent passage of liquid or watery stools. It is associated with a quarter of all child deaths, most occurring in the first 2 years of life. In developing countries it is more frequently caused by bacterial pathogens such as enteropathogenic *Escherichia coli* rather than the viruses prevalent in the industrialized world (see Ch. 5). It may be acute or persistent (lasting for 2 weeks or more). Repeated attacks of diarrhoea lead to undernutrition and poor growth as a result of anorexia, malabsorption and increased nutrient requirements (the malnutrition–infection cycle).

Dehydration is graded according to clinical signs which reflect the amount of fluid lost. As dehydration worsens, this is shown by thirst, irritability, dry mucous membranes, decreased skin turgor and sunken eyes; when severe, the child may show evidence of hypovolaemic shock with no urine output and impaired consciousness.

Acute diarrhoea in all age groups can be safely and effectively treated by oral rehydration solution (see Ch. 5), a mixture of glucose, sodium chloride, sodium bicarbonate and potassium chloride, or by a starch-based rehydration solution which replaces glucose with a common local starchy food such as rice or maize.

The essential principles of management of acute diarrhoea are:

- Prevention of dehydration by promotion of suitable oral fluids, especially breast milk
- Treatment of dehydration by correcting the estimated fluid deficit, replacing ongoing losses and providing normal daily requirements
- Feeding during and after diarrhoea, to prevent nutritional damage.

Antimicrobials are rarely indicated, except for dysentery, cholera, amoebiasis and giardiasis. Antidiarrhoeal medication, though widely prescribed, has no practical benefit in children.

Tuberculosis

Over 150 000 children die each year from the two most severe forms of the disease – tuberculous meningitis and disseminated miliary tuberculosis. Tuberculosis is increasing in most developing countries because of poverty, urbanization, the neglect of tuberculosis control programmes and the spread of HIV. Signs and symptoms of tuberculosis in children are often non-specific such as fever, cough, prolonged diarrhoea, weight loss or swelling of lymph nodes. Diagnosis of tuberculosis is more difficult than for adults because sputum is difficult to collect, most cases are sputum negative anyway, and skin tests may be unreactive as a result of malnutrition or HIV infection. Treatment involves an initial intensive phase of three or more drugs for at least 2 months, and a continuation phase of two drugs for at least 4 months. The BCG vaccination given at birth is protective against disseminated disease. Preventive chemotherapy is used for young infants whose mothers have active pulmonary tuberculosis and for asymptomatic children aged under 5 years living in the same household as a person with infectious tuberculosis.

Malaria

In sub-Saharan Africa most deaths from malaria occur in childhood. Severe malaria (usually caused by *Plasmodium falciparum*) may present differently in children than in adults, with rapid onset after symptoms for only 1–2 days and convulsions, which may indicate cerebral involvement or hypoglycaemia. Neurological sequelae after cerebral malaria occurs in about 10% of cases. Children usually respond rapidly to treatment.

The principles of management of severe falciparum malaria are:

- Early suspicion and referral to the highest level of care available
- Early parenteral antimalarial therapy using optimal doses of an appropriate agent
- Prevention of complications (e.g. convulsions, hypoglycaemia)
- Correct fluid–electrolyte balance
- Proper nursing care.

The principles of prevention are:

- Prevention of insect bites using insect barriers, e.g. DEET (diethyltoluamide) lotion, permethrin-impregnated bed nets, insect sprays or burning mosquito coils.
- Chemoprophylaxis: a suitable drug regimen will depend upon the country and the pattern of chloroquine resistance. For young children, dosage should be carefully calculated, and mefloquine avoided. For travellers, drugs should be started 1 week before departure and continued for 4 weeks after return.

HIV

Over 1 million children are infected with HIV worldwide (see also Ch. 14), and more than 5 million have been orphaned through HIV infection of their parents. Most children are infected by perinatal transmission during pregnancy, birth or breast feeding. More rarely, infection occurs through contaminated blood products (see Ch. 14). In developing countries, more than half of HIV-infected children die before they are 12 months old.

Key principles of care for HIV-infected children are:

- Monitor growth and maintain good nutrition
- Treat common childhood infections early
- Immunize as usual, except those with clinical HIV infection who should not receive BCG vaccination
- Watch for tuberculosis in children and family members
- Treat the child as normal, and give comfort and medication when in pain or distress.

Although breast feeding carries a significant risk of HIV transmission, breast feeding in developing countries should still be strongly promoted where HIV prevalence is high, and alternatives advised only when a mother known to be HIV-positive has been counselled and the risks of breast feeding are judged to outweigh the risks of not breast feeding. New drug treatments to reduce transmission in pregnancy are available, but still too expensive for use in most developing countries.

Common childhood diseases

Common childhood diseases such as measles, poliomyelitis, pertussis and diphtheria have been substantially reduced as a result of the Expanded Programme of Immunization led by the WHO and UNICEF. In 1980 only 15% of children were immunized against vaccine-preventable diseases; in 1997 this had increased to over 75%.

Vaccine-preventable diseases
The following diseases are targeted by the WHO Global Programme for Vaccination:
- Diphtheria
- Pertussis
- Polio
- Tetanus
- Tuberculosis
- Measles
- Hepatitis B.

In industrialized countries, vaccination against mumps, rubella and *H. influenzae* type B is often included in national programmes. Vaccines of proven effectiveness are available for particular high-risk groups against pneumococcal disease, typhoid fever, cholera, hepatitis A, chickenpox, rotavirus, yellow fever and rabies.

Polio has now been eliminated from the Americas, and mortality due to neonatal tetanus and epidemics of measles substantially reduced in developing countries. However, problems remain. Less than 1% of African children receive hepatitis B vaccination despite it being recommended for routine immunization programmes by the WHO. In the states of the former Soviet Union, falling immunization coverage has led to extensive epidemics of diphtheria (Fig. 20.1) and pertussis. Approximately 75% of all global polio cases are reported from south Asia, where the standard immunization regimen produces lower than expected herd immunity.

CHILDREN IN DIFFICULT CIRCUMSTANCES

In 1997, 80 countries had major conflicts or serious political violence, 65 in the developing world. It is estimated that child victims as a result of warfare during the last decade include 2 million killed, 5 million disabled, 12 million left homeless, over 1 million orphaned, and over 10 million psychologically traumatized. As many as 200 000 children have been used as soldiers. Children are especially vulnerable to landmines; an estimated 110 million of these devices are still lodged in the ground.

Sexual and physical abuse of children is increasingly recognized as a problem. Urban poverty and the breakdown of traditional family structures has led to rising numbers of street children and child prostitutes. The UN Convention on the Rights of the Child (see Table 1.1), adopted by most countries in 1990, provides guidelines for monitoring the activities of countries in protecting children in difficult circumstances.

FURTHER READING

Chambers R 1997 Whose reality counts? Putting the first last. Intermediate Technology Publications, London
Costello A, Tomkins A 1997 Child health in developing countries. Medicine, 3–7
The World Bank 1997 Health, nutrition and population sector strategy paper. The World Bank, Washington, DC
UNICEF 1999 The state of the world's children. Oxford University Press, Oxford

Index